Health Communication in Africa

Contexts, Constraints and Lessons

Edited by
Andy O. Alali
B. A. Jinadu

University Press of America,® Inc.
Lanham · New York · Oxford

4720 Boston Way
Lanham, Maryland 20706
UPA Acquisitions Department (301) 459-3366

PO Box 317
Oxford
OX2 9RU, UK

Printed in the United States of America
British Library Cataloging in Publication Information Available

ISBN: 978-0-7618-2407-7

∞™ The paper used in this publication meets the minimum requirements of American National Standard for Information Sciences—Permanence of Paper for Printed Library Materials, ANSI Z39.48—1984

Contents

Preface

When our discussions started about editing a book on health communication in Africa, we did not seriously consider the amount of time and work that was required to complete a project of this magnitude. We thought our educational training and professional experience in communication studies (Andy O. Alali) and medicine (B.A. Jinadu) provided the skills required to edit this book. No sooner did we start the project that we realized our expertise in these two distinct disciplines was not enough to complete this book. We soon realized that the input and encouragement of a network was necessary if we were going to finish this book in a timely manner. It is with this in mind that we acknowledge those who, directly and indirectly, created the environment for us to complete this book. We must say, though, that as much as the support network helped us during this project, we take full responsibility for the content in the book.

First, we wish to thank our colleagues here in the United States and Africa whose contributions form the chapters for this book. We believe your multidimensional approach and the interdisciplinary perspectives presented in your respective chapters illuminate for our readers and enhance the discussions about health communication and promotion in Africa. We also wish to thank our editorial staff at University Press of America, Inc., particularly Stephen H. Ryan, for their guidance, support, and patience during the preparation of this work. We would be remiss if we did not acknowledge the assistance of our copy-editor, Ms. LaVonne Taylor, for her constructive comments on an earlier version of the chapters that constitute this book.

We are grateful to the Subsidiary Rights Department at Elsevier Science for granting us permission to use the following two articles: E.S. Ataudo, "Traditional Medicine and Biopsychosocial Fulfilment in African Health," *Social Science & Medicine,* Volume 21, Number 12, pp. 1345–1347 (1985) and Bernice N. Ezeilo, "Psychology and Health in Africa," *Social Science & Medicine,* Volume 31, Number 6, pp. 705–710 (1990).

(1990).

We thank the editors of two other journals; the *South African Journal of Sociology* for granting permission to publish the article, "A Sociological Contribution to the 'New Public Health' in South Africa," by Leah Gilbert, that appeared in Volume 26: 1–10 (1995); and the *Journal of Psychology in Africa*, for permission to republish K. Peltzer and V.I. Cherian's article, "Health Promotion on HIV/AIDS in Sub-Saharan Africa," that previously appeared in Volume 9: 148–160 (1999).

Finally, we acknowledge our indebtedness to our family, friends, and colleagues who offered daily encouragement and support for us to complete this project. They include: Shakirat Jinadu, Folasade Jinadu, Baahir Jinadu, Clinton and Claudia I. Orugbani, Enighe Kiri-Kalio, Eunice Alali, and Akari Alali.

Andy O. Alali
B.A. Jinadu

Part I

Overview

Chapter 1

Health Communication in Africa: An Overview

Andy O. Alali
California State University, Bakersfield

B.A. Jinadu
Department of Public Health, County of Kern, California

During the last decade, Africa has witnessed a myriad of health problems, ranging from substance abuse to the AIDS, or acquired immunodeficiency syndrome, pandemic. Africa has also been confronted with how to deal with the deadly Ebola virus, smoking-related illnesses, and a host of other health problems that jeopardize maternal and child health. As with most problems, some African countries have devised a variety of ways - including traditional and nontraditional methods - to ensure the health of their people. Some of these public health efforts and disease prevention strategies are, unfortunately, conspicuously absent in the health communication literature.

Equally neglected in published works are the challenges health promotion experts face in their attempt to communicate healthy lifestyles and wellness strategies in urban and rural areas of Africa. As a result, public health specialists interested in health promotion in Africa are unable to point to a text or a collection of published work that documents current experiences as well as articulates ways to navigate some of the challenges they are likely to face on the continent.

To fill this void, we have assembled an impressive list of scholars and practitioners whose contributions form the chapters for this book. Collectively, these chapters address a variety of subjects that include: existing and innovative health promotion programs; outcome evaluation and effectiveness studies; health communication in refugee settings and among displaced communities of Africa; and examples of collaborative programs among international, national, and regional agencies that have been successfully implemented. Because each chapter is written from a multidimensional and interdisciplinary perspective, we believe the book fills a void that currently exists in health communication in Africa, as well as reflecting the numerous research findings and practical application of health promotion activities on the continent. We hope the book would serve as a road map for those interested in the study of health communication, health promotion, and disease prevention strategies in Africa.

An Overview of the Chapters

The book is organized in five parts, comprising 20 chapters. Part I of the book includes two chapters that begin with an overview on health communication in Africa, written by the editors. Chapter 1 deals with the purpose of the book, highlights for the reader the relevant issues about health communication in Africa, and articulates the rationale for the current project. In Chapter 2, we discuss some of the current public health crises facing peoples of Africa. Here, we elucidate for the reader some of the sources and major factors that create health problems in Africa. In the process, we also identify some of the roles African scholars dedicated to health communication and health promotion can play in improving the health status of Africa and its peoples.

Part II expands on some challenges and considerations in Africa's health contexts, particularly, as it relates to research, campaign strategies, and planning required to encourage healthy lifestyles, as well as promote disease prevention. This section starts with Chapter 3, "Research Considerations for Effective Health Communication in Africa." Here, the author provides a road map for health communication research and examines some of the theoretical constraints that impede health communication in Africa. The discussion focuses on two key proposals for research: developing appropriate methodology for health communication research; and creating evaluation tools that would enable assessment of health communication campaigns at three stages - planning, program operations, and program outcomes. Additionally, the author provides specific recommendations for ethical standards that should guide responsible health communication research in Africa. In Chapter 4, "Health Promotion Challenges in Nigeria: Globalization, Tobacco Marketing and Policies," Dr. Igbo N. Egwu of the University of Calabar, Nigeria, articulates the challenges inherent in antismoking campaigns in a typical African country, Nigeria. Here, the author talks about the role of globalization in Africa's health context and the extent to which it contributes and constrains attempts to address the harmful effects of tobacco consumption in most African countries. And, even though the author's analysis is based on the Nigerian case study, he argues for an Africa-specific health communication modality where approaches to health communication would move beyond "administrative" or "organizational" levels to an "operational" or "field level" approach. Such a model, according to the author, entails the analysis of how both traditional African and contemporary (multi) media can be used as well as situationally adapted to communicate vital health promotion messages to the most affected African publics in the 21st century.

In the next chapter, "Health Communication in Africa's Rural Communities: Navigating Emerging Social and Cultural Challenges," the authors present some new understandings of social and cultural issues in planning health communication and disease prevention campaigns in Africa's rural communities. The main thrust of the argument here, the authors observe, is that current approaches to health communication and campaigns for disease prevention in Africa's rural communities do not take into account some of the social and cultural issues identified in this chapter. Consequently, Dr. Andy O. Alali and Dr. Ogom Peter Nwosu suggest ways to effectively integrate Africa's unique social and cultural issues in health communication and disease prevention campaigns, especially in rural areas with no access to adequate health care.

The seven chapters that comprise Part III deal with social and institutional support systems as well as the cultural dynamics that play a role in Africa's health context. In this section, we begin with a discussion of the important roles of communication among health care professionals, patients, and their support networks in influencing health decisions and determining access to health care. The authors argue that the dominant paradigm that emphasizes a biomedical approach to health communication should be abandoned for a new strategy that "requires an integrative, overarching theory of health (that is) built on sound, contemporary theories of communication." They conclude with suggestions of some elements we should consider in this new strategy.

In Chapter 7, the focus shifts to the role of communities in health promotion. Here, the authors argue that contemporary community-based strategies for health promotion in Africa need a new approach to ensure campaign success. This new approach is necessary because the late 20th century marked the beginning of a shift and erosion in the "concept" of community that characterized most African societies. This new perspective in Africa's conception of what constitutes a community, they argue, offers no alternative community-based approach that is inclusive to sustain an interactive health communication and disease prevention campaigns in Africa. In light of this new development, the authors of this chapter suggest that the strategies and community partnership initiatives for prevention and rehabilitation in Kigali, Rwanda, could serve as models for solving some of the major health problems that African countries would face in the 21st century.

An equally important topic that is often ignored in most discussions about health care and disease prevention relates to the role women ought to play in the health of peoples of Africa. The focus of this next chapter is on the role of women in health promotion. This is crucial in the African context of health because societal beliefs and cultural practices often relegate women to passive roles in decisions about sex and sexuality. This has implications on health, particularly as it relates to HIV infection and AIDS. Consequently, the health of a nation is intrinsically linked to the extent women are involved in health promotion and disease prevention efforts.

The next two chapters deal with traditional medicine and the psychology of health, respectively. In Chapter 9, "Traditional Medicine and Biopsychosocial Fulfillment in African Health," the author examines the role of traditional medicine in the promotion of biopsychosocial fulfillment in African health, and argues that every society has its own methods of managing illness and of controlling the environment. It discusses how African societies deal with health issues within the constraints of its own unique system of social structure, language and communication, belief and customs, attitudes, and behaviors and cultural facts. The addition of this chapter is indicative of the importance placed on Africa's belief system and oral tradition on health decisions. Therefore, Africa's diverse traditional belief systems should be incorporated in any agenda aimed at shaping the communication objectives of the African scheme of health.

The terrain of discourse about health in Africa often excludes issues related to psychology because its complex culture and traditional belief systems are perceived to be incongruous to psychological interpretations of health issues. For some Africans, interpretations of ill-health and wellness are indexed and contextualized by identifiable cultural and traditional fields that cannot be explained by psychological perspectives. However, the author of this chapter, Bernice N. Ezeilo, argues for a redirection of the African mindset so as to embrace contemporary psychological arguments that are crucial in the interpretations of health and wellness in the African society. Consequently, the author suggests ways psychological services can be fully and effectively integrated into Africa's healthcare delivery system with the goal of improving patient care.

It is our conviction that a discussion of health communication in Africa should also be situated in sociological contexts. In this chapter, Leah Gilbert, explores the dimensions of this new public health in general and particularly, in South Africa's context of health, and the role the that field of sociology can play in public health research, training, and practice. We hope our readers agree with us that we can make sense out of the complex health issues facing Africa today by integrating sociological perspectives in the overall scheme of health communication. We conclude Part III with a discussion on how interpersonal communication and social support influence health decisions in an African health context.

We also believe that our discussion of health communication in Africa would be incomplete without analyses of specific health contexts, the constraints in dealing with these health issues, and the lessons that were learned from them. Part IV addresses these issues through analyses of current health problems and the complexities associated with achieving a healthy Africa. This section begins with an assessment of the UNAIDS/PennState Framework for HIV/AIDS Communication and the promises it holds for African AIDS communication management. The authors conclude by presenting other frameworks that deserve attention from health communication researchers and practitioners in various regions of the world.

The next chapter deals with health promotion on HIV/AIDS in Africa. Here, the authors deal with epidemiological information relating to HIV/AIDS in Africa, as well as how the information can contribute to the effective role health promotion can play in increasing awareness of the need for an array of national and international strategies that would decrease the pandemic in Africa. The authors also discuss needed information concerning at-risk sexual behaviors and other possible correlates for HIV infection, and increasing self-efficacy, especially among at-risk groups such as women and adolescents. Along these lines of discussion is an equally important analysis (Chapter 15) of the comprehensive and integrated strategies used for HIV/AIDS campaigns for the South and Southern African region of the continent. With their collective experience in applied health communication research, the authors suggest specific strategies to combat HIV/AIDS in that region of the continent.

Another interesting feature of this book, which is absent in most works, is our discussion (Chapter 16) of the public health issues that affect refugees and internally displaced persons (IDPs) in Africa. Included in this discussion are some of the factors that create refugee status, displacement and poor health in Africa, economic and health consequences of displacement, and health communication approaches to the acute health care needs in nomadic settings.

We hope any reader of this book would agree that the power of health communication is evident in some of the discussions presented so far. We add to that discussion an analysis of a silent, but public health problem in Africa, onchocercal skin disease. Onchocerciasis, which occurs in some rural areas of Africa, manifests itself in the form of reactive and nonreactive skin lesions. It triggers several effects, including itching, which is particularly troubling for the affected. The author examines a set of prevention ideas held by some local communities in Ghana that is a growing problem where onchocerciasis is endemic.

Besides emerging infectious diseases that are devastating Africa, one of the most crucial public health issues that significantly impacts the continent is infant health and child mortality. Research indicates that the major factor that contributes to this public- health problem is micronutrient deficiency or malnourishment. In the next chapter we analyze the magnitude of micronutrient deficiencies in seven African countries, the factors that contribute to these deficiencies, and recommendations for communication strategies to reduce malnutrition and the infant mortality rate in the continent. We conclude Section IV with an excellent discussion on current trends and future directions of mental health care in a specific African country. Here, the authors argue that the introduction of democracy in South Africa has led to restructuring of its mental health services so as to enable rural communities to have access to services they were previously denied. The authors suggest ways current public health care infrastructure could be used to significantly improve mental health services in rural areas of South Africa.

One of the reasons we decided to work on this project is to elucidate for our readers some of the health communication efforts in Africa. Equally important is the need to provide Africanist scholars the resources they need to facilitate future research. In this age of digital divide, most researchers in the continent do not have easy access to Internet research resources. When available, connectivity is expensive and unaffordable for most academics and researchers. To reduce the time required to browse the Internet, we conclude this book with a chapter on "Selected Internet Resources for Health Information and Communication in Africa." Even though we may not have captured resources that cover all health issues in Africa, we are confident that the comprehensive list of websites and the summary of information provided in this chapter would be useful to those who study health issues in Africa, especially in the realm of disease surveillance and health communication.

In conclusion, we hope this book would attract a wide range of readership, including students of world health issues and health communication, public health and community medicine specialists, health educators, counselors, researchers, and non-governmental organizations (NGOs). In our opinion, this book would be an excellent addition for health departments, universities, and libraries. More important, we hope it would provide readers with the appropriate information they need to function in their respective fields and to conduct scholarly research on issues related to health communication in developing countries, particularly in Africa. We hope our contribution to this issue would help to improve the health status of Africa and its people.

Chapter 2

Public Health Crises in Africa: Initiatives for Improved Health in the 21st Century

B.A. Jinadu
Department of Public Health, County of Kern, California

Andy O. Alali
California State University, Bakersfield

An analysis of the health status in most African countries would indicate that the public's health has become an increasingly critical issue in the economic development of the continent. Epidemiological data, research and surveillance reports from national and international health agencies show that, over the past two decades, there has been a downward shift in the health status of the peoples of Africa. The deteriorating health of most Africans has imposed hardships and created unanticipated effects on development and the economic viability of the region (Nagarajan, 2001; WHO, 1996; Stock, 1986; Hughes & Hunter, 1970). Poor lifestyle habits and a host of other factors, including sociocultural beliefs, have put the lives of most of the work force in danger. It is also clear that policy issues and environmental conditions contribute to the poor health status in most African countries. Some of the prevailing conditions in Africa today include decreasing budgets for health agencies and infrastructures, a distant gap between health care that is available to the poor versus the affluent segment of the population, and the rising aggression and conflicts in the continent.

These trends have led to the neglect of critical health needs, such as malaria control, nutrition, expanded program on immunization, and health care infrastructures. Consequently, these have created a major public health crisis that has serious implications on development in Africa. Some of the public health crises, which result from these prevailing factors, are by way of preventable diseases that are commonly referred to as "diseases of poverty" (Kibirige, 1997, p. 249). Amongst these are airborne, vector-borne, and water-borne diseases. Whereas, the most prevalent waterborne disease in Africa is cholera, reports show that influenza, tuberculosis, measles, whooping cough, and chicken pox are the most persistent airborne diseases. Likewise, vector-borne diseases, such as malaria, pose a public health problem for Africa. WHO estimates that "80 percent of malaria mortality in the world occurs in Sub-Saharan Africa" (Kibirige, 1997).

Equally important is the burden posed by the ominous HIV/AIDS that has affected every aspect of the African life. Also, a high incidence of cardiovascular disease, and a number of other infectious diseases have emerged, or re-emerged, during the past few years.

In this chapter, we focus on some of the issues we believe have contributed to public health crises in Africa, as well as the sources and major factors that create these health problems. In the process, we identify some initiatives for improved health in Africa in the 21st Century.

Compelling Issues Impacting Public Health in Africa

There are obvious differing perspectives on the causes of ill health in Africa. None is more convoluted than the argument that poverty, not HIV, is the main cause of AIDS. For many years, this perspective was strongly endorsed and amplified in his speeches by South Africa President Thabo Mbeki. By the end of 2001, however, under national and international pressure, President Mbeki reluctantly abandoned his reckless and disturbing pronouncement.

We introduced this issue here to suggest that Mbeki's short-lived perspective on AIDS points to an often ignored reality: that by analyzing the rhetoric about causes of ill health in Africa, one can fully understand how intricate traditional beliefs, socio-cultural practices, lifestyle changes, and their experience impact on people's notions of healthcare, illness, and how these ideas mediate discussions about health. In other words, the "African concept of health" or ill-health is often conditioned by traditional beliefs or ideas and how these assumptions are indexed by others in the attempt to explain why a specific individual is afflicted by a disease. This is to say that cultural practices and traditional belief systems are prevailing constructs in the definition and analysis of health or ill health in most African health contexts. Illustrative of this notion is the fact that illness is sometimes defined within the relational distance or connectedness between the afflicted individual, his or her ancestors, and the deity they worship, or their religion. Thus, an illness may be viewed as punishment for one's disrespect of an elder or that the condition may have been brought about by one's enemies. It is this view that helps to legitimize the role that the traditional medicine man plays in health outcomes.

Clearly, while these personal perspectives and traditional belief systems do influence discussions about the causes of illness, we argue here that Africa's public health crises ought to be recognized as an event or process resulting from a complex interaction between socio-economic, political, environmental, and behavioral factors that have become an associated part of life in most African societies. Among these factors are unhygienic conditions in urban and rural communities, inadequate infection control practices in health facilities, proliferation of counterfeit and degraded medical products, underfunding of the public health sector, and political instability, violence, and war. We discuss these critical factors and their implication on the health status of Africa in the next section.

Unhygienic Conditions

Africa's health status is heavily influenced by the living conditions found in most communities. Large-scale population shifts and displacements, due to ethnic conflicts and war, have altered the living conditions of a vast majority of Africans. Consequently, unhygienic living conditions have become an associated part of life in most rural settings and urban centers of African countries. Unfortunately, these conditions now serve as a host and the breeding grounds for microbes that promote an epidemic of diseases with catastrophic impact on the health of Africa. This is not to suggest that unhygienic conditions are unique to Africa alone, however, we contend that some of the conditions in the rural-urban corridor of most African countries serve as enabling environments for infectious diseases, most of which had re-emerged in the past two decades.

For example, in the urban metropolis of Lagos, Nigeria, where overcrowding and improper sewage disposal and illegal waste dumpsites are the norm, it is not uncommon for unhygienic conditions to facilitate the exchange of organisms and resistant genes among bacteria. These conditions breed antibiotic-resistant strains such as E-coli (Lamikanra & Okeke, 1997). Also, it is not unusual that small towns and villages with contaminated water; ill-ventilated housing and improper waste disposal are breeding grounds for infectious and parasitic diseases, such as tuberculosis (TB), Ebola virus, and malaria. For example, a WHO study estimates that two-thirds of the South African population is infected with the TB germ and an estimated 180,000 new cases each year (WHO, 2001a). Additionally, it is well documented that the shantytowns in South Africa also serve as breeding grounds for malaria (WHO, 2001b).

Further, it is evident that a link exists between poor sanitation and public health. Yet, 80 percent of residents of developing countries, including countries in Africa, have no sanitary facilities for sewage disposal (WHO, 1992). For example, in western Kenya, with a population of about 400,000, "only 5 percent of the homes have toilets" (Green Africa, 2001). In the situation described above, sewage and wastewater are let into streams and rivers, thereby contaminating the only source of domestic water. The locals, with no other source of fresh water supply, have no choice but to consume the contaminated water that is now host to waterborne diseases, such as cholera - a leading cause of illness and death in these areas and in most of Africa (WHO, 2001b).

Inadequate Infection Control Practices in Health Facilities

Infection control practices in health facilities in most Africa countries often compromise the health of patients. There is no doubt that health facilities are supposed to create the infection-free environment for patients to receive adequate medical care and attention from trained medical professionals. Yet, it is not the case in some African health facilities. Evidence from studies suggests that inadequate infection control practices are prevalent in some African health facilities; both at out- and in-patient care facilities (Okello et al., 1997; Meers, 1988). As in most cases, these conditions facilitate the breeding of organisms that infect patients and are subsequently transmitted to the larger population. For example, in Uganda, it was found that "untreated hospital waste was often dumped into public sewers or thrown into rubbish heaps ravaged by scavengers" (Okello et al, 1997). While no correlative evidence of contact and infections was documented in the Ugandan case, it is possible for scavengers to be infected with some diseases from repeated contact with contaminated hospital waste. A case in point is the Lagos metropolis of Nigeria were inadequate infection control practices were responsible for the spread of resistant organisms, such as the E-coli strains, within the urban population (Lamikanra & Okeke, 1997).

Additionally, hospital-acquired infections are responsible for maternal and neonatal deaths more than puerperium hemorrhage or congenital malformations, respectively. Improper ventilation and air-exchange in hospitals contribute to spread of communicable diseases and inhalation of unhealthy particles. The situation is also worsened because linens are not routinely changed and most health facilities are infected with all types of vectors and formites.

Proliferation of Counterfeit and Degraded Medical Products

The commercial availability and proliferation of drugs have led to misuse of antibacterial products in most of Africa. With over 700 brands of antibiotics marketed to the public via licensed and unlicensed pharmacies, a great number of these antibacterial products are prescribed by unskilled practitioners and misused by the public at large (Okeke, Lamikanra, & Edelman, 1999). It is equally significant to note that instances of counterfeit pharmaceuticals are more prevalent in the developing world than in other areas. Estimates indicate that 65 percent of the instances of counterfeit pharmaceuticals reported to WHO or Interpol from 28 countries were in developing nations (McGregor, 1997). This raises questions and concerns about the quality and standardization of medical products that are dispensed in these areas, as well as the risk posed by the therapeutic failure and impact of these products.

Clearly, the source and quality of a majority of the medical products found in most African countries is suspect. In some cases, medical products, such as drugs, do not contain the concentration of active substances stated on their labels (Adjepon-Yamaoah, 1980; Land, 1992; McGregor, 1997). There is cumulative evidence suggesting linkages between counterfeit and degraded medical products and deaths in both Anglophone and Francophone African countries (see Lee, et al., 1991; Land, 1992; Alubo, 1994; Couper, 1997). Ironically, a pharmacist once pleaded for genuine intravenous medication while lying on a surgical table in preparation for elective surgery.

Some noteworthy cases involving death include situations in Nigeria where "products for which excipients have been replaced by less expensive alternatives, e.g., substitution of ethylene glycol for propylene glycol in pediatric puracetamol formulations" (Alubo, 1994). In another case in Nigeria, it was reported that a traditional healer admitted to "augmenting herbal preparations with tetracycline from commercially available capsules" (Ogungbamila & Ogundaini, 1993).

Also, during a visit to Nigeria in 1979 by one of the authors of this chapter, he asked a street peddlar what was contained in a big clear plastic bag full of capsules, which the peddlar was advertising as a cure for hemorrhoids. His response was, tetracycline, an antibiotic. While these cases are not unique to Nigeria, there is ample evidence to suggest that it is a problem endemic in Africa, and it has public health implications.

The problem of the proliferation and counterfeiting of drugs is compounded by the lack of knowledge and corruption within law enforcement agencies who are either unable to detect the counterfeit drugs or are paid to protect the counterfeiters. To counteract this, some African governments have now instituted measures aimed at informing the public and punishing the perpetrators of such crimes. For example, the Nigerian government recently embarked on an innovative program, through its drug enforcement agency, to identify and publicize fake pharmaceutical products. Unfortunately, the publicity is done in specialized media, particularly in newspapers, that are disseminated to urban settings and inaccessible to those who cannot afford to purchase a newspaper on a daily basis.

In addition to the problem of drug proliferation and counterfeiting, climatic conditions and inadequate storage facilities contribute to the degradation of drugs in most African countries. Noteworthy are cases in Guinea-Bissau and Nigeria where climatic conditions and inadequate storage facilities account for excessive degradation of active ingredients contained in antibiotics, particularly the often-used tetracycline (Ballereau, et al., 1997; Shakoor, et al., 1997). In the Guinea-Bissau case, for example, evidence suggests that most of the drugs that lost their active constituents as a result of inadequate storage facilities were anti-microbial drugs that are often prescribed for infections. Without the benefit of the active constituents in antimicrobial therapy, an infected patient and those he or she comes in contact with can be a source of infection for the community at-large.

Underfunding and Neglect of the Public Health Sector

Another problem area that contributes to health crisis in Africa is the underfunding of the public health sector. For example, over the last 35 years the military budget of most African countries has outstripped all other medical or social spending. Analysis of World Bank data shows that "developing countries spent $41 per person on health in 1990, compared with the $1,500 per person spent by industrialized countries" (Okeke et al., 1999). When the expenditure on the public health sector is analyzed within the health-care and delivery contexts, it is clear that the gross underfunding of this sector is bound to handicap efforts aimed at providing adequate health care in Africa. An ancillary part to this is the dismal salary structure and the living conditions of health-care workers in Africa, which is a consequence of misplaced priority in most national health policies. And, because health-care workers and medical practitioners are underpaid in most African countries, it has led to the extortion of patients who cannot afford the "hidden fees" needed for adequate medical examination and treatment. What we are suggesting here is that the underfunding of the public-health sector contributes to inadequate medical care, as well as high rates of mortality in Africa. To us, this is a peculiar public-health crisis that African governments should address urgently.

Compounding these problems is the fact that the effective public health system that was in place during the colonial era has now been overrun by years of neglect, with consequential effect on public health. Illustrative of this is the fact that during colonialism, houses and apartments were routinely visited by sanitary inspectors, or what the Yorubas in Nigeria call wole-wole, who had enforcement powers to cite landlords whose properties were neglected and were deemed a health hazard. These inspectors made routine housecalls looking for infectious agents such as maggots in water pots, rats, and roaches; also and ensuring that bathrooms were scrubbed clean. The streets were regularly swept and public drainage systems were also routinely cleaned. Also, open swamps were routinely sprayed and there were collection points for household garbage. The colonial health system also ensured that meats sacrificed during religious or social ceremonies were inspected and devoid of infection. Unfortunately, the abandonment of these health practices by most African governments has contributed to the public-health crisis in Africa.

Political Instability, Violence, and War

Here, we argue that human-made catastrophes - violence, conflicts, and war in Africa - have serious implications on public health. It is not a far-fetched notion to suggest that the most significant factor that impacts on public health in Africa is the armed struggles that result from ethnic conflicts and the breakdown in political institutions. Clearly, any student of Africa knows that this is a continent ravaged by war and conflicts. There is no doubt that Africa has been a breeding ground for insurrections, most of which have dislocated families and created countless number of refugees in displaced settings. Overcrowding in refugee settings tends to breed unsanitary conditions that facilitate the rapid dissemination of contagious diseases. It is not uncommon for refugees and displaced persons to be victims of disease outbreaks, such as cholera, bacillary dysentery, and Ebola virus, in the refugee settings of sub-Saharan Africa. Typical examples are the African countries of Rwanda, Uganda, Sudan, Sierra Leone, Liberia, and Zaire, where armed conflicts have relocated families into refugee camps, thereby created new unhygienic settlements that create health problems (Dodge, 1990; Goma Epidemiology Group, 1994). (See Chapter 16 for further reading about refugees and public health).

Clearly, because the concept of accountability is not fully practiced and the rule of law is relative in most African countries, rising aggression of war and political instability also engender a culture oriented toward the mismanagement of public funds that were appropriated for the health sector. It is a routine and acceptable orthodoxy for African leaders and their cronies to illegally amass wealth while essential health infrastructure and resources are neglected. With these observations as background, we offer a few ideas on how to improve public health in Africa in the 21st Century.

Initiatives for Improving Africa's Public Health in the 21st Century

The preceding discussion indicates that most of Africa's health is negatively affected by conditions that are mostly human-made: unhygienic conditions; inadequate infection control practices in health facilities; proliferation of counterfeit and degraded medical products; underfunding of the public health sector; and political instability, violence, and war. It is unacceptable that Africa, with only about 12 percent of the world's population, accounts for 80 percent of the world's deaths due to AIDS and over 90 percent of the world's deaths due to malaria (Africa Action, 2002). There is no doubt that HIV/AIDS has socioeconomic impact on Africa, vis-à-vis its workforce, economy, and the displacement of children and adolescents. Similarly, WHO estimates Africa's economic losses due to malaria alone at $2.2 billion a year (Africa Action, 2002). Clearly, these figures about HIV/AIDS and malaria indicate an urgent need for African countries to develop priority initiatives aimed at improving public health.

The goal of improving public health in Africa requires priority initiatives guided by the Jakarta Declaration (WHO, 1997), which states that: "Health is a basic human right and is essential for social and economic development." We contend that public health initiatives in Africa must be sensitive to the premises that "peace, shelter, education, food, income, a stable ecosystem, sustainable resources, and social justice, and equity" are the prerequisites for health, a notion that is the core of the Ottawa Charter for Health Promotion (WHO, 1996). Consequently we offer the following suggestions:

First, we suggest that public-health issues in Africa should no longer be taken lightly, or left solely in the hands of corrupt governments and underpaid medical personnel. Rather, public health must be approached from a framework that encourages active community participation or local initiatives, through the efforts of nongovernmental organizations (NGOs). In this public health context, citizens should be empowered through adequate and accurate health information, education, and communication (IEC) at the community level. It is what we refer to here as a contextual approach to health promotion, a process that focuses more on the community than the individual. In this model, health promotion campaigns must treat individual perceptions and health behavior as an event that is connected to, and not isolated from, the larger context of community influence. This is one way to recognize the individual as a product of the community. Consequently, specific local initiatives should be aimed at accomplishing the following: provide information on community-based resources and strategies for health; enable locals to know where to find information regarding health; train locals to become respected agents of social change in their respective communities; develop and encourage locals to participate in activities that improve their lives; and recognize the importance of informal networks and mobilize traditional sources that interact with health decisions in the local community. All of these initiatives would have no meaningful effect if they are not linked directly with local health organizations, or if they do not receive the necessary institutional or governmental support and an unqualified involvement by the public.

Second, we need to develop a mechanism to identify some of the most vulnerable groups to disease epidemics in African countries and respective communities. By plotting the urban-rural axis of most countries and determining the characteristic of the most likely groups that are susceptible to communicable diseases, we can develop and organize structures to respond to some of these health problems before they reach epidemic proportions.

Third, in most African communities where interpersonal communication, social support, and health decisions are contextually bound, it is important to determine the extent to which discussions about health enable or disable health-related behavior. The result of such inquiry would help health educators determine how an existing social relationship and the interaction that takes place within the relationship can be merged and ethically manipulated to achieve health promotion objectives. We say this to suggest that the affiliative relationships found in Africa's health context influences information acquisition because most Africans tend to confide in those they trust and, in times of crisis, turn to them for advice about their health. As Cline and Boyd (1993) observed, "people in crisis, particularly those with serious illness, rely on social support as a preventive agent" (p. 131). Therefore, campaigns aimed at health promotion must consider the context of social support.

Lastly, we must try to plan more effective campaigns that assist people to seek reliable and accurate health information from informed sources. The one way we can achieve the goal of a healthy society is to recognize that health promotion is transactional. It is transactional in the sense that health promotion requires us to understand the rules that govern a communication event, environment, and the cultural variables that impede the particular health promotion objectives. By such understanding, we can design pre-campaign research that seeks to determine whether there are similarities and/or differences in how the peoples of Africa would respond to a specific health campaign. What this means is that we must begin to recognize that Africa's development is tied to the health of its people, and our efforts should be aimed at eliminating these emerging infections and tropical diseases, the main contributors to morbidity and mortality in Africa, particularly among children and adolescents. Consequently, emphasis must be placed on health education that ensures a healthy society. The alternative, which is the extinction of Africa, appears least desirable.

References

Africa Action (February 2, 2002). *Africa's right-to-health campaign: background on Africa's health.* Location: *http://www.africapolicy.org/action/health.html.*

Alubo, S.O. (1994). Death for sale: A study of drug poisoning and deaths in Nigeria. *Social Science & Medicine,* 38:97–103.

Ballereau, F., Prazuck, T., Schrive, I., Lafleuriel, M.T., Rozec, D., Fisch, A., et al. (1997). Stability of essential drugs in the fields: Results of a study conducted over a two-year period in Burkina Faso. *American Journal of Tropical Medicine & Hygiene,* 57; 31–36.

Cline, R.J.W., & Boyd, M.F. (1993). Communication as threat and therapy: Stigma, social support, and coping with HIV infection. In E.B. Ray (ed.), *Case studies in health communication* (pp. 131–147). Hillsdale, NJ: Lawrence Erlbaum Associates, Publishers.

Couper, M.R. (1997). Strategies for the rational use of antimicrobials. *Clinical Infectious Diseases,* 24 Supplement1: S154–S156.

Dodge, C.P. (1990). Health implications of war in Uganda and Sudan. *Social Science & Medicine,* 31:691–698.

Goma Epidemiology Group (1995). Public health impact of Rwandan refugee crisis: What happened in Goma, Zaire, in July 1994? *Lancet,* 345:339–344.

Green Africa Network & Rachuonyo Medical Centre (2001). Sustainable rural healthcare programme: Medical care for all. Location: *http://www.memberss.spree.com/ greenafrica/Rural_Healthcare.html.*

Hughes, C.C., & Hunter, J.M. (1970). Disease and 'development' in tropical Africa. *Social Science & Medicine,* 3:443–493.

Kibirige, J.S. (1997). Population growth, poverty and health. *Social Science & Medicine,* 45; 2:247-259.

Lamikanra, P., & Okeke, I.N. (1997). A study of the effect of the urban/rural divide on the incidence of antibiotic resistance in E-coli. *Biomedical Letters,* 55; 91–97.

Land, J. (1992). Combating counterfeit drugs. *Nature,* 355:192.

Lee, P.R., Lurie, P., Silverman, M.M., & Lydecker, M. (1991). Drug promotion and labeling in developing countries: An update. *Journal of Clinical Epidemiology,* 44 Supplement 2; 49S-55S.

McGregor, A. (1997). Counterfeit drugs flood developing world. *Lancet,* 350: 1690.

Meers, P.D. (1988). Infection control in developing countries. *Journal of Hospital Infections,* 11 Supplement A:406-410.

Nagarajan, P. (2001, July 4). Sub-Saharan Africa – Toward health-led economic development. *The Hindu Business Line* (Internet edition). Location: *http://www.hindubusinessline.com.*

Okeke, I.N., Lamikana, A., & Edelman, R. (1999, January-February). Socioeconomic and behavioral factors leading to acquired bacterial resistance to antibiotics in developing countries. *Emerging Infectious Diseases,* 5; 1:18–27.

Okello, D., Konde-Lule, J., Lubanga, R., Arube-Wani, J. (1997). Waste disposal in private medical clinics in Kampala, Uganda. *Journal of Clinical Epidemiology,* 50; Supp. 1:45S.

Ogungbamia, F.O., & Ogundaina, A.O. (ed.) (1993, January 21–23). Traditional healing methods in the control and treatment of infections diseases: Report of a workshop on traditional healing methods in the control of infectious diseases. Obafemi Awolowo University, Ile-Ife, Nigeria.

Shakoor, O., Taylor, R.B., & Behrens, R.H. (1997). Assessment of the incidence of substandard drugs in developing countries. *Tropical Medicine & International Health,* 2:839-845.

Stock, R. (1986). 'Disease and development' or 'the underdevelopment of health': A critical review of geographical perspectives on African health problems. *Social Science & Medicine,* 23; 7:689–700.

World Health Organization (2001a). Menaces of Africa: Tuberculosis. Location: *http://www.clas.ufl.Edu/users/bmcdade/GroupDakar/tb.html.*

World Health Organization (2001b). Menaces of Africa: Malaria. Location: *http://www.clas.ufl.Edu/users/bmcdade/GroupDakar/malaria.html.*

World Health Organization (1997, July 21–25). *The Jakarta declaration on leading health promotion in the 21st Century.* Fourth International Conference on Health Promotion, Jakarta. WHO/HPR/HEP/41CHP/BR/97.4.

World Health Organization (1996, March 14). *UN special initiative on Africa: The health dimension.* Press Release WHO/18.

World Health Organization (1992). *Implementation of the global strategy for health for all by year 2000, second evaluation: and eighth report on the world health situation.* Geneva: WHO.

World Health Organization (1986, November 21). *Ottawa charter for health promotion.* First International Conference on Health Promotion, Ottawa. WHO/HPR/HEP/95.1.

World Health Organization (1978, September 6–12). *Declaration of Alma-Ata.* International Conference on Primary Health Care, Alma-Ata, USSR.

Part II

Challenges and Considerations

Chapter 3

Research Considerations for Effective Health Communication in Africa

Andy O. Alali
California State University, Bakersfield

The emergence of health communication as a discipline has stimulated scholarly interest about the importance of communication in healthcare, especially in the promotion of healthy lifestyles. As a relatively new discipline, health communication has significant and universal implication to medical encounters. The theories derived from research activities are capable of stipulating the appropriate ways to present accurate, up-to-date health information to the public so as to achieve specific health promotion goals.

As with most new disciplines, health communication is faced with a distinct challenge: how to provide health information in simple and understandable terms so that the public can act on it. This challenge, however, is compounded by some theoretical constraints that impede health promotion objectives. The impact is felt in developing nations where current research activities have not developed indigenous health communication theories that, if integrated with available health knowledge, will serve as persuasive injunctions to unhealthy behavior and destructive lifestyles. What we are omitting here is that even though current studies in the field of health communication have produced what Pettegrew (1988) calls "theoretical pluralism," they are not sufficiently embodied in the African contexts of communication nor are they aimed at developing effective health promotion and disease control programs in Africa. This is due, in part, to how the African context of communication has been relegated to the Western notion of communication process (Nwosu, Taylor, & Onwumechili, 1995). The issue is further developed in another section of this article.

The purpose of this article is to determine some of the theoretical constraints in health communication research in Africa, and to provide some research direction that would facilitate health communication campaigns in this region of the world. In the process, specific ethical culture for health communication research in Africa is discussed.

Focus on Health in Africa

The focus on health communication research in Africa is due, at least in part, to the population explosion as well as the pandemic outbreak of communicable diseases in the continent. It is widely discussed that Africa's population of nearly 500 million is growing at a yearly rate of 3.3 percent, and that such increase has produced a host of health concerns for people who reside in the urban and rural areas of the continent. An analysis of some of the health concerns follows.

HIV Prevalence

The pandemic explosion of communicable diseases such as the human immunodeficiency virus (HIV) that causes AIDS, or acquired immune deficiency syndrome, is a case in point. It is estimated that two-thirds of the roughly 16 million people infected with HIV live in the AIDS belt, a region comprising a chain of countries in eastern and southern Africa. Medical evidence and surveillance reports suggest that 23 percent of those who reside in major cities and 10 percent of those who live in the rural areas of the AIDS belt may be infected with HIV (Caldwell & Caldwell, 1996). In South Africa alone, 2.2 million people, including an estimated 13 percent of its pregnant women, have HIV. The most recent surveillance reports suggest that between 1988 and 1997, the infection levels reported in South African clinics increased from less than one percent to over 20 percent. Clearly, the AIDS epidemic in Africa deserves some health communication research attention.

Substance Abuse

Another health concern is substance abuse. In most African countries alcohol has important social and cultural functions, which has encouraged its abuse. Alcohol abuse is particularly evident "during ritual ceremonies, communal planting and harvesting, and spirit media celebrations" (Acuda, 1995, p. 24). Even though some abuse problems may be less publicly visible, health care practitioners have reported an alarming rate of alcohol abuse among their patients.

For example, a busy health care clinic in Harare reported that "66 percent of the men and 48 percent of the women who drank were getting drunk on each occasion" (Acuda, 1995, p. 24). Because alcohol use is socially sanctioned and culturally accepted in most parts of Africa, the aggressive marketing of this substance seems to legitimize its use in social functions; causing a situation that fosters abuse. Interestingly enough, the production and social marketing of alcohol in most parts of Africa have not been equaled by health campaigns aimed at reducing its abuse.

A more troubling concern regarding substance abuse in Africa is that most parts of the continent are experiencing an increase in the use of psychoactive substances, such as tranquilizers, cannabis, stimulants, and more recently cocaine and heroin. Like alcohol abuse, the use of psychoactive substances may alter the user's state of mind and possibly lead to life-threatening behavior, such as the sharing of needles by intravenous drug users that facilitates the spread of HIV infection (Bergendahl & Hsu, 1995).

Smoking

The growing literature on tobacco research has provided abundant evidence that smoking is a health hazard. Descriptive epidemiological findings on cancer occurrence correlates with levels of exposure to cigarette smoking, a suspected agent in cancer of the lungs, larynx, esophagus, and oral cavity (Page, Cole, & Timmreck, 1995, p. 220). Recent studies show that "one in 10 heavy smokers is likely to get lung cancer" (Perera, 1996, p. 54). Similarly, smoking is known to increase the chances of heart disease, stroke, and chronic obstructive pulmonary disease.

In spite of the convincing evidence that smoking poses a series of health risks, cigarette tobacco continues to be one of the most common substances used in Africa. A case in point is South Africa where one in every three adults smoke cigarettes, 28-34 percent of whom are 16 years of age or older (Alali, 1997). Nearly 50 percent of South African males and 18 percent of females are cigarette smokers. And, even though over 25,000 South Africans die each year of smoking related causes, cigarette smoking is present in 83.1 percent of South African coronary heart disease patients (McKibbin, 1994). Clearly, aggressive cigarette advertising in the South African case has not been met with strong anti-smoking campaigns that provide long-term effect.

Major Morbidities

AIDS, substance abuse, and smoking illnesses are not the only health problems that threaten life in Africa. Malaria, for example, accounts for more than one million deaths every year. Recently, the World Health Organization (WHO) announced that 1996 was the worst year on record for cerebrospinal meningitis (an inflammation of the lining of the brain and spinal cord) in Africa, with around 150,000 reported cases and 16,000 deaths. These health problems as well as the outbreak of cholera and Ebola in some regions of Africa, have far reaching implication, especially within the context of life expectancy in the affected countries. It is estimated that by the year 2010, the life expectancy in countries such as Zambia would be lowered by the AIDS epidemic from 66 to 33 years, Zimbabwe from 70 to 40 years, Kenya from 68 to 40 years, and Uganda from 59 to 31 years (Alali & Nwosu, 1996).

Theoretical Constraints in Effective Health Communication Research

The magnitude of the health problems in Africa has prompted urgent attention among national governments and international donor agencies to address the crisis. Agencies such as WHO, the United Nations Children's Emergency Fund (UNICEF), the United Nations Educational, Scientific, and Cultural Organizations (UNESCO), the United States Centers for Disease Control and Prevention (CDC), and a number of European-based organizations provide funding and technical assistance for research, education, and disease prevention efforts.

Yet most of the research aimed at health promotion and disease prevention efforts in Africa appear to be casually-linked to the public's health. Hence, the communication models developed by those who study health issues have not fully addressed the individual and societal factors that interact with public health compliance; neither do their studies create linkages between theory and practical issues in health promotion and disease control in Africa. This is not to suggest that health communication research be more diagnostic to replace medical experts and those trained in epidemiology. Rather, health communication research should be treated, not merely as an isolated event that is intermittently studied, but one that associates health and wellness with culture, values, attitudes, and behavior. It deserves a higher level of scholarly commitment from those of us who study the field because our research findings are expected to stimulate and guide the direction of future health promotion efforts and subsequent research endeavor.

Unfortunately, much of the health communication research out of Africa is anecdotal and does not assist in the production of campaign programs that deal with health issues from realistic perspectives. This, in the author's view, is attributable to the bradytelic nature of health communication research in Africa. Consequently, the dominant paradigms affecting theoretical and methodological issues in health communication research have failed to offer the value of their constructs on health communication practices.

There are three basic issues that may help to further this argument. First, the field of health communication, particularly in Africa, has not advanced efficacious theories, and it is evident that the current theoretical constructs of health communication are not sufficiently embodied in the African contexts of health beliefs to enable explanations of the systematic elements that shape health campaigns and, in the long run, predetermine health outcomes. A good example is the AIDS campaigns in Africa where health communication efforts have disappointing results of compliance. The health communication research out of Africa tends to focus more on the end-result or effectiveness of a specific health message without fully understanding the target audience, how they interact with health providers, and the socio-cultural variables that impede compliance of campaign messages (Alali & Nwosu, 1996). Let us examine, further, the issue of health care provider interaction within the context of public health.

Health care providers are crucial instruments of change for people in medical contexts. They are trained to carry out primary health care, health education, and to execute intervention programs in their communities. In most cases, their encounters with patients create an opportunity for on-the-spot discussion of health issues and counseling for at-risk individuals. In this context, they are an important link that can affect patient compliance with health messages. However, current health communication research efforts in Africa are yet to yield evidence that would help clarify the impact of health provider interaction on patient compliance, and whether such interaction serves to benefit them or to reduce compliance. What do we need to know about the interaction that takes place between the health care provider and the patient that is not presently addressed in research?

Some of the questions research about communication and health care should seek to answer are: What type of interaction takes place between health professionals and the patients with whom they have contacts? Does the interaction center around the patients' health status and treatment, or does it deal with generalities? How much do we know about the patients' perceptions of health care providers' interaction with them? Is the interaction between health care providers and patients to provide emotional support more than as source of information? Does the patient perceive the care provider to be an authority figure? Does the patient consider the care provider as having a caring attitude toward the patient? Do health care providers use go-betweens, such as nurses, community health workers, or in the case of imminent death, the priest? Lastly, what is the patient's preference for health care provider/patient communication? Do patients prefer to delegate decisions to their doctors? Do the health provider and patient make health decisions alone or jointly? These are communicative acts that impact on health and patient compliance and, therefore, must be fully explored by research.

Second, it is clear that one of the basic philosophical objectives of conducting health communication research is to develop theories and models that would foster social health. As health communication scholars, our research efforts are expected to make an impact on disease prevention and control, a socially important issue. Yet, most of the health communication research and the ill-defined sociological expectations that result from them may, actually, produce ineffective results that have dangerous health consequences. For example, there are questions about the rate at which health campaigns in Africa are declared "successful" and are immediately applied to other health communication contexts and disease prevention efforts. There is a litany of such health campaign efforts that have been feverishly declared successful without the benefit of a constructive evaluation tool which can produce meaningful and significant results that have benefits to other health campaigns.

The problem for health communication campaigns is that the theoretical armamentarium that results from research in this field has become ineffectual in evaluating the African contexts of health. This is also true of the research methodologies that are used in African contexts of communication. Discussions about the appropriateness of research methods used in African contexts have been an age-old issue in the academy. (For further discussions see Boafo & George, 1992; Mukasa & Becker, 1992; Taylor, 1991; Nwosu, 1990; Okigbo, 1985; Ugboajah, 1985). However, most recent discussions offer a more practical insight to the problem inherent in the universal application of research methods, especially those developed by Western scholars for Western societies, to evaluate African communication phenomena. Researchers argue that the African contexts and the Western contexts of communication are two distinct and unconnected processes that cannot be evaluated with the same research methodologies (Nwosu, Taylor, & Onwumechili, 1995). Nwosu et al. suggest that the Western models are not sufficient tools for evaluating African communication phenomena because the Western contexts of communication tend to focus on "the individual as the primary source and receiver of information as opposed to the African context where the community and community values are central to communication interactions and decision-making process" (p. 398).

Lastly, the third constraint deals with the interdisciplinary nature of the field that demands collaborative research effort. Health communication is an interdisciplinary field that draws from biomedical and the social and behavioral sciences. The current environment in which personal and public health is at jeopardy requires collaborative efforts to assist professionals in these fields to navigate through treacherous waters where voluntary patient behavior and recklessness contribute substantially to disabilities and deaths. Understanding human behavior (a difficult variable to measure) is the key to the design of effective campaigns aimed at health promotion and disease prevention. Research efforts in health communication are not collaborative enough, hence their inability to understand the multiplicity of factors that affect human behavior and unhealthy lifestyles in Africa.

The day of the independent researcher is over and health communication researchers must recognize that this is an interdisciplinary field. Health communication researchers must work together with scholars from other fields. For example, biomedical researchers and medical associations in Africa should establish linkages with health communication scholars to develop ideas that would encourage healthy lifestyles and educate people on how to prevent communicable diseases and chronic conditions, such as alcoholism.

The issues articulated here have far reaching implication on health.

Clearly, a multidisciplinary approach to health communication research can yield concrete data about the traditional and cultural issues that affect health campaigns, political and social realities that frame national health policies, and how these policies shape health promotion, disease prevention efforts, and affect patient compliance. The peculiar nature of the contexts within which health communication research are framed in Africa need to be revisited to produce a shift in paradigm.

The discussions about theoretical and methodological constraints provide the backdrop for developing effective research and, perhaps, identifying some ethical issues that health communication researchers in Africa should consider. To the extent that there are serious challenges for health communication research, the question here is how do we navigate through the so-called "treacherous waters" of health communication without imposing ineffective models that exacerbate health problems in Africa? More specifically, we need to determine on what areas of empirical study health communication researchers should focus. What this chapter does is to provide a road map for a health communication research agenda in Africa as well as some of the ethical considerations for researchers. It is expected that this endeavor would usher in some important directions for health communication research in Africa.

Research Considerations

The crucial role communication plays in health care has forced the exhaustive use of communication constructs that were in place before the epidemic of diseases in Africa. Communication scholars, especially those who study health, desperately need to understand the variables that render health campaigns ineffectual. We believe that the quality of measurements employed in research would, ultimately, lead to the development of theories and constructs that can facilitate effective health promotion campaigns. There are two areas for research considerations that demand immediate attention. Let us examine each of these.

Appropriate Research Methodology

For health communication research in Africa to have credibility, an appropriate research methodology for each health context must be employed. The appropriateness of a research methodology can be further determined by evaluating the *sources of information*, *measurement instruments*, *data collection*, and *analysis of information*.

Health communication researchers are duty bound to clearly describe their sources of information so as to enable interpretations within the context of the source(s). This is not to suggest that issues of confidentiality and anonymity should violated or compromised by the researcher. Profiles that violate the confidentiality of sources must meet established guidelines for human subject research.

Another important element researchers must consider is the measurement instruments used for the research. In fact, it is an acceptable orthodoxy in research that "the measurement instruments used for the purpose of data gathering must possess relevant psychometric evidences for the particular purposes being used" (Torabi, 1993, p. 59). Therefore, it is an appropriate research method for the researcher to produce evidence for validity and reliability of the instruments used in their research. (For further discussions of measures of validity and reliability within the African contexts of communication, see M'Bayo, 1996; Nwosu, Taylor, & Onwumechili, 1995). The selection and development of appropriate research tools are crucial to the validation of health communication research findings.

If the culture of health communication research demands that the sources of information and the instruments used to measure information be clearly articulated, then the health communication researcher must monitor the data collection process to reduce, if not minimize, human errors that may lead to biased interpretations. The data generated from any research should be of the highest quality and health communication research should not be exempt from this standard.

Clearly, the methodological soundness of research is not complete without an appropriate statistical tool to use in the analysis of the quantitative information collected. This is especially crucial when a small sample is used to draw inference on a larger population. If the expertise in statistical analysis is not available within the team of researchers, use statistical consultants.

Evaluation Tools for the Health Campaign Process

Ultimately, health communication research efforts should lead to the development of evaluation tools that would be directly useful to people and health promotion programs. The evaluation tools should focus on three basic areas: *planning*, *program operations*, and *program outcomes* (Pirie, 1990).

Planning

During the planning stage, the measurement tools that result from the research effort ought to have the ability to evaluate key elements of a health program, such as existing data about the health problem, the budget available for the specific health campaign, political realities and institutional constraints, religious and ethnic concerns that may affect the campaign, and the target audience (in terms of its demographics).

The target audience is one of the most important elements in public health campaigns; a target audience defines the ways a public health educator should design, conduct, and implement a campaign. The challenges posed by differences in audiences, as well as the different approaches and perspectives in health communication, require the development of appropriate evaluation tools to measure areas that are crucial to campaign success. For example: Who is the target audience? Would the campaign identify the relevant categories of at-risk population for the health problem? What personal characteristics, values, and ideological beliefs are likely to increase or impede the target audience's chances of compliance? What are the target audience's previous experiences? And most importantly, is the campaign culturally appropriate and sensitive to the target audience's sensibilities?

Clearly, the target audience defines the nature of the campaign. An evaluation tool that carefully assesses these elements at the beginning of the campaign can illuminate the dark alleys public health educators occasionally stumble into as they attempt to inoculate the public with messages that are aimed at changing their attitudes, beliefs, and behavior toward a health issue.

Program Operations

Research efforts may, in fact, assist public health educators with the tools to best define objectives of their programs, particularly those that relate to the design, message objective, medium of communication, and channel selection.

The contents of a health campaign are a measure of their impact on learning and behavior. To determine whether the contents of a health campaign can produce the desired impact on learning and behavior, an evaluation tool should be capable of:

1. assessing the accuracy, relevance, and currency of health informa-

tion in the campaign;
2. determining the appropriateness of the information for the target audience;
3. assessing the readability level of the health message;
4. determining its objectivity, or lack of bias;
5. determining whether the health information is authoritative and supported by scientific evidence;
6. determining whether the health information is free of all controversial religious, political, or ideological views; and
7. determining whether the health promotion objectives can be accomplished through the specified campaign.

Program Outcomes

Lastly, the health communication research in Africa that may result from these considerations are expected to focus on the development of an evaluation instrument for assessing health campaign effectiveness. Such an evaluation tool should ask the right questions about the effectiveness of the program, the direction of the program (continue/discontinue, expand/reduce), the shifts in behavior that affect the campaign, and policy initiative resulting from the campaign. The aim here is to develop evaluation measures that document short-term results of the campaign, and determines whether the program objectives were met and how well each stage of the campaign process was handled.

Ethical Considerations

Responsible research on health communication in Africa must be governed by specific ethical standards that are couched on six climate types: *professional*, *caring*, *role oriented*, *instrumental*, *efficient*, and *independent* (Victor & Cullen, 1990). The generally acceptable belief that ethics govern the moral acceptability of behavior in different contexts will have no value if those within a social context have no shared perception of how issues in their environment should be addressed, and to some extent, what is ethically acceptable behavior. Clearly, health communication research should not be made exempt from such precepts.

In health communication research, issues of ethics should revolve around specific objectives such as: the use of information to promote health and prevent the spread of diseases. And, because health communication depends on information, it should not be value laden. This is to say that ethical standards in health communication research should be governed by the six climate types articulated earlier (Victor & Cullen, 1990). There is no doubt that the challenges for health communication research can be further complicated by the ethical issues that confront researchers, however, we also believe that not knowing about ethical systems and ethical principles may inhibit the success of health communication research.

Additionally, as health communication researchers, we must position ourselves as equal participants in the development of appropriate framework for health promotion and disease prevention programs in Africa. Consequently, we must begin to consider the adoption of some ethical standards to guide our research agenda. Following are a few ethical issues health communication researchers should consider.

Define Ethical Obligations of Researchers

In developing an appropriate agenda for health communication research, it is important to define specific ethical obligations for researchers, especially as it relates to their motivation for pursuing the research. Recently, some scholars in the medical community have accused communication researchers of being attracted to health communication research because there is money to be made through extramural funding (Burgoon, 1995). To render such criticisms mute, it is imperative that we establish ethical standards for researchers in this field so as to validate the findings of those who are committed to the objectives of health communication. This is to say that researchers in this field are ethically bound to do the right thing by developing information that is not value laden and, yet, is valuable to health promotion and disease prevention efforts. Therefore, to anticipate ethical problems in our research is the starting point for delineating ways to handle the ethical issues that confront researchers.

Goal Oriented

Health communication research efforts should be goal oriented and realistic enough to offer effective solutions to problems as well as anticipate future concerns for health campaigns. It must establish a premise for a coordinated effort to promote healthy lifestyles for individuals and prevent the spread of diseases to the larger population. Again, such efforts must not be value laden.

Examine Cultural and Religious Contexts

Health communication researchers in Africa must recognize and respect the cultural and religious sensibilities that interact with the health issue being studied. Elements of culture and religion are not easily divorced from all aspects of life in Africa. Therefore, health communication researchers should examine carefully the cultural and religious contexts that serve as a backdrop for each health issue, and act in ethically appropriate ways that recognize such issues yet, preserve the public's health.

Distinguish Between Research and Policy Paper

Ethical research culture demands disclosure to enable readers to distinguish between a research and a policy paper that is aimed at advancing a particular perspective. It is a particularly acceptable ethical practice for a researcher to identify the sponsors of their research and the interest being represented in their paper. It is possible that the our sources of research funding have a stake in the outcome of the studies they fund. We must declare our position and identify those who sponsor our research to eliminate any suspicion that may be associated with our findings.

Explicit and Open Communication

While research on health matters should encourage explicit and open communication about health, we must also exercise restraint over the extent to which researchers talk to patients about a potential disease. We are not physicians and, as such, should not be involved in epidemiological or clinical/diagnostic aspects of the disease or patient. Our lack of training in the pathology of diseases may create situations that panic the public into adopting unhealthy therapy.

Accuracy and Truth

Responsible and effective health communication depends upon accurate and unbiased research. Accuracy and truth in information gathering, analysis and reporting would provide decision-makers with the necessary information, and reduce misunderstanding by the public.

Timeliness

Health communication researchers must share their findings with the appropriate sources in a timely manner. Because of the nature of the subjects being studied, delaying the release of any findings may cost lives and, in the long-run, would diminish the importance of the research findings.

Summary and Conclusion

Health communication is a global issue that is real and inescapable. As customs of the world spread across cultures so do health issues. There is a consensus among epidemiologists that no one country is immune from diseases of the world. Research efforts aimed at health promotion and disease prevention in Africa must be articulated with a perspective that also recognizes diseases as a global issue with local implications. At the same time, health communication researchers must work within the political realities and institutional influences that determine the research agenda, directions, contexts, and outcome.

Health communication researchers should spearhead efforts to understand variables which interact with health promotion and disease prevention campaigns. And because the findings that result from such research have immediate and important impact on people's lives, health communication research requires a measure of variables which would be included in theoretical models for health promotion and disease prevention in Africa.

The challenge here is for health communication researchers to find ways to work collaboratively with allied fields to develop and disseminate accurate, up-to-date health information to the public so as to serve as persuasive injunctions that influence behavioral and lifestyle changes. There is a role in health communication research for all disciplines, particularly medicine, health education, communication, sociology, psychology, political science, philosophy, and anthropology. The health communication research that results from this fusion would ultimately help researchers to provide the public with health information in simple and understandable terms so they can act on it and, in return, reduce the probability of infection.

In conclusion, it is fitting here to cite Becker (1995), who sums up the role of health communication scholars best:

> We can do our society a tremendous amount of good by bringing our special expertise to bear on getting people to lead healthier lifestyles. In the process we will also help the public and institutional perception of our field quite considerably when they see us and our colleagues helping to solve problems that they recognize important - especially if our efforts are successful (pp. 19-20).

The health communication research that comes out of Africa has the potential to make contributions to the continent. Collectively, communication scholars and researchers in allied fields can create a research agenda for effective health communication in Africa.

References

Acuda, S. W. (1995, July-August). An African example. *World Health*, 4:24.

Alali, A. O. (1997). Health warnings and content disclosures in cigarette advertisements: The case of South Africa. Unpublished research data.

Alali, A. O., & Nwosu, P. (1996). Social and cultural considerations in planning AIDS education and campaigns in Africa. Paper presented at the 10th Bien nial African Council for Communication Education Conference, Cape Town, South Africa, November 15-22).

Becker, S. L. (1995). Improving the nation's health: The role of communication scholars. Paper presented at the 1995 Speech Communication Association Summer Conference on "Communication and Health" (July 19-23, Washington, D.C.).

Bergendahl, P., & Hsu, L. (1995, July-August). Women and substance abuse. *World Health,* 4:12.

Boafo, S., & George, N. (eds) (1992). *Communication research in Africa: Issues and perspectives*. Nairobi: African Council on Communication Education.

Burgoon, M. (1995). Navigating the treacherous waters of health communication: Dawning of the age of Aquarius or rule of Proteus? 1995 SCA Summer Conference Proceedings and Prepared Remarks, July 19-23, Washington, D.C. Annandale, VA: Speech Communication Association.

Caldwell, J. C., & Caldwell, P. (1996, March). The African AIDS epidemic. *Scientific American*, 62-68.

M'Bayo, R. (1996). Methodological considerations in the study of communications and information policies in Africa. *Journal of Research Methodology and African Studies*, 1;1: 1-33.

McKibbin, E. C. (1994, August). An analysis of the risk factors for coronary heart disease in patients aged 55 and younger with proven heart disease. *South African Journal of Nursing*, 17;3: 51-56.

Mukasa, S., & Becker, L. (1992). Toward an indigenized philosophy of communication: An analysis of African communication educational resources and needs. *Africa Media Review*, 6;3.

Nwosu, P. (1990). Communication and agricultural development in Swaziland: Toward a need-based integrative model. Unpublished doctoral dissertation, Howard University.

Nwosu, P., Taylor, D., & Onwumechili, C. (1995). Search for appropriate research methods in the African context. In Nwosu, P., Onwumechili, C., & M'Bayo, R. (eds), *Communication & the transformation of society: A developing region's perspectives* (pp. 397-426). Lanham, MD: University Press of America.

Okigbo, C. (1985). Is development communication a dead issue? *Media Development,* 4:23-25.

Page, R. M., Cole, G. E., & Timmreck, T. C. (1995). *Basic epidemiological methods and biostatistics: A practical guidebook.* Boston, MA: Jones and Bartlett Publishers.

Perera, F. P. (1996, May). Uncovering new clues to cancer risk. *Scientific American*, 54-62.

Pettegrew, L. S. (1988). Theoretical plurality in health communication. In J. A. Anderson (ed.), *Communication Yearbook II* (pp. 298-308). Newbury Park, CA: Sage.

Pirie, P. L. (1990). Evaluating health promotion programs: Basic questions and approaches. In N. Bracht (ed), *Health promotion at the community level* (pp. 201-208). Newbury Park, CA: Sage.

Taylor, D. S. (1991). Application of the uses and dependency model of mass communication to development communication in the western area of Sierra Leone. Unpublished doctoral dissertation, Kent State University.

Torabi, M. R. (1993, July/August). General standards for educational evaluations. *Health Values*, 17;4: 57-59.

Ugboajah, F. O. (1985). Oramedia in Africa. In F. O. Ugboajah (ed), *Mass communication, culture and society in West Africa.* London: Hans Zell Publisers.

Victor, B., & Cullen, J. B. (1990). A theory and measure of ethical climate in organizations. In W. C. Frederick & L. E. Preston (eds), *Business ethics: Research issues and empirical studies.* Greenwich, CT: JAI Press.

Chapter 4

Health Promotion Challenges in Nigeria: Globalization, Tobacco Marketing and Policies

Igbo N. Egwu
University of Calabar, Nigeria

The growing literature on tobacco research has provided abundant evidence that smoking is a health hazard. Research findings on cancer occurrence correlate with levels of exposure to cigarette smoking, a suspected agent in cancer of the lungs, larynx, esophagus, and oral cavity. The health problems associated with smoking are more acute in developing nations were aggressive marketing of tobacco products is sanctioned by government policies. In this chapter, we tackle the notion of globalization and marketing as complex challenges in the attempt to address the harmful effects of tobacco products in Nigeria. However, in order to fully address the issues discussed in this chapter, it is necessary to define some of the key concepts.

Definition of Concepts

Health Promotion. The concept of health promotion is not new. What is new is its redefinition by the *Ottawa Charter on Health Promotion* in

1996 (WHO, 1986). The Charter expanded the concept of health to include peace, adequate economic resources, food and shelter, and a stable ecosystem and sustainable resource use. This inevitable expansion of the original definition of health promotion is consistent with the need to move towards a *new* public health in the 21st century.

Under this perspective, health promotion is the process of enabling people increase control over and to improve their health. Put differently, health promotion enables individuals and populations to increase control over the determinants of health. These interactive factors include personal, social, economic and environmental influences on health status: health behaviors and lifestyles, income and social status, education, employment and working conditions, access to appropriate health services, and physical environments. Health promotion is therefore, fundamentally concerned with action and advocacy which address potentially modifiable determinants of health. In subsequent sections of this essay, and in relation to moving health promotion into the 21st century, as defined in the *Jakarta Declaration* of 1997 (WHO, 1997), *health literacy* or learning provides access to education and information which are essential to the achievement of effective participation (involvement) and empowerment of individuals and communities.

Accordingly, the *Jakarta Declaration* specifies five areas of priority: promotion of *social responsibility for health*; increase in *investments for health development*; expansion of *partnerships for health promotion*; increase in *community capacity and empowerment of the individual*; and *securing an infrastructure for health promotion.* A discussion of these areas of priority follows.

Social Responsibility for Health: Social responsibility for health is reflected by the actions of decision-makers in both public and private sectors to pursue policies and practices which promote and protect health. Such policies and practices should not harm health of individuals; they should restrict the production of trade in harmful goods and substances as well as discourage unhealthy marketing practices (WHO, 1997).

Investment for Health Development: Investment for health development refers to resources which are dedicated to the production of health and health gain (improved health outcomes). Investment for health strategies is based on knowledge about the determinants of health.

Partnerships for Health Promotion for Health: Partnership for health promotion for health represents a voluntary agreement between partners–e.g., government and corporate/non-governmental organizations to work cooperatively towards shared health outcomes. Such partnerships may take the form of intersectoral collaboration or alliances for health promotion.

Community Capacity and Empowerment of the Individual: The concept of community empowerment means a community in which individuals and organizations apply their skills and resources in collective efforts to address health priorities to meet their needs.

Securing Infrastructure for Health Promotion: Human resources, organizational and administrative structures, policies, regulations and incentives which facilitate the organized health promotion response to public health issues and challenges. Infrastructure includes not only tangible resources and structures, but also the extent of public and political awareness of health issues and participation (involvement) in actions that address health concerns.

Globalization: The notion of 'global village' is closely associated with the 20th century; with it comes the increasing realization that the health of populations is dependent on numerous external factors. Market forces, environmental hazards, access to mass communications and technology, and cultural influences (WHO, 1997). Globalization is characterized by increasing economic and social interdependence. It can also be viewed in two dimensions: as a threat to health of population or as providing some major opportunities to work together for a healthier world (Potter, 1997; WHO 1997).

There are several health implications of globalization: (a) There is globalization of health risks and diseases as well as opportunities such as diffusion of ideas and technology; (b) the need for intersectoral action through transnational cooperation and partnerships: (c) an enhanced role of international legal instrument/regimes, standard setting, and global norms; (d) the need for new intersectoral forms of global vigilance, monitoring and assessment. Information on health status and the global determinants of health are vital for defining future actions in a rapidly changing policy environment.

One of the consequences of increase in transnational trade, travel and migration is the risk of cross-border transmission of infectious diseases. As the world becomes more interconnected, diseases are disseminated more rapidly and effectively. The HIV/AIDS pandemic is a vivid example of the globalization of infectious diseases. Another example of significant international health problem arises from food-borne disease, traceable to a tremendously large number of movement of person traveling across national borders – about 400 million every year (WHO, 1997).

Trade Promotion Versus Health Promotion

Despite the positive opportunities provided by globalization (a few are mentioned above), there are negative influences of globalization on health. Some of the products and lifestyles/habits exported to developing countries clearly affect health negatively- e.g. international tobacco trade and associated advertising of tobacco products. In the last 20 years, the

Figure 4.1: ***Effects of Control and Advertising on Tobacco Consumption in Developed Countries***

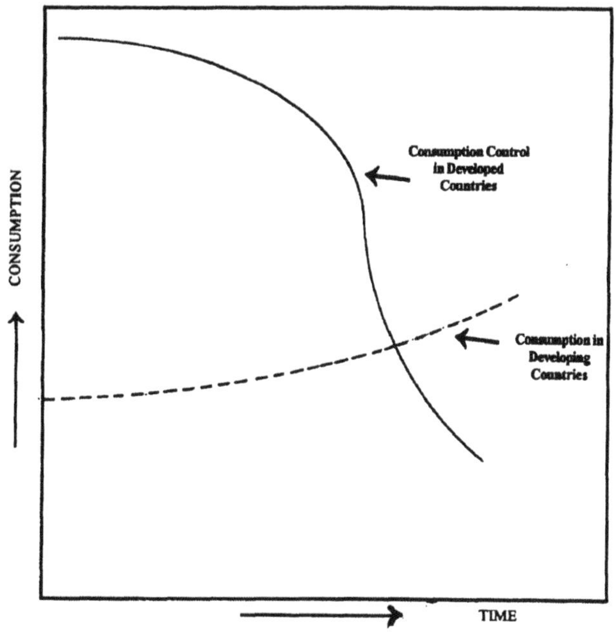

world's consumption of tobacco has increased by about 75 percent; and much of this increased consumption has occurred in developing countries. Here, the multinational corporations aggressively advertise their products as an inexpensive way of appear Western, sexy, adventurous and successful (Potter, 1997). It is estimated that by 2020, over 70 percent of tobacco related death might be occurring in developing countries (Potter, 1997). The effect of dumping tobacco advertising in developing countries, including Nigeria, is hypothetically depicted in Figure 4.1. It shows an inverse relationship between tobacco consumption in developed and developing countries: as developed countries increase controls over tobacco consumption through policies and legislative means, and lawsuits (e.g. in the United States of America), tobacco manufacturers and their marketing agents are exporting and intensifying their marketing strategies to drive up consumption of tobacco products in developing countries.

Globalization of Tobacco and its Harmful Effects

A harmful consequence of globalization is associated with the negative effects on health by exporting harmful products/lifestyles through international trade, and advertising by multinational corporations (Potter, 1997). Tobacco related diseases are preventable. Smoking is associated with increased risk of different cancers, including lung, bladder, ischemic heart disease, bronchitis and emphysema, and perinatal mortality of infants whose mothers smoked during pregnancy (Potter, 1997). Environmental exposure to tobacco smoke poses health risks of *passive smoking* to nonsmokers exposed to such an environment.

It has been stated that tobacco consumption has been increased by aggressive advertising methods of multinational tobacco conglomerates that have increasingly targeted women and adolescents in developing country markets. Connolly (1992) revealed that tobacco companies encountered declining sales in developed country markets and therefore, looked for alternative markets to penetrate in Asia, Africa and other developing countries. This practice has been pursued in recent years with greater intensity. Correspondingly, the vulnerable populations of the target groups in these countries have proven to be eager consumers of tobacco products. The harmful effects are obscured by the sophisticated promotional strategies which portray smoking as an inexpensive way to buy into glamorous lifestyles of the upper or successful social class (Stebbins, 1992).

Tobacco Marketing in Nigeria

Tobacco marketing in Nigeria rests on an unhealthy 'triad' made up marketing versus law; smoking versus law and government versus economic gains. This positive or negative relationship is portrayed here as the Triad Model in Figure 4.2.

Figure 4.2: ***The Tobacco – Marketing, Sales and Consumption (Triad) Model***

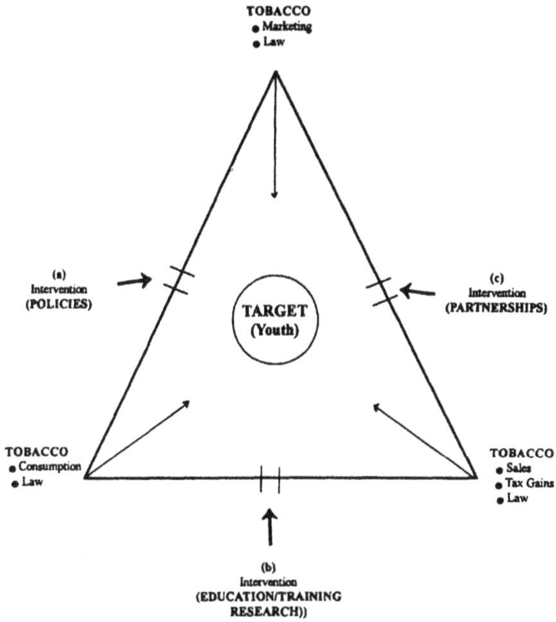

Tobacco Marketing vs. Law

Six transnational tobacco companies – two British and four American, dominate the international trade in tobacco. Together, they control 85 percent of the world's tobacco market (Frankel, 1996). These powerful transnationals also operate in Nigeria. Decree 20 of 1990 was put in place as an enabling law to fight tobacco promotion. Eight years later, a new nongovernmental organization – Nigerian Anti-Tobacco Alliance

(NATA) was still calling for enforcement of Decree 20; the organization even called for the elimination of direct and indirect tobacco advertising promotion and sponsorship. At the same time, the Health Minister condemned the use of advertising by tobacco manufacturers to recruit new smokers who are made to believe that smoking leads to success. Examples include Rothmans, Pall Mall, the Nigerian Television Authority (NTA), sports program and Golden Tone musical concert; all defy the law on tobacco. Some of these tobacco companies also erect bus stops where their advertisements are conspicuously displayed without the warning: ***THE FEDERAL MINISTRY OF HEALTH (OF NIGERIA) WARNS THAT TOBACCO SMOKING IS DANGEROUS TO HEALTH.*** Yet the tobacco smoking (control) Decree No. 20 of 1990 (section 2 [2]) provides that:

> ...no tobacco industry, firm or association of individuals or any other body corporate shall sponsor or promote any of their products at any sport event sponsored or promoted by them.

Smoking and Law

On the legitimacy of advertising, proponents of sustained advertising, represented by local agents of American Association of Advertising Agencies (AAAA) pretend that the global advertising industry supported efforts to curb smoking by minors. At the same time, it opposed banning of advertising of tobacco to adults. Ebissemiju and Okungbawo (1988) quoted a spokesman of the transnational advertising organization recently as saying: "We oppose the advertising regulations, not the restrictions on sales."

The logic of this position is a fallacy because the argument advanced by the pro-advertising group recognized that the government has the legal right to protect its citizens from harmful products. Yet the advertisers insist that the legal right to produce tobacco and its products also confers on them the right to promote tobacco products. From their position of strength, the only concession that tobacco advertisers are willing to make (if seriously threatened) is to devise alternative promotional and marketing strategies available in their marketing and communication mix. It appears that tobacco marketing and the laws are deliberately in conflict, leaving the vulnerable targets of advertising and marketing of tobacco, particularly the youth, defenseless (Figure 4.2). In an apparent reference to the vulnerable target group, Decree No. 20 (1999) adds that:

> ...no package containing tobacco products meant for smoking shall be sold in Nigeria, unless...rotating warnings are inscribed on the package....Smokers are liable to die young.

Most observers view this only as a mere caveat.

Government Tax Gains and Law

Economic considerations of gross national product (GNP), tax gains from the sale of tobacco products and alcohol define the official/government stance on the advertising, marketing and sales of these harmful substances. For example, the defunct Tobacco Advisory Council of Nigeria (TACON) had argued that tobacco is a legal product. It also cites a study of the Nigerian Institute of Social and Economic Research (NISER) which showed that in 1993, tobacco industry injected ₦40 million naira (US $1 = ₦22 at 1993 rate), into rural economy and provided 10 million jobs. Distributors of the products also made an annual turnover of ₦482.6 million, while annual tax gains for the government was about ₦300 million. In 1996, tobacco industry taxes were 700 million (Ebissemiju & Okungbawo, 1988). Advertisers' position (supportive of sustained advertising of tobacco products), seems to make poverty-induced deaths statistics and tobacco-induced death less significant. More sinister arguments from advertisers interpret the unenforceable government restrictions and anti-tobacco campaign, as neither deep-rooted nor genuine, notwithstanding the inaction of the government and Decree No. 20 (1990).

It would appear then, that Decree 20 of 1990 could have been an effective control or even banning of tobacco advertising, but the law ambivalently provides tobacco companies and advertisers a loophole. This loophole is contained in section 3(1a) which implies that merely warning smokers satisfies the law and potential targets on the packages that "tobacco smoking is harmful and in section 3(1b) that smokers are liable to die young." There is widespread belief that this law is flagrantly disregarded.

Ironically, some key members of the Advertising Council of Nigeria (ACON) blame foreign mass media e.g., *CNN* for the exportation into Nigeria of the U.S. model of advertising restrictions. This implies that Nigerian advertisers are more than ready to import glossy and sleek images of U.S. advertising strategies but not U.S. effective control/restrictions against the promotion and marketing of tobacco products.

Profile of Youth: The Target of Tobacco Advertising and Marketing

Although there are obvious socio-cultural differences among young people in different countries, they tend to respond, in some global way, to carefully packaged tobacco advertising and marketing messages. Targeting of youth comes in different forms including heavy investment in promotional activities. Examples, are sponsorship of concerts, sporting events, public entertainment: distribution of specially items which cigarette logo – e.g., *Benson and Hedges' Golden Tone, Rothmans Mega Groove* concert, and sponsorship of English Premier (soccer) League.

Youth are also targeted through advertisement in popular magazines. *The News* and *Tell* magazine advertise *St. Moritz* menthol cigarettes with the enticing words: "The cool, smooth choice;" or "enjoy smooth fresh taste." *Webster's* cigarette "selected Virginia tobacco" is attractively and colorfully displayed in *Tell* magazine as "the freedom to be you!" The word "international" is underscored on the package in red, suggestive of globalization.

Similarly, *Benson and Hedges'* appeals to the youth and other vulnerable people to "turn to Gold," as they are encouraged in an advertisement to link cigarette smoking with a bar window that is overlooking a beach full of youth and leisure boats. In its most daring appeal, *Rothmans* shows a jubilant young soccer coach with a cheering full stadium and the catch phrase: "There is nothing better". In another version of its magazine advertising *Rothmans* also displays two young men who are rejoicing with a gold trophy winner – obviously emphasizing *success.*

In each of these advertisements the caveat "the Federal Ministry of Health warns that Tobacco smoking is dangerous to health (Decree 20, 1990) is inserted," almost as an after thought, and in small prints. These are a few samples of the youthfulness vigor, sexual attraction and independence and success portrayed by tobacco adverts in news magazines and billboards in Nigerian cities. Other tactics include gift specialty like T-shirts, key chains, calendars etc. with cigarette logos. In addition, non-factual reassuring images of glamour make tobacco appealing to young people. Comparable observations have been made in other African countries.

Observations from the Field

A recent survey in the University of Calabar in seven faculties, is informative. A total of about 18 percent of those interviewed were smokers 15 percent were male and 3 percent were female. The ages of the students ranged from 15-30; with the age of onset of smoking, in 4 percent of the student between 5-10 years, while 56 percent started smoking between ages 16-21. Awareness about the harmful effect among smokers was 80 percent, indicating that awareness did not deter smoking.

By year of study, the prevalence was 5 percent in year One, 31 percent in years Two and Four, respectively, indicating increase in smoking in the final years of college. If this is even slightly suggestive of the trend in other universities in Nigeria, then children and young adults are potentially vulnerable to globalization of tobacco advertising/marketing in Nigeria.

Challenges, Gaps and Strategies

The challenges of health promotion in Nigeria, and indeed Africa, are as varied as they are complex. The need to address this problem in most countries in the continent was apparent during an African 'group forum at the 4th International Conference on Health Education in Jakarta, Indonesia in 1997. The need for communication among health promotion professionals at the inter-regional and intra-national levels, as a clear choice and means of enhancing health communication in Africa, was identified. Some laudable initiatives, as a follow-up to Jakarta 1997, have been made Africa countries, particularly by those in the East Central region of the continent.

Beyond such 'administrative' or 'organizational' level of health communication, African countries need to move towards to the 'operational' or 'field' level – i.e. communicating vital health promotion messages to their population, in the 2lst century using multimedia strategy, mass media, traditional media or contemporary media. Here again, there are varying degrees of efforts at selective or a 'mix' of these strategies in Africa: Zimbabwe is a good example of the later.

Policy, Economic and Political Environment of Health Promotion in Nigeria

Before we proceed with further discussion, the policy economic and political environment of health promotion in Nigeria should be kept in its proper frame. This is because of the pivotal importance of environments, planning, implementation and evaluation of health promotion programs.

Policy

Nigeria's national health policy is based on the principles of Primary Health Care (PHC) as enunciated at Alma-Ata in 1978 (WHO. 1978). As Dr. Karch aptly comments, "...it is a very rare exception if you don't find some reference to health promotion in the health policy documents of countries throughout the world" (Karch, 1998). In the case of Nigeria's Health Policy of 1988, it briefly stipulates that there shall be redistribution of financial allocation to ensure that more emphasis is placed on health promotion and preventive services. In Nigeria, secondary and tertiary levels of care absorb more than 80 percent of health care budgetary allocation.

Given decentralization policy, which is in place, which leaves local governments with responsibility for PHC services (including health promotion), this situation means that health promotion is one of the most neglected aspects of primary health care sub-system development. It can be argued that this financial challenge is traceable to dwindling resources from the health system due to global economic recession, debt burden and declining commodity prices. These, in turn, led to decrease in national health budget with concomitant low preventive services and low health service utilization. Under these adverse conditions, in all sectors of the economy, the *Structural Adjustment Program* (SAP) was adopted as a preferred policy shift presumably to obviate the strains of economic recession. Donor agencies believe that this policy was an appropriate policy to reverse the adverse effect of global recession through "refocused" primary health care services. Yet there is a total lack of emphasis on health education in general and health promotion in particular.

The concept of health promotion in Nigeria–both in policy and practice remains a rudimentary one, although PHC is relatively well organized. As a consequence, health promotion in Nigeria – its policy, planning or practice, has not been influenced by the positive wave of international conferences relevant to strategies in health promotion, including healthy public policy. In Ottawa, Canada 1986; Adelaide, Australia 1988; and Jakarta, Indonesia, 1987 these strategies were examined. The 1997 conference is a crucial one because it reflected lessons learned from effective health promotion, reexamination of determinants of health, and identification of directions and strategies.

Preconditions – First Things First

In Nigeria, tobacco marketing or globalization is a 'model' of the challenges of health promotion. The Nigerian experience raises a number of fundamental issues. The first is that it seems to contest the Ottawa Charter definition of health promotion. The people seem to have lost "control over" and cannot therefore "improve" their health. In this single example alone, promotion of harmful products has aggressively displaced the promotion of health. Owing to such orchestrated *economic oppression*, Nigerian government is unable to define health promotion within its global perspective. The second concomitant issue is that health promotion/health education professionals may face a very difficult task of health promotion in the 2lst century.

Of special interest in this regard, is the fact that policy makers will be unable to (a) "avoid harming the health of individuals" and (b) "restrict production of and trade in inherently harmful goods and substances – e.g. tobacco and alcohol, as well as marketing practices…" Thirdly, Nigeria may fail to fulfill these priorities in the 21st century (less than 1/2 year away). This will certainly leave Nigeria on the start-line of the race towards global health promotion in the 2lst century.

To counter this scenario, this author advocates changes through fiscal policy in support of health promotion as an enabling politico-economic environment. These are the minimum conditions that ought to be met before any solutions to some of the challenges including the tobacco 'model' can be addressed.

Solutions

Reforming PHC Policy

In general, the national health policy which is based on the principles of PHC makes a cursory reference to health education and health promotion. This theoretical concept needs to be concretized. The notion of health matters in general, PHC activities and health education/promotion are on the concurrent list of state governments. This means that the Federal government allows states to have preeminent authority over implementation of PHC. But the direct funding of health programs controlled by local governments can provide a control mechanism for effective funding. Policy changes to focus specifically on health promotion activities can be fostered through local governments (LGAs). In fact, this is more logical, and more effective, since the population base is at the LGA – the tier of government nearest to the people.

Potential Options for Financial Health Promotion Programs

If the policy adjustments are put in place, then we can identify supplementary sources of funding to sustain health promotion programs. They include:

Health System Fund (HSF): This is an innovative means of financing the health sector through wholesale banking of health services. It involves arrangement with the World Bank in which the Federal and State governments are expected to participate. The *modus operandi* is not clear.

Petroleum Trust Fund (PTF): PTF funds are generated from petroleum tax proceeds under the trusteeship of an independent Board. The funds have been applied to a number of capital projects...roads, capital building project – e.g. hospitals etc., the PTF recently embarked on massive financing health infrastructures and drug revolving projects. It is a good candidate for financing projects in PHC in general and health promotion, in particular. It should also be considered in any partnership approach to health promotion programs. PTF may be disbanded.

Fiscal Policies – Taxes and Duties: imposed directly on income or sales of luxury goods and consumer products which have adverse effect on the health of people, e.g. tobacco and alcohol. It has already been pointed out above that the tobacco industry in Nigeria that taxes from tobacco industry in 1996 alone amounted to $8.2 million. Some approaches to the maximization of this source were examined during the Jakarta Conference of Health Promotion in 1997. Unless partnership is involved, there is the possibility of shift to high-tar homemade products. Other examples are budgetary allocations, private financing, community financing and charitable voluntary donations (Egwu, 1998).

Strategies to Meet Challenges: We return, once again, to the Tobacco 'Triad' model proposed above in Figure 4.2. It was applied earlier to explain the complex, negative and interactive relationship between tobacco marketing, tobacco advertising/sales and tobacco consumption, and the ambivalence of law and regulations/restrictions at each angle of the triad. This model is also useful in proposing possible strategies to control the harmful health effects of tobacco-related economic activities described. *Intervention* – using the triad model, three broad categories of intervention on tobacco are conceivable: (a) policy intervention; (b) education, training and research intervention; and (c) partnership intervention. The approach is to coordinate knowledge, technology and skills to break the 'bonds' between the key negative factors that sustain tobacco-induced health challenges.

(a) Policy Intervention

This is the responsibility of federal, state and local government who must act in concert ("concurrent list" notwithstanding), to take firm legislative action to ban advertising of tobacco products in *all* media; ban consumption of tobacco products in public places (Decree No. 20, 1990 is a good start but needs expansion and enforcement): (i) policies which support diversified funding base to ensure flexibility and ability to withstand political changes; (ii) policies that recognize the determinants of health – social, economic and environmental. This means governments' readiness to address the impact of health factors, adoption of comprehensive health promotion strategy, assessment of impact of public policy on health and recognition of communities as significant foci for health action; (iii) policies should facilitate intersectoral action and coordination; and (iv) Policies to establish a focal point for health promotion.

(b) Education/Training and Research Intervention

Adequate and continuing training to provide manpower is a crucial strategy. Academic and scientific communities should adhere to highest professional scientific and ethical standards in embracing research on the harmful effects of tobacco products.

(c) Partnership Intervention

A partnership for health promotion is a voluntary agreement between two or more partners to work cooperatively towards a set of shared health outcomes. Partnerships may be part of *intersectoral collaboration* for health or be based on alliances. As a strategy for tobacco products, promotion and consumption, it may be the most effective strategy. It may involve local, national, regional and global partners.

Partnership may be built from private sector, government or public sector, nongovernmental organizations (NGOs) and a combination of the above. Some of the principles for health promotion partnership include: definition of eligibility for partnership, development and management; freedom of partners to respond to opportunities while protecting their image, interest, independence and flexibility to adapt to changing environment (WHO Working Papers for 4th International Conference on Health Education. Jakarta, Indonesia, 1997).

(d) Communication

Before we conclude this discussion, it is highly necessary to mention that the main technical 'lubricant' for health education/health promotion is communication – health communication. In any joint campaign for healthy lifestyles, against tobacco sales or consumption, there is an enormous scope for such partnerships with the communications industry. Globalization of tobacco products is an example of negative health communication in Africa; positive health communication is desirable.

Conclusion

Health promotion in Nigeria is challenged by a number of factors, not the least of which is the vagueness of total unfamiliarity with the concept in Nigeria. The notion of globalization is discussed as a complex challenge which constrains attempt to address the harmful effects of tobacco products in most African countries. But the focus is on Nigeria where the prevalence of tobacco product consumption is reaching epidemic proportions due to globalization of the advertising, marketing and consumption. Globalization has other advantages and positive influences. However, its application to target young people in Africa gives it a label as negative health communication in Africa. The health problems associated with tobacco products including cancer and other diseases that can destroy the youth. The irony of this insidious danger is that the same government, which presumably would defend its citizens against foreign invasion, helplessly watches its citizens, being consumed by the flame of transnational tobacco companies. This is negative the effect of globalization.

In Nigeria, there are controls aimed at smoking in public places, as provided in Decree No. 20 of 1990. Young people easily obtain tobacco products. The most important economic consideration is the huge taxes which tobacco companies pay to government. Promotional activities are the earliest strategy for "catching" prospective smokers young.

Health promotion challenges in Nigeria in the 21st century should address three broad categories: policies, education/training and partnerships. Public policy options for health education/promotion should be intersectoral, diverse, determined by epidemiological and risk studies and aimed at the most vulnerable. Governments have the responsibility to ensure comprehensive control strategies for the prevention of tobacco-related diseases, in Nigeria and elsewhere in Africa.

References

Connolly, G. (1992). Worldwide expansion of transnational tobacco industry. *Journal of National Cancer Institute: Monographs*, 12: 29-35.

Ebissemiju, B., & Okugbowa, A. I. (1988, July 5). Tobacco marketing under threat? *The Guardian*, p. 9.

Egwu, I. N. (1998). Financing health promotion programs in Nigeria: Gaps and options. *Health Promotion: Global Perspectives*, p. 1, *4-5*.

Egwu, I. N. (1996). *Primary health care in Nigeria: Theory, practice & perspectives*. Lagos: Ehmore Publishers.

Katch, B. (1998, May/June). Health promotion economies. *Health Promotion: Global Perspectives*, 1:1.

Frankel, G. (1996). How tobacco firms and U.S. smashed barriers to the East International Frileure, Zurich, November 18, 1996.

Katch, B. (1998). Health promotion economics. *Health Promotion: Global Perspectives*, 1:1.

Potter, I. (1997). *Health promotion: A global challenge*. Paper presented at the 4th International Conference on Health Promotion, Jakarta, Indonesia, July 21, 1997.

Roemer, R. (1993). *Legislative action to combat the world tobacco epidemic*. Geneva: WHO.

Stebbins, K. (1992). Politics and economics: Implications for global health. *Social Science & Medicine*, 33: 1317-1326.

Tobacco Smoking (Control) Decree (1990). Lagos: Federal Military Government of Nigeria.

WHO (1997). *Health promotion glossary*. Geneva: WHO, p. 17.

WHO (1978). *Primary health care – Alma Ata*. Geneva: WHO.

WHO (1986). *Ottawa Charter for health promotion*. Geneva; WHO.

WHO (1997). *Jakarta Declaration*. WHO: Geneva.

WHO (1997). *Think and act globally and intersectorally to protect national health*. WHO: Geneva, p.3.

Yatch, D. (1996). Tobacco in Africa. *WHO Forum*, 17: 29-36.

Chapter 5

Health Communication in Africa's Rural Communities: Navigating Emerging Social and Cultural Challenges

Andy O. Alali
California State University, Bakersfield

Ogom Peter Nwosu
California State University, Sacramento

In a major speech at the opening ceremony of the "World Summit on Social Development" held in Copenhagen, Denmark, in 1995, the Director-General of the World Health Organization (WHO), Dr. Hiroshi Nakajima argued that "there can be no social development or sustained economic growth without health" (WHO, 1995a). In sum, "the development and prosperity of any society directly depends on the strength and creativity of its people, that is on their health," Nakajima stated.

While current development literature have not adequately addressed the link between health and the "development and prosperity" perspective articulated by Nakajima, there seems to be no question that health and wellness issues are important variables in the process of national development. However, the difficulty associated with realizing the hopes and aspirations of the Nakajima perspective is more acute for Africa because of the considerable amounts of complexities that shape *the contexts* in which health and wellness take place, especially in rural communities. These contexts are embedded in the social and cultural folkways that interact with the decisions people make and, to a large extent, affect their health status. For the most part, there are emerging challenges, in addition to existing ones, that health educators must recognize and find ways to address if the goal is to help people in rural parts of Africa to comply with the prescriptive measures necessary for healthy lifestyles.

To the extent that there are social and cultural challenges for health promotion in rural communities of Africa, the question here is, how do health educators navigate through some of these challenges that shape the way rural people view health and adopt procedures aimed at healthy lifestyles? What this paper does is two-fold: (1) to begin some dialogue on some of the emerging challenges to health promotion in rural Africa, and (2) to provide a road map for health educators and planners for navigating some of the social and cultural contexts that shape collective discourse, individual behavior, and personal decisions about health and wellness in rural communities of Africa.

First, we begin with a discussion of some of the prevalent and emerging challenges to health promotion in rural Africa. Second, we examine some of the constraints that thwart current health promotion, and disease prevention and control efforts. Finally, we identify specific ways that health educators can navigate through the social and cultural challenges to effect appropriate changes for more healthy lifestyles in rural communities of Africa.

Some Major Health Concerns in Rural Africa

Much has been written about health education and wellness in Africa (Riley, 1995; Soola, 1995, Alali & Nwosu, 1996, Alali, 1997a). With a population of nearly 650 million, Africa continues to experience a host of health concerns. The population explosion of the last decade, with a yearly rate of 3.3 percent and the movement of people across rural, national, and regional boundaries has not slowed the tide of communicable diseases in the continent. Within the last few years, Africa's urban centers have witnessed a myriad of health problems ranging from the AIDS virus which has ravaged Eastern and Central Africa; the deadly Ebola virus which wreaked considerable havoc in parts of Central Africa, in particular The

Republic of Congo (formerly Zaire); substance abuse, increasingly emerging as a major health challenge in Africa; smoking-related illnesses; and issues pertaining to maternal care, among others. The impact of these health concerns in parts of rural Africa is far-reaching. Let us address each of these health concerns.

HIV

The pandemic explosion of communicable diseases such as the human immunodeficiency virus (HIV) that causes AIDS, or acquired immune deficiency syndrome in Africa in the last decade continues to task the resources of national governments and healthcare providers and educators in the continent. It is estimated that two-thirds of the roughly 16 million people world-wide infected with HIV live in the AIDS belt, a region comprising a chain of countries in eastern and southern Africa (see Table 5.1). Medical evidence and surveillance reports suggest that 23 percent of those who reside in major cities and 10 percent of those

TABLE 5.1: ***Percentage of Population with HIV by Country***

23%* 10%** *(AIDS Belt)*	15%	5%* 4%**	4%* 3%**	1%* 1%**
Central African Republic	Abidjan	Mali	Chad	Senegal
Southern Sudan		Burkino Faso	Cameroon	Gambia
Uganda		Parts of Ivory Coast	Equatorial Guinea	Guinea-Bissau
Kenya		Ghana	Gabon	Sierra Leone
Rwanda			Congo (Zaire)	Liberia
Burundi			Angola	Niger
Tanzania			Namibia	Togo
Zambia			South Africa	Benin
Malawi			Swaziland	Nigeria
Zimbabwe			Lesotho	
Botswana			Mozambique	

*Major City
**Rural Area

Source: John C. Caldwell & Pat Caldwell. The African AIDS epidemic. *Scientific American*, March 1996, pp. 64-65.

who live in the rural areas of the AIDS belt may be infected with HIV (Caldwell & Caldwell, 1996). In South Africa alone, 2.2 million people, including an estimated 13 percent of its pregnant women, have HIV. The most recent surveillance reports suggest that between 1988 and 1997, the infection levels reported in South African clinics increased from less than one percent to over 20 percent. Clearly, the AIDS epidemic in Africa deserves some health communication research attention.

Ebola Virus

The Ebola virus hemorrhagic fever is Africa's next deadly threat. Discovered in 1976, the virus is named for a river in Congo, where it was first detected. Ebola, a filovirus, is transmitted through bodily fluids and secretion. An infection from the virus causes massive internal bleeding, diarrhea, vomiting, abdominal pain, sore throat, and chest pain. It is estimate that 80 percent of infected patients die of intractable shock from the virus.

For Africa, the threat of Ebola is clear. It has generally struck in tropical, often remote, regions of Africa where a significant number of people reside. In most cases, those who reside in rural communities of Africa have no ready access to medical facilities, which are often located several miles away. And, because the virus is spread through close personal contact with a person who is very ill with the disease, secondary infection often occurs in hospital workers and family members who are aiding the infected person or transporting them to medical facilities for treatment. The African experience with Ebola so far suggests that thousands of people, if not millions, would die from the disease. Most affected countries of Africa are Zaire, Gabon, Sudan, Cote d'Ivoire, and most recently, an isolated case in South Africa. The most current demographic and health indicators suggest that the outbreak of Ebola has resulted in more than 800 deaths in Africa.

Clearly, we wish to impress upon policy makers that the threat of Ebola is serious and it hastens the wake-up call for Africa to institute an active surveillance effort and to implement health promotion programs in rural communities where Ebola is most likely to surface. It is crucial that these programs be culture-specific, people-centered and emphasize self-protection, sanitary issues, and an established capacity to detect antibodies associated with the deadly Ebola virus infection.

Substance Abuse

Substance abuse has become an emerging national health concern for African governments, who are conflicted between the need to preserve the social and cultural functions embedded in substance consumption and the need to prevent abuse. Consider alcohol, for example, which has important social and cultural functions in rural communities across the continent. Yet we find that alcohol abuse is particularly evident "during ritual ceremonies, communal planting and harvesting, and spirit media celebrations" (Acuda, 1995, p.24).

Even though some abuse problems may be less publicly visible, health care practitioners have reported an alarming rate of alcohol abuse among their patients. A busy health care clinic in Harare, Zimbabwe reported that "66 percent of the men and 48 percent of the women who drank were getting drunk on each occasion" (Acuda, 1995, p. 24).

The critical point we make here is because alcohol use is socially sanctioned and culturally accepted in most parts of Africa, the aggressive marketing of this substance seems to legitimize its use in social functions; causing a situation that fosters abuse. Interestingly enough, the production and social marketing of alcohol in most parts of Africa have not been equaled by health campaigns aimed at reducing its abuse. Besides, the culture of alcohol abuse in Africa is nurtured by the lack of legislative controls that prevent young people under the age of 18 from having unfettered access to alcohol.

Maternal Health

In recent years, attention is being focused on the problem of maternal health in rural Africa. The literature in the area is clear: that maternal health has implications for children and the viability of the household.

Current statistical data suggests that African women are increasingly vulnerable to a host of diseases because of inadequate nutrition during pregnancy. Nemapare (1989) found that most pregnant and nursing women in Africa get only 52 percent of the calories they needed. Consequently, malnutrition is on the rise, particularly in the rural communities of Africa. Illustrative of this notion are the findings during a maternal health and nutrition survey of pregnant women in Masvingo Province of Zimbabwe which concluded that 70 children die out of every 1,000 births (Nemapare, 1989). This is attributed, in large part, to maternal malnutrition.

Similarly, maternal mortality is a problem facing Africa. A report issued by the World Bank (1994) suggests that maternal mortality in Africa is at 700 women per 100,000 live births. This figure mirrors the findings of an earlier study that 500,000 women die of pregnancy complications every year in Africa (Nemapare, 1989).

Clearly, maternal health is a problem that has implications for Africa, particularly as it relates to the vertical transmission of diseases such as HIV - via the placenta, at delivery or postnatally - from mother to child.

(Re)emerging Infections and Major Morbidities

AIDS, the Ebola virus, substance abuse, smoking illnesses, and maternal health are not the only health problems that threaten life in rural Africa. There are a host of other emerging or re-emerging infections that health promotion efforts must now address.

One of the major infections that is re-emerging in African communities is cholera. Generally, the spread of cholera is associated with lack of water and poor sanitation that result from crowded living conditions and poor hygiene. As people migrate from one region to another, outbreaks follow that path. This is more acute along the river and road routes that people travel.

Most cases of cholera are found in four West African countries – Burkina Faso, Mali, Niger, and Nigeria. Nigeria has the largest number of cholera cases. If not treated adequately, cholera fatality rate can go as high as 24 percent. In 1996 alone, 14,000 cases of cholera and 9,000 deaths were reported in Africa (WHO, 1996).

Other health concerns for Africa include malaria, which accounts for more than one million deaths every year. Recently, the World Health Organization (WHO) announced that 1996 was the worst year on record for cerebrospinal meningitis (an inflammation of the lining of the brain and spinal cord) in Africa, with around 150,000 reported cases and 16,000 deaths. These health problems as well as the outbreak of Ebola, polio, tuberculosis, and yellow fever in some regions of Africa, have far reaching implication, especially within the context of life expectancy in the affected countries. It is estimated that by the year 2010, the life expectancy in countries such as Zambia would be lowered by the AIDS epidemic from 66 to 33 years, Zimbabwe from 70 to 40 years, Kenya from 68 to 40 years, and Uganda from 59 to 31 years (Alali & Nwosu, 1996).

Some Constraints That Impede Current Health Promotion Efforts

The question we tackle here is: What are some of the constraints that impede current health promotion and disease prevention strategies in the Africa? We know that the magnitude of disease epidemics in Africa has focused the attention of health specialists from Ministries of Health, from universities and research institutions in Africa, and from the non-governmental sector and international donor organizations to support an African agenda to finding new ways to solve health problems. Most support initiatives for health improvements have been at the urban level. These initiatives provide funding or technical assistance for research, education, and prevention efforts. Most research efforts focus on identifying the sources of epidemics, while the education and prevention efforts have been directed at changing the attitudes and behaviors which shape the health status of individuals.

Even though disease prevention activities have included multi-pronged strategies involving the use of various forms of interpersonal channels of communication and the mass media, there are a number of constraints that stymie these efforts. Let us review some of these constraints.

Language

There are over 1,000 indigenous languages spoken in African today. In some parts of Africa, one has to be multilingual to function, while other countries have a national language that facilitates communication amongst its people. In areas where multilingualism is the norm, dozens of languages are spoken within an area of a few hundred square miles. Because it is not possible for most people to speak all of the languages in their country, it becomes difficult to accomplish nationwide tasks, such as public education and health promotion campaigns that are based on language that is not theirs. In fact, some people tend to resist messages that are not language specific or appear to be alien to their regional communication pattern or dialect. Consequently, public health campaigns face the initial obstacle of resistance to the extent that the key constituents for whom the messages are designed may actually exclude themselves from the campaign. Often, these individuals become the prime candidate for HIV infection because they are either unable to comprehend prevention messages because of linguistic differences or they are simply resistant to messages that are not spoken with their dialect or accent. In planning health communication campaigns, national governments and donor agencies must take into consideration the challenges that linguistic variations may pose to effective health education efforts.

Circumcision

Another challenge to health education campaigns in Africa has to do with circumcision. Circumcision involves the surgical removal of the foreskin on the penis or the clitoris. In most parts of Africa where it is practiced, circumcision of men is done for medical or hygienic reasons and in some cases for religious reasons; for women, however, circumcision is a "tribal" ritual often performed to reduce the sexual desires that is believed to lead to promiscuous lifestyles.

With regards to AIDS, it has been argued that lack of circumcision itself makes men more susceptible to AIDS due to the prevalence of chancroid infection among such men. Chancroid causes large, soft sores on the genitals of uncircumcised men, which may easily facilitate HIV infection.

Even though no conclusive evidence has been advanced about this issue by researchers, preliminary findings suggest a linkage between lack of circumcision and HIV infection. In a study by Caldwell and Caldwell (1996), it was found that 53 percent of HIV cases in Kenya were uncircumcised men with chancroid, as opposed to the 2.5 percent cases of HIV infections attributed to circumcised men with chancroid. The study also shows that "certain sexually transmitted diseases tend to occur more frequently among uncircumcised men in poor areas where monitoring personal cleanliness is difficult" (Caldwell & Caldwell, 1996, p. 66).

These observations dovetail with research findings which suggest that "the regions across sub-Saharan Africa with high levels of HIV infection among local peoples corresponded remarkably well with the areas where men were typically uncircumcised" (Moses et al., 1990; Bongaarts et al., 1989). Clearly, the difference in AIDS rate among the Luo migrants of western Kenya and the Kikuyu from central Kenya is evidence of this notion; the Luo ethnic group, who tend to be uncircumcised, have greater rate of HIV infection than the circumcised Kikuyu group. This is supported by more recent research that concludes that male circumcision is associated with lower HIV prevalence in rural Tanzania (Quigley et al., 1997).

Condom Use

Another critical factor which we believe impedes health education and prevention campaigns in Africa is the resistance associated with the use of condom by men as a protective measure during sexual intercourse. Oftentimes, to suggest to a man that a condom be used during sex is to evoke responses in men that seem conditioned by social attitudes and cultural beliefs. In the male dominated African society, women have little control over the sexual behavior of the men folks. For a woman to suggest to her husband or partner that he use a condom is perceived as evidence of the woman's infidelity, or it is felt by the man as defiance or insolence. Additionally, those who are in polygamous relationships believe that it is the man who makes decisions as to the place, time, and manner of sexual activity. More critical to health promotion efforts is the fact that many men in rural Africa perceive condom use as unnatural; and that it reduces their ability to enjoy sex. To these individuals, health promotion campaigns that are aimed at safe-sex may not be effective; for them, condom is used generally against pregnancy not protection against AIDS. In the African cultures where the married woman is traditionally expected to bear many children, insisting on safer sex or refusing to engage in sexual relationship is impossible. Additionally, religion is an obstacle to public health campaigns aimed at preventing HIV infection in Africa. Religious beliefs sometimes create incompatible gulfs that impede healthy lifestyles. Why safe sex? Why family planning? Why condoms? AIDS education and prevention efforts constantly must work to balance these question, religious beliefs and the need to save human lives.

Socio-Economic Conditions

As more people leave their villages for the cities, some are faced with the financial burden and social hardship that is associated with a demanding urban lifestyle. Most of these individuals particularly women, tend to be unemployed and have less access to adequate health care. Yet, as poverty sets in, there continues to be the social expectation that women should look "good" and remain "attractive" for their men. Often times, such pressures result in antisocial behavior that encourages some women who do not have the financial means and resources to resort to promiscuous lifestyle so as to get money from men. Of course, the richer the men the better for the women, and the more the men, the greater the chances of getting more money through multiple partners. The economic inequalities which reduce women to promiscuous lifestyle serve as an impediment to AIDS education and prevention campaigns in Africa.

Prostitution

An ancillary factor to the socioeconomic conditions that impede health education in Africa is prostitution. In most urban centers of Africa, prostitution is rampant, and it is not a regulated behavior. Clearly, both men and women who engage in the activity expose themselves to infection with HIV, and subsequently become carriers who may infect others they have sexual contact or with whom they share IV-drugs. The problem for health promotion efforts lies in the fact that prostitution is not regulated, and, therefore, no supportive environment exists for compulsory testing of individuals caught or convicted of prostitution. While there is no available data on actual AIDS cases attributed to prostitution, there is no doubt that HIV infection and prostitution are closely connected, and those who participate in this behavior increase their chances of infection with HIV and other sexually transmitted diseases. These infections may multiply tenfold as the sexual partners increase.

Refugees

The problem with refugees is a matter of politics and socio-economic displacement. There is no doubt that political instability and ethnic controversies have displaced many Africans, particularly in the sub-Saharan regions of Africa. Recent skirmishes in Liberia, Burundi, Rwanda, Somali, Zaire, Sierra Leone and the Ethiopian-Eritrean conflicts are a few examples. Clearly, there are public health concerns such as sanitation problems, low nutritional intake and lack of immunization that result from the refugee problem, and we believe these concerns ought to be addressed. Certainly, the health care industry, particularly those that are managed by the government, can begin to put in place health campaigns and disease prevention programs to assist refugees maintain healthy lifestyles in their new, yet uncertain, environment.

While political decisions which contribute heavily to the refugee problem in Africa may influence government attitude toward refugees, these decisions must not influence health promotion efforts aimed at the health of refugees. Governments must realize that, in most part, the politics of displacement does not, in itself, prevent sexual activity.

Nomadic Communities

There appears to be an apparent omission in health care and preventive services in Africa as they relate to nomadic communities, a people on the move. Any program designed for this community must not only be culturally appropriate, but should be structured to include their beliefs and practices. In addition, these programs should draw from tested traditional health practices as they currently exist. Consider, for example, the Woodaabe people, a sub-group of West Africa's large Peul community who live in the arid lands of the Sahel bordering the Sahara Desert. Because of their lifestyle, their dispersed living arrangements, they "developed a health system which is an essential component of their strategy of life" (Aliou, 1995, p. 24) or rural communities in Africa.

> Sickness or accidents may occur at any time, so before seeking specialist help, every adult male or female needs to be able to do something about it. They invariably carry with them materials such as powders, tree-backs or roots with which to make medicines for emergency treatment. Recipes, knowledge and practices are handed on among members of the group as basic elements of the apprenticeship for adult life (Aliou, 1995, p. 27).

Community health educators can learn to integrate modern health practices with this traditional approach, as modern health structures, on their own, rarely succeed in meeting the health needs of the Woodaabes (Aliou, 1995).

Navigating Through Social and Cultural Contexts for Health Promotion at the Community Level

The value of learning about a people's way of life is that health educators are able to incorporate such knowledge in the design of a health care system that is sensitive to that community's way of life. In the process, health educators would actually receive the support of the target population as well as create the environment that may restore confidence in the health message and in the messenger. An ancillary outcome of this strategy is that preventive services can be made readily available and accessible to the specific community.

In the years since disease epidemics have become a matter of public health concern for most African governments, the social and cultural contexts of health have not been adequately considered when community health educators design disease prevention campaigns. The importance of these factors are premised on the belief that sociocultural theories correlate with the notion that the health and ill-health of a people are attributed, in part to social beliefs and ideological mind-set of a society. Consequently, to design a health campaign, one must fully understand how that society functions and the dominant values and belief system that would create supportive environment for the promotion of new social norm, such as the use of condoms during sex.

Additionally, to effectively educate the African rural public about modern medicine requires an understanding of the basic relationship between culture, lifestyles (physical and social) and health, and how to navigate through the interaction that takes place. For example, what culture fosters beliefs about safe sex and children? What role does religion play in the sexual relationships of the target audience? Other important considerations include the patriarchal nature of the society and the availability as well as the affordability of health care.

Indeed health educators must first understand the sociocultural factors that interact with health to effectively design campaigns that are credible for local consumption and are able to navigate through existing social and cultural belief systems in rural Africa. We say this to suggest that community health educators ought to give adequate consideration to inhibiting factors, such as beliefs and attitudes; the skills and resources that enable the reception of messages and compliance; and the social support system that may reinforce the new social norm. These issues are the reasons why current community health education and prevention campaigns have not been effective in Africa. Serious considerations should be given to these sociocultural factors because adequate integration of people's attitudes and values in the planning, design, and dissemination of campaign materials could enhance campaign success (Nwosu, 1990; Nwosu & Megwa, 1993).

There are, in our view, existing support systems which can be utilized to navigate through social and cultural contexts in the effort to promote a more healthy lifestyle in rural communities in Africa. These systems include traditional healers, community leaders and role models, community health workers, school-based programs, market health agents, community-based health education, family health approach, mobile/community based theater and support networks. We identify below the mechanisms for achieving this.

Traditional Healers

Traditional healers, or medicine men, play a crucial role in the health belief system of African peoples. The opinions of traditional healers are often revered because they are the first place of call for health advise for most people in rural communities. These medicine men often diagnose and provide cure for illnesses. Indeed, they are critical to the health dynamics of a community. It is, therefore, important that health educators guard against the assumption that people in rural areas are homogeneous and would easily embrace a modern health education model that, for them, may be alien to their traditional beliefs and in conflict with the predictions of the "medicine men."

In their analysis of peoples of the nomadic communities, Omar and Omar (1995) determined that much of the curative effects of the traditional healers' skills "is primarily psychological and based on magical practice and the enormous prestige and confidence people bestow on the medicine man" (p. 25). In most cases, they tend to "function as a kind of psychiatrist" (Omar & Omar, 1995, p. 5).

Undoubtedly, most of health behavior is "anchored on existing practices" (Soola, 1995, P. 310). Traditional healers may therefore serve as conduit for the health behavior and attitude adjustment that is needed to achieve an effective health education and disease prevention campaign in rural Africa. We agree with Omar and Omar (1995) that amongst other important variables, the role of traditional healers in the health beliefs of a people should be understood before any health care intervention is planned. Furthermore, traditional healers can be used in ways that supportive roles that include dissemination of modern health information in Africa's rural communities.

Community Leaders and Role Models

In general, community leaders and role models have not been given adequate role in any plan aimed at health education and disease prevention at the community level. As leaders and role models, they can be considered as support network that assists in creating an identity for the campaign, and as a means of developing a following which ultimately would establish trust amongst their kinfolk.

To increase compliance and engender healthy lifestyles in people, the role community leadership must play should not be overlooked. Reed (1994) suggests that community involvement affirms the relationship between health care officials and the community itself. Reed argues that "when our programs were geared solely toward a health problem that *we* sought to address, we were less successful in getting the community's participation than when the community played an integral role in shaping the program" (p. 27). Clearly, knowledge of a community may not ensure campaign effectiveness. It would seem that a more effective health promotion approach would be community participation, especially through role models and leaders. Accordingly, Bracht (1990) suggests that the community "must be involved early and have a real, not token, role in decision making for implementing health promotion activities" (p. 254). A much more effective way of ensuring community participation is to involve community leaders from the inception of program planning all through program implementation.

Community Health Worker

An important interpersonal channel which has been used in the fight against emerging infection and disease epidemics is the Community Health Worker (CHW). Also called "Community Health Agents" in some African countries, these are "men and women who are trained and supported by the health sector to work in their own communities" (Kahssay, 1996, p.6) and to help bring about change in health behaviors. Their participation in the promotion of health and disease prevention campaigns has been amplified by recent epidemics, such as AIDS and Ebola.

They are trained to carry out primary health education and execute intervention programs in rural communities. Most of their work consists of on-the-spot education and counseling of patients and at-risk individuals.

The CHW is an important link between medicine (science) and culture. They tend to serve as liaison between the community and the health sector, primarily illuminating the community's attitudes, beliefs, and practices for health practitioners. Clearly, they are best positioned to involve people who reside in their community in healthy lifestyles and to embrace health promotion efforts.

Besides their role in campaigns about healthy lifestyles, the CHW is not viewed by the general population as alien to the community, even though they serve as agents of a health sector that may not have credibility amongst certain groups. This type of arrangement is beneficial to the health sector because through the CHW they are able to understand the linkages between the health of that community, their culture and environment. Additionally, they are able to monitor a peoples' living conditions and relate that to their health status, thereby generating data that, theoretically, would assist in the formulation of health care policy. International agencies working on the AIDS epidemic have found this group to be a vital link between them and the community in AIDS education and prevention efforts in Africa. The major disadvantage here is coverage– the inability of the CHW to reach larger and wider audiences, especially when there are just few CHWs. Ultimately, not many communities receive the benefit of health advisory critical to their survival. Given the success of CHW, there is a need for African governments to provide adequate resources to extend the reach of this approach to rural communities.

School-Based Programs

Schools have become an important venue for the dissemination of health education and disease prevention information in Africa. Here positive health information is made available to school-age children. Some health information is integrated in the curriculum while some are disseminated through other means. In Nigeria, for example, UNICEF has used drama, as a tool, in disseminating disease prevention information in some Nigerian secondary schools. This kind of approach has had tremendous success in reaching young people, and in fact can be replicated in rural communities.

Market Health Agents

The effectiveness of Market Health Agents (MHAs) in Africa is evident, particularly in campaigns aimed at population control and other health issues. The one case that illuminates this method of health promotion is the Ibadan Market Based CBD Program, an operation research project of the Fertility Research Unit at the College of Medicine, University of Ibadan, Nigeria. This program, which was funded, in part, by the United States Agency for International Development (USAID), was designed to assist in the campaign for distribution of contraception for population control.

The uniqueness of this program is in its utilization of women as MHAs to mobilize people for health promotion activities in the marketplace. The MHAs use different strategies in their health promotion activities, some of which include the distribution of leaflets, public announcements about the importance of disease prevention, the use of songs in their dialect to enable the target audience to sing along, and the distribution of T-shirts inscribed with health awareness and disease prevention messages.

Perhaps, the most important aspect of this program is that illiterate women are actually trained to use their local dialects to educate other market women, their neighbors, and the entire community to accept health promotion programs, and to look at health in relations to their community. Public awareness of health issues has improved dramatically in local markets. The marketplace is ideal for one-on-one information about AIDS, and a place to distribute condoms to insure some compliance to safe sex practices, and we recommend wider use of this in health promotion efforts in rural Africa.

Community-Based Health Education

The community-based health education strategy utilizes the expertise of existing community resources, including trained health personnel, to develop a health education program that has practical utility to the specific community. The aim is to: 1) develop health promotion and disease prevention programs; 2) mobilize the community, including advocacy and constituent building, for a specified health and behavior outcome; 3) select and recruit community-based workers for health promotion campaigns; 4) train workers at three levels (management, training-of-trainers, and training of workers or the agents of change); 5) supply materials for campaigns; 6) deliver services such as health education and prevention; 7) keep records and report information; 8) monitor and supervise activities; and 9) evaluate impact of project, needs and resources. Community-based participation in all phases of program development promotes and strengthens firm links between the community and the formal health sector. In most parts of Africa, the level of compliance to prevention messages seem to increase with the community-based health education approach.

Family Health Approach

Africans subscribe to a more expansive definition of family. The concept of the family in Africa goes beyond the Western notion of the nuclear family, and is all-inclusive of extended relatives, friends, peers, neighbors, the village, and the community. To understand the role of the family in African contexts of life, one must have a knowledge of how the African definition of family frames their attitudes and belief systems. Health educators must realize that while the family is the basic unit of society and the primary setting for human development, the individual, in the African context of being, exists because of the group. That, in turn, affects health behavior. It is therefore no coincidence when the World Health Organization recognized that the family is an "entry point for health promotion, disease prevention and care" (World Health Organization, 1995b, p. 6).

The family is important to health outcomes for several reasons. Apart from sharing genes, family members share: lifestyles, dietary habits, exercise, and the same environment (and frequently infections). Africans believe that health begins in the family, and the family has influence on the health outcomes of their members: bad family influences results in bad health. Consequently, issues of health care are considered an integral part of the family. The following are some of the usefulness of familial health strategies in the African context:

1. It facilitates the acceptance of health services to families.
2. It enables health services to be accessible to all.
3. It increases providers' understanding of the patient's expectations.
4. It creates an opportunity for understanding the factors that determine health: those linked with the environment (open-air wood burning); psychological; behavioral; and cultural, economic, and social factors together define the way patients are taken care of by the family.
5. It ensures that the burden of care is not placed on women alone; but should involve the whole family.

Mediated Forms of Communication

Mediated forms of communication–radio, television, newspapers and other printed matter–have also been used in efforts to reach large numbers of the population. Soola (1995) has presented several examples of the use of the mass media in addressing the AIDS problem in Africa. In Zaire, for example, the government in conjunction with the United States Agency for International Development (USAID) mounted a multi-media AIDS education and prevention campaign in 1992. The campaign was targeted at young people between the ages of 12 and 30, a population group considered by public health research to be more at risk with the

AIDS virus in Zaire. The multi-media campaign on radio and television was supplemented by folk media. According to Soola, post-campaign research findings revealed a considerable shift in attitude among the targeted population as more people moved towards compliance with the campaign messages.

In other areas of Africa, such as Nigeria, while only one percent of the population is reported to be infected by the virus, the government has embarked on a massive education and prevention campaign using multimedia channels. Soola (1995) reports that AIDS education and prevention efforts in the country have involved the use of fear appeals as well as more persuasive messages rendered in the popular pidgin language. The following message in pidgin is an example of the content of the Nigeria AIDS education and prevention efforts:

> Man and woman wey no dey waka waka no get AIDS disease if them meet, na im be say make man and woman dey put eye for one place, and if man and woman no wan get AIDS at all at all, make dem dey use dat small rubber abi rain coat wey oyibo dey call condom, any time wey dem want meet (Soola, 1995, p. 317).

Translation

> Man and woman who are not promiscuous do not get AIDS when they meet. That is why it is important to remain monogamous. And if man and woman do not want to get AIDS at all, they should use the small rubber the whiteman calls condom anytime they want to meet.

Clearly, the language is plain, not offensive, and at the same time punchy.

Mobile/Community Based Theater

A unique arrangement which has served well in integrating cultural values in targeted information delivery programs is the use of community theater. Armed with valuable information about a community's social needs and cultural values, community theater as currently used by UNICEF in Nigeria has been an effective instrument of social change.

> Not only does it entertain, it also makes a great impact on the people by telling them the causes and solutions to their problems in a way no other method could do. It enables the audience to identify with the characters on stage, and through the resolution of the problems of the characters, the people learn to solve their problems. A good play has the power of making the audience feel that everything happening on stage is real and they react as

such to the characters on stage (Okechukwu-Nwosu, 1995, p.1).

Working with Double Barrel Theater, a Non-Governmental Organization, UNICEF has since 1993 used this tool in delivering information on different health issues, especially in guinea worm endemic communities in the eastern part of Nigeria with huge success. The need to reach many communities and to make the program sustainable has prompted UNICEF to now provide training for drama groups selected at the local government level to help disseminate health information to rural communities. The trained local drama groups prepare the message taking into account the cultural idiosyncrasies of their communities, and eventually present the information on any specific health problem in the language(s) of the communities they serve. Songs are also composed to go along with the performance. Difficult subject matter such as sex and the attendant health implications are discussed in a serious, yet entertaining manner. We know from experience and research that a communication strategy for the dissemination of innovations is incomplete, until it includes indigenous modes of interaction in the continent such as songs, dances, folklore. (For a detailed discussion of indigenous modes of communication in Africa, see Njoku Awa in Nwosu et. al, 1995, *Communication and the Transformation of Society. A Developing Region's Perspective*).

Support Network

We no longer should underestimate the role support network can play in public health promotion and disease prevention efforts. While there are expectations that the strategies and approaches to health campaigns, particularly in Africa, may differ from country to country (Soola, 1995), it is generally accepted that a well structured support network may link community beliefs and attitudes with public health expectations, beliefs and attitudes. This is to say that a well integrated support network can build a support group that can be linked with the health status of people. The assumption here is that the support network has more understanding of the local history, tradition, and communication dynamics of peoples in their communities. Therefore, their input, their presence, and their resources are equally important in health education and disease prevention at the community level.

Critical to this process are three groups–the primary support network, the social support network, and the health agency support network. In practice, the network has on-going impact on the individual; the social support network includes professional and social organizations the

FIGURE 5.1: *Proposed Health Promotion Support Network*

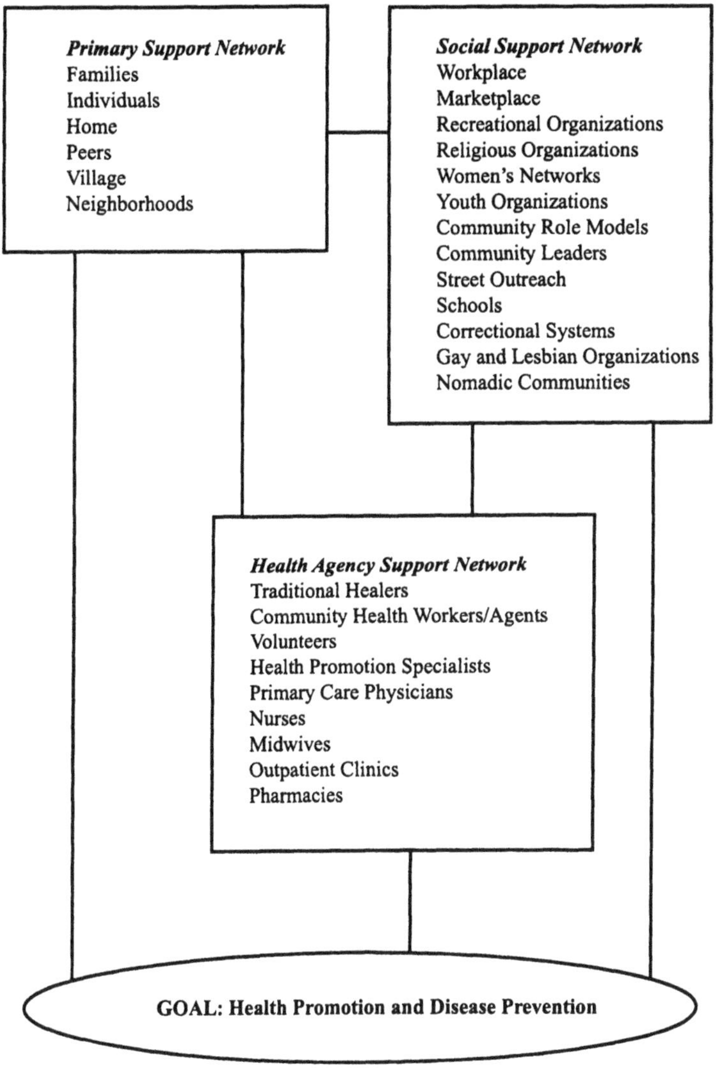

individual belongs to, and are influential in their life decisions. The health agency support network are individuals who, by virtue of their professional training, have daily contacts with patients. We have identified a list of individuals and community groups that are essential to the effective functioning of the support network proposed here. (See Figure 5.1.) The point we make is that public policies on health should integrate the support network identified here in all efforts to promote healthy lifestyles.

Conclusion

An important element in the process of navigation and integration is collaboration. No doubt efforts aimed at health education and disease prevention in Africa have not always been successful because there is no collaborative agenda in place to network agencies that provide services to communities and those who study such services. Clearly, collaborative efforts between the academic sector that produces research, the government that makes policy, volunteers who assist in the campaigns, donor agencies, and regional and international organizations would enhance the campaign planning process, its implementation, and the evaluation of program effectiveness. In fact, we believe such collaboration would ensure that health campaigns are culturally sensitive, culturally competent, developmentally appropriate, and linguistically specific. With such characteristic features of a campaign, it should enhance social and cultural acceptance of programs and confer credibility to a specific health campaign, including AIDS education and prevention campaign.

Stemming the tide and the toll of the disease epidemics remains a major health challenge for African governments. Throughout this paper, we have discussed health issues which paint a picture of the impact of disease epidemic in the continent. Numerous national and international conferences have been held to discuss the global impact of disease epidemic, and there are on-going efforts to find a treatment for them. In the absence of such treatment or cure, there is no better way of controlling disease epidemics except through education.

We have presented information here that point to a lack of understanding of some of the deep-rooted socio-cultural forces which impede health education and disease prevention efforts. We have also offered some ways to integrate these contexts in on-going/future education and prevention campaigns and, in the process, to navigate through them for effective health promotion at the community level. It is equally important that there is an effective local and community leadership to support initiatives for health improvements at the community level. And, unless national governments and international donor agencies take serious consideration of the social and cultural contexts of health in the communities they serve, any effort to stem the tide of disease epidemics in rural Africa is merely elusive and wasteful.

References

Acuda, S. W. (1995, July-August). An African example. *World Health*, 4:24.

Alali, A. O. (1997a). Research considerations for effective health communication in Africa. *Gazette*, 59;4-5: 365-377.

Alali, A. O. (1997b). Health warnings and content disclosures in cigarette advertisements: The case of South Africa. Unpublished research data.

Alali, A. O., & Nwosu, P. (1996). Social and cultural considerations in planning AIDS education and campaigns in Africa. Paper presented at the 10th Biennial African Council for Communication Education conference, Cape Town, South Africa, 15-22 November.

Aliou, S. (1995, November-December). People on the move. *World Health*, 6: 26-27.

Awa, N. E. (1995). The role of indigenous media in African social development. In Nwosu, P., Onwumechili, C., & M'Bayo, R. (eds.), *Communication & the transformation of society: A developing region's perspectives* (pp. 237-251). Lanham, MD: University Press of America.

Bergendahl, P., & Hsu, L. (1995, July-August). Women and substance abuse. *World Health*, 4: 12.

Bongaarts, J., Reining, P., Way, P., & Conant, F. (1989). The relationship between male circumcision and HIV infection in African populations. *AIDS*, 3;6: 373-377.

Bracht, N. (1990). Applications to special populations: Case studies. In Neil Bracht (ed), *Health promotion at the community level* (pp. 253-256). Newbury Park, CA: Sage.

Caldwell, J. C., & Caldwell, P. (1996, March). The African AIDS epidemic. *Scientific American*, 62-68.

Kahssay, H. M. (1996, March-April). Building on local health culture. *World Health*, 2: 6-7.

McKibbin, E. C. (1994). An analysis of the risk factors for coronary heart disease in patients aged 55 and younger with proven heart disease. *South African Journal of Nursing*, 17;3: 51-56.

Moses, S., Bradley, J. E., Nagelkerke, N. J. D., Ronald, A. R., Ndinya-Achola, J. O., & Plummer, F. A. (1990, September). Geographical patterns of male circumcision practices in Africa: Association with HIV seroprevalence. *International Journal of Epidemiology*, 19;3: 693-697.

Nemapare, P. (1989). Maternal health and nutrition survey for Masvingo Province, Zimbabwe: An appraisal of pregnant women. *Nutrition Report International*, 39;20: 265.

Nwosu, P. (1990). Communication and agricultural development in Swaziland. Toward a need-based integrative model. Unpublished doctoral dissertation. Howard University.

Nwosu, P., & Megwa, E. (1993). Communication and development in Swaziland. *Africa Media Review*, 7;1.

Okechukwu-Nwosu, N. (1995). Training approaches for CSD information delivery through community theater. The Zone A experience. (Paper presented to the Summer 1995 meeting of UNICEF, Kano, Nigeria).

Omar, M. A., & Omar, M. M. (1995, November-December). Nomads in the horn of Africa. *World Health*, 6: 25.

Quigley, M., Munguti, K., Grosskunth, H., Todd, J., Mosha, F., Senkoro, K., Newell, J., Maynard, P., ka-Gina, G., Klokke, A., Mabey, D., Gavyole, A., & Hayes, R. (1997, February). Sexual behavior patterns and other risk factors for HIV infection in rural Tanzania: A case-control study. *AIDS*, 11;2: 237-248.

Page, R. M., Cole, G. E., & Timmrack, T. C. (1995). *Basic epidemiological methods and biostatistics: A practical guidebook.* Boston, MA: Jone and Bartlett.

Perera, F. P. (1996, May). Uncovering news clues to cancer risk. *Scientific American*, 54-62.

Reed, J. (1994). Health promotion: A community-based perspective. *Medicine in the Twenty-First Century: Challenges in personal and public health promotion* (Supplement). *American Journal of Perspective Medicine*, 10;3: 26-29.

Riley, M. (1995). Development communication and health care in Ghana. In P.
Nwosu, C. Onwumechili, & R. M'Bayo (eds), *Communication & the transformation of society: A developing region's perspectives* (pp. 321-332). Lanham, MD: University Press of America.

Soola, E. O. (1995). Development communication and health campaigns in Africa. In Nwosu, P., Onwumechili, C., & M'Bayo, R. (eds.), *Communication & the transformation of society: A developing region's perspectives* (pp. 307-319). Lanham, MD: University Press of America.

World Bank (1994). *Better health in Africa–Experience and lessons learned.* Development in Practice Series. Washington, DC: World Bank.

World Health Organization (1996, April 12). Growing concerns over health situation in West Africa. Press Release WHO/31. Geneva: WHO.

World Health Organization (1995a, March 11-12). Health is central to social development. Speech by Dr. Hiroshi Nakajima at the "World Summit on Social Development," Copenhagen, Denmark. Press Release, WHO/18. Geneva: WHO.

World Health Organization (1995b, March-April). Interview: Health begins with the family. *World Health*, 2: 6-8.

Part III

Social Support, Institutional Roles and Cultural Dynamics

Chapter 6

Provider-Patient Communication in the African Health Context

Sonja Verwey
Andrea Crystal
Rand Afrikaans University, Johannesburg, South Africa

"The state of the art of health communication is embryonic, to say the least... By applying communication theory and research as well as interpersonal and group skills, communication specialists can enhance interactions in medicine, health-care delivery systems, and health care in general" (Cassata, 1991, p. 583). Health communication arose as a response to the growing pragmatic and policy interest in health promotion and disease prevention, especially in developing countries like South Africa. Many developing countries have limited manpower and financial resources and many inhabitants live in Third World conditions (Goosen, 1988, p. 3).

Statistics highlight the challenges that face health-care providers in developing countries. The *World Health Report* (1996) indicates that of all the births in 1995, almost 16 million were in the developed world, almost 25 million in least developed countries, and over 98 million in developing countries. Of the more than 11 million deaths among children under five, in the developing world about nine million were attributed to infectious diseases, 25 percent of them preventable through vaccination.

The issue that needs to be analyzed is the relationship between health care, health communication, and development. Communication strategies between health-care professionals, patients, and their support groups play a key role in determining and assessing health outcomes. According to Kreps (1988), effective health care and health promotion are guided by relevant health communication. Communication is thus clearly the primary process used in health care to gather and disseminate health information. Communication is essential in the provision of social support (by health-care provide participants in formal and informal support groups, family, and friends). Communication is also fundamental in coordinating health-care treatment and activities of various interdependent providers and consumers (Kreps, O'Hare, & Clowers, 1994, p. 429). According to Kaplan (1997, pp. 75–82) communication is perhaps the most essential ingredient in effective health care.

What constitutes health care in developing contexts may vary from that which has evolved in developed contexts as part of a wide network of social and welfare infrastructure and societal processes. According to Freimuth, Edgar, and Fitzpatrick (1993, p. 509), health promotion challenges the medicalization of health, stresses its social and economic aspects and portrays health as central to flourishing life. The definition of health within developed contexts is, according to Phillips (1990, p. 2), often a technocratic view that health is the absence of disease (both organic and mental). In contrast the World Health Organization (WHO) indicates that health encompasses a "state of complete physical, mental and social well-being, not merely the absence of infirmity in an individual." It is therefore essential to review health-care provision in the developing societies in light of the fact that it is today widely agreed that health as a technical measure, thus the absence of diagnosed illness is insufficient for most purposes (Feacham, Graham, & Timaeus, 1989, pp. 133–191).

Health-care provision in developing contexts should not just be viewed from a focus on its modern technical components using quantitative measures of epidemiological characteristics to express health status. Rather more useful, according to Lachenmann (1982) and Stewart (1985) is the objective of the basic human needs approach to provide a full life in which healthy individuals live in caring, well-provided, and intellectually stimulating communities. Nevertheless, there is still a tendency in the developing world as elsewhere, to regard health care in a rather narrow technical light, although this has now been challenged by the WHO and in many other quarters (Phillips, 1990, p. 21). Barker and Turshen (1986) contend that "health" is often regarded as something determined or created by the delivery of health services, rather than by overall development. Paradigms of development and underdevelopment impinge to some extent on the views of health and the nature of health programs. However, the concept of development has many meanings, which are not always clearly specified in practice or research. In the 1970s and early 1980s ideas of dependency had come to the fore with theorists such as Frank (1971) suggesting that "Third World Development" was being prevented, and underdevelopment even being exacerbated, by dependent relations with developed countries. According to Phillips (1990, p. 8) the debates about the causes of underdevelopment and health have progressed considerably in recent years. The debate has since shifted in theoretical and political terms to a growing conviction that some market liberalization can mutually benefit both the developing world and developed world. The debate therefore tends to be between dependency and free-market thinkers (Elson, Harris, & Sen, 1989). According to Phillips (1990, p. 3) there appears to be a reciprocal relationship between development and health in the broader sense, although this relationship is not simple or one-way. Development affects health both favorably and unfavorably. While development generally brings improved diets, housing, social change and reductions in infectious diseases, it is also usually associated with rises in degenerative diseases, mainly apparently of noninfectious etiology (so-called Western diseases) (Hutt & Burlutt, 1986). In this regard Phillips (1990, p. 5) states, "While it appears that many so-called 'Western' diseases did actually exist in traditional societies, modernization with increased expectation of life has brought epidemiological change and such conditions are growing in importance, health-care needs change and new health-resource problems, both replace and stand alongside the old." Broader-based development for health demands considerable intersectional collaboration, which is often difficult to achieve. Pluralistic health-care systems are common in many developing societies, although they are by no means confined to the developing world. Cultural, social, and psychological acceptance of health systems other than the modern scientific paradigm has long been established and recognized in the majority of developing societies. This contrasts with the tendency in the developed world for health care to be sought largely from formalized biomedical outlets (Phillips, 1990, p. 69). The ethnomedical system encompasses the total medical resources that are available to, and might be utilized by, a community and society including its biomedical and traditional forms of therapy. Good (1987a) summarizes an ethnomedical system as comprising three main spheres, although the weight of each will vary from culture to culture. These include:

1. The popular sphere that consists of knowledgeable sources (lay) referrals that are believed to be authoritative).
2. The biomedical sphere which consists of formal sources such as physicians, nurses, and midwives; and
3. The traditional sector that may be more or less discrete entities such as folk healers and alternative therapists who may have some overlap with scientific medicine.

According to Good (1987a), an ethnomedical system encompasses folk knowledge and beliefs, traditions, symbols, and values related to health, illness, and disease: a society's causal theories and taxonomies of sickness, supportive social institutions (groups, families, dispensaries, hospitals, recognized specialists [traditional, modern, professional, and paramedical]) and the spatial arrangements and interaction between various physical settings in which various phases and elements of illness and therapy are diagnosed, evaluated, and administered. The existence and use of a wide range of sources of medical care, traditional and modern, static and evolving, are generally known as medical pluralism. Illich (1976) provides a critique of modern medical care in developing context, while Phillips (1990, p. 5) suggests that enormous improvements in healthcare can and should be gained without the use of high technology. According to Phillips (1990, p. 5) there has been a shift in philosophy globally from favoring large scale, top down, technology oriented development projects to smaller scale, bottom up or grassroots approaches to development and the provision of human services such as health care. The focus of public health has also shifted from treating infectious diseases to preventing chronic ones such as AIDS, heart disease, and cancer. According to Freimuth *et al.* (1993, p. 503) health research reflects this change by focusing on behavioral and psychological variables that might enhance prevention and adoption of healthier behaviors, as well as on family and social systems that could strengthen or weaken these changes. Downie, Fyfe, and Tanahill (1990, p. 28) define this process as communication activity aimed at enhancing positive health and preventing diminishing ill health in individuals and groups through influencing the beliefs, attitudes and behavior of those with power and of the community at large. The challenge for development practitioners and researchers is to relate development communication and information regarding health-care issues to individual and community empowerment (Malan, 1998, p. 70). What is required is an understanding and appreciation of the issues underlying health communication.

Communication strategies between health-care professionals, patients, and their support groups play a key role in determining and assessing health outcomes. According to Kreps (1988) effective health care and health promotion are guided by relevant health communication. Communication is thus clearly the primary process used in health care to gather and disseminate health communication. Communication is essential in the provision of social support (by health-care provider participants in formal and informal support groups, family, and friends). Communication is also fundamental in coordinating health-care treatment and activities of various interdependent providers and consumers (Kreps, O'Hare and Clowers, 1994, p. 429). According to Kaplan (1997 pp. 75–82) Communication is perhaps the most essential ingredient in effective health care.

Shifting Paradigms in Health Communication

Kaplan (1996) and other health communication scholars, such as Sharf and Street (1997) identify two approaches to the management of health care, namely:

(i) the traditional biomedical model also referred to as the "find it - fix it" model; and
(ii) the outcomes model where the ultimate outcome is not a measure of the disease process.

The Biomedical Model

According to the traditional model, diseases have a clear biological basis. The role of the physician is to identify illnesses and to provide remedies. Once the problem is identified, an arsenal of effective medical treatments is available. The appropriate remedy is selected and the patient cured (Kaplan, 1997, p. 75).

In this type of interaction, communication is limited to a mechanistic view where the emphasis is on the transfer of information as opposed to the establishment of mutual understanding through dialogue as opposed to monologue. Rimal, Ratzan, Arnitson, and Freimuth (1997, p. 62) note that traditional illness centered models assume health professionals 'know' what is in the patient's best interests, and research questions center around factors that inhibit or promote rates of compliance. Communication is conceptualized as a one-way flow (from the doctor to the patient) in which information is used as an instrument to bring about change (compliance).

This results in the desocialization of the health setting, undermining the human-environment (ecological approach) relationship. The biomedical approach negates the manner in which medical beliefs and behavior are linked to cultural contexts in which they appear. Ackerknecht (cited in Landy, 1997, p. 23) stated that, "Medicine is nowhere independent and following its own motivations. Its character and dynamism depend on the place it takes in every cultural pattern; they depend on the pattern itself." Furthermore, the perception of how disease is imagined and how disease is represented is not taken into account.

Health issues need to be looked at in a holistic manner, as socially organized responses that constitute a cultural system (Kleinman, 1980, p. 24). This cultural system is made up of organized schemata relating to the arrangement of social institutions and patterns of interpersonal interactions. Illness and healing should thus be regarded as culturally constituted experiences and activities. However, even though modern medicine has a significant biological orientation, a concern with social and cultural aspects and their impact on health issues is deeply rooted in medical history. Landy (1977, p. 14) even refers to references that show medicine at one time was conceived as a social science. Biomedicine has thus been criticized as being ethnocentric and reductionist. To quote Kleinman (1980, p. 32) in this regard, "The ingrained ethnocentrism and scientism that dominates the modern medical and psychiatric professions follows the paradigm of biomedical science to emphasize in research only those variables compatible with biological reductionism and technological solutions, even if the problems are social ones."

Health issues are socially and culturally constructed. They are forms of social reality. This social reality is established, learned, and expressed in clinical settings. For example, Singer (1990, p. 179) criticizes the notion of doctors and patients being regarded as equals, citing class and other power relations that are embedded in the clinical setting as being a primary factor that will govern doctor-patient interactions. "Beliefs about sickness, the behaviors exhibited by sick persons, including their treatment expectations, and the ways in which sick persons are responded to by family and practitioners are all aspects of social reality" (Kleinman, 1980, p. 38). This constructionism results in culturally constructed meaning. Singer (1990, p. 80) writes that from this perspective illness is seen as a symbolically rich text. It needs to be read if the deeper meanings especially the cultural ones, are to be comprehended. Good and Good (1981, p. 175) argue that all clinical practice is inherently interactive. They also state that, "Biomedicine's failure to recognize that physicians and patients inhabit different semantic worlds and are ensnared in different webs of significance is said to be one of it major shortcomings."

Health-care settings involve matrixes containing several levels that provide the context of meaning. As the individual moves through and encounters different levels they will be exposed to different medical languages (discourses) and will need to translate from one language to another. The problem could arise that there could be different interpretations in these transactions (Kleinman, 1980, p. 53). Landy (1977, p. 21) states that in some instances phenomena considered to be symptoms of disease by some groups may be regarded as signs of health or without medical significance by others. These interrelated structural components also provide legitimization of health-related issues.

Keesing (1987, p. 161) argues that cultures do not only constitute webs of significance but ideologies too. According to Lull (1995, p. 6) ideology represents organized thought. For example, non-Western ethnomedicine is viewed within the biomedical framework as a component of culture while biomedicine is seen as scientific (Singer, 1990, p. 181). Singer refers to the work of Beson that highlights biomedicine's' role as a mechanism of cultural hegemony. Hegemony refers to the process through which dominant ideology is transmitted, consciousness is formed and social power is exercised (Lull, 1995, p. 6). Simply stated it is the power that one social group holds over another and is also a means for gaming and maintaining power. Social power finds its origins in institutionalization. The biomedical community is heavily institutionalized. Kleinman (1980, p. 54) refers to Freidson who states how the modern medical profession, using legal and political means, gained professional dominance in the health-care field by forcing all other healing traditions to disband, submit to its professional control, or retreat into the quasi-legal folk fringe." Another quote from Kleinman (1980, p. 56) also reinforces the argument about the dominance of the biomedical profession, namely. "Research by physicians and public health personnel, in most instances, is systematically limited to problem-frames defined by biomedicine; the solutions offered fit professionally sanctioned solution-frames and are evaluated only from that standpoint...Professional socialization of modern health professionals causes them to regard their own notions as rational and to consider those of patients, the lay public, and other professional and folk practitioners as irrational and 'unscientific.'" Singer (1990, p. 183) also refers to the impact of the political economy on the theory, practice, organizations and history of biomedicine.

Even the metaphors used in health issues reflect cultural meaning. Kleinman (1980, p. 108) shows how the metaphors of war are commonplace. These include "fighting" infection; "defenses" and "invaded" by pathogens.

The Outcomes Model (Bio-Psychosocial Model)

At the heart of this approach is the assumption that health behaviors can be changed only to the extent that individuals are empowered with effective psychological tools that promote learning of appropriate health behaviors. According to Rimal *et al.* (1997, p. 62) recent thinking presents a much more dynamic role for both the provider as well as the consumers of health information. According to Arnston (1989) it recasts health as a wellness-centered phenomenon by conceptualizing health as a multi-faceted concept that includes biomedical, psychosocial, and environmental determinants. According to Rimal *et al.* (1997, p. 62) a wellness-centered approach is adaptive to problems faced by the population in the latter half of the century, especially as it relates to chronic diseases. Sharf and Street (1997, p. 7) view this model as one in which health outcomes are defined not only from the mortality and morbidity perspectives of medical and public health practitioners, but also in patient initiated terms that give more attention to dimensions such as quality of life, respect and advocacy, physical and psychological well-being, and attention to individuals' preferences, values, and expanded choice making. According to Lambert, Street, Cegala, Smith, Kurtz, and Schofield (1997, p. 31) the physician is viewed as the interactional partner with the greatest potential impact on the patient's well-being and health. Research still takes place in predominantly medical settings and outcomes are often of more interest to providers (e.g. adherence, utilization) than to patients. According to Lambert *et al.* (1997, p. 32) interaction approaches maintain that health is created and sustained in interaction. Similarly, interpretations and meaning are interactional creations. Health behavior is mediated by meanings and interpretations, behavior is therefore a consequence of symbolic interactions. Lambert *et al.* (1997, p. 32) view identity as the prime mover in health cognitions and behaviors, and because identity is itself the product of communicative interactions, communication must be at the very core of what it means to be healthy.

Reasons for the Shift in Paradigm

Clearly medical providers may need to shift their form of storytelling from an emphasis on technical knowledge (what technology does to the body) toward social knowledge (what technology does to the person) (Hyde, 1990).

Lammers and Geist (1997, p. 56) note, however, that curriculum in medical schools persists in the advancement in biotechnological knowledge to the exclusion of sociocultural knowledge.

Individuals dissatisfied with and critical of the progressive ideology and biomedical emphasis of traditional medicine generally, and managed care specifically, may see self-care and holism as less expensive, more humane medicine. The progressive ideology that permeates medicine is that many participants have become blind subjects of technology, legitimating and privileging technical knowledge over social knowledge. In Hyde's (1990, p. 120) view "the machine has become the physician; the definitive advisor." Thus, for example, patients find that their sociocultural characteristics have no place in the managed health-care world and under these circumstances the patient may feel dehumanized. Furthermore, the biomedical model reinforces the power imbalance that is propagated between the physician and the patient. It therefore highlights the power of the practitioner relegating the patient's experiences and interpretations to a secondary role. Unfortunately, in this kind of medical setting, the social concerns of patients related to their health status are repeatedly marginalized and ignored. As previously mentioned this creates a context where the structural and cultural hegemony implicit in health related discourses are to a large degree ignored. Sharf and Street (1997, p. 20) suggest that the hierarchical power ascribed to physicians needs to be shared with the patients. This will result in a more active and co-equal role for the patient. The traditional imbalance of power also results in an imbalance of control. As previously mentioned, this creates a context where the structural and cultural hegemony implicit in health-related discourses are to a large degree ignored. The power imbalance of the biomedical model is once again reinforced, as power is often conceptualized in a vertical manner (the dominance of the biomedical model has led to a one-sided power baseline with the physician and the institutions of medicine). Malan (1998, p. 51) writes that if development is seen as the process of improving the individual's material, spiritual and similar conditions then development should include capacity building, education and improvement. The biomedical model does not recognize this building human capability perspective and functions more in terms of the medical practitioner acting as a benefactor and the recipient as a beneficiary. This is an outdated perspective of development.

Traditionally emphasis was placed on acute medical care where the fix-it models were used regularly. Kaplan (1997, p. 76) suggests, however, that we are now faced with problems for which this medical care system was not designed. With the progress toward the elimination of infectious acute illness, came the era of long-term chronic illness. By definition, chronic illness cannot be cured. The chronic care model requires long-term interactions between providers and patients. Dialogue is the nucleus of communication and also of cultural interaction. Outdated approaches to development were characterized as top-down, one-way and anti-traditional (Malan, 1998, p. 60). Self-management including goal setting is central to this model. Furthermore, psychological and sociocultural factors have a profound influence on the cause of the problem. As Kaplan (1997, p. 76) states, "One way communication could suffice in acute care, but two-way communication is the central component of chronic care. Our health care system, grounded in the acute care paradigm, is poorly equipped for this interaction." In chronic illnesses, the exchange of information will influence the patients' outcomes as much as their medicines and surgeries. Thus, the key element here is the building of relationships that is totally dependent on the presence of transactional communication or what is referred to as participatory communication.

According to Rimal *et al.* (1997, p. 62) one of the primary criticisms that can be leveled at the bio-medical approach is that the multiple goals present in the physician – patient encounter are ignored. Sharf and Street (1997, p. 4) highlight the need to reposition the concept of "patient" in order to achieve an increased understanding of the patients' role and influence in health related interactions. This would ensure that the direct and indirect factors that shape an individual's health will be take into account as opposed to focusing on the individual only. An exclusive focus on the individual places the responsibility of change on individuals and disregards the wider societal-level factors that can inhibit change. By implication, those who do not practice healthy behavior are perceived to be irresponsible, unmotivated or incompetent. Rimal *et al.* (1997, p. 63) believe that if the environmental constraints are not taken into account, then we run the risk of "blaming the victim."

Lammer and Geist (1997, p. 45) reinforce this belief of Rimal *et al.* by writing that managed care is a factor that further inhibits a dialogue between health provider and health receiver. They believe that this managed care can be characterized as a paternalistic view of communication where there is "an inability to capture the context, complexity and consequence of communication, and a narrow focus on the biology of health that excludes the psychological, social, cultural and spiritual." It is imperative to acknowledge the impact of the integrated environment on the health of the individual.

The traditional biomedical approach has also failed to take cognizance of the fact that the patient of today is very different to the patient of five/ten years ago, thus their expectations will also be significantly different. The range of information that is available to patients has increased dramatically due to:

- the emergence of specialized self-help groups
- increased media coverage of medical research
- patients making use of multiple physicians for basic and specialized care (Vanderford, Jenks, & Sharf, 1997, p. 22)
- the empowerment of patients to become informed about their own ailments. Vanderford *et al.* (1997, p. 14) adds that individuals are playing a more active role in their own medical care and decision-making.

The problem is that physicians do not know and do not ask what the patient knows (from other sources) about specific ailments and health in general (Vanderford *et al.,* 1997, p. 22). The physician does not take the time or effort to sort through information which the patient already has pertaining to health care, but that may be confusing conflicting or misleading. The health provider needs to expand their understanding of how individuals experience and make use of health information. In the words of Vanderford *et al.* (1997, p. 22), "knowing the ways in which patients use information and create meaning can help the medical community to guide that process more fully, clarifying differences that may hamper mutual understanding and cooperation." Patient-centered research will thus help the physician to understand how the patient moves through and uses a variety of sources. This would go a long way in recognizing the impact of the patient's perceptions in the health decision-making process, minimizing the degree of misunderstanding and dissatisfaction that is often the outcome of doctor-patient interactions.

What is needed therefore, is a shift in orientation to one that acknowledges and heightens the understanding of the patient's role and influence in health related interactions. Sharf and Street (1997, p. 5) assert that it is important to draw a distinction between making the patient a central construct, versus the patient as the central construct. With the importance of the patient being recognized, the opportunity for making choices and decisions is created (Bennett & Irwin, 1997, p. 87) as patients will be more active, knowledgeable and informed. This will ensure that the cultural codes associated with institutionalized medicine do not result in the marginalization and disempowerment of the recipient. Elements such as literacy, education, elitism, and technological expertise further act as cultural codes that structure communication in a slanted manner. Hegemony is maintained via these cultural codes. This would result in greater patient participation in the health care process. There is a growing body of research that suggests that once patients' preferences and involvement in determining therapeutic regimes and related forms of decision-making have occurred, there is a resultant increase in the improvement in health outcomes and a reduction of health care costs (Sharf & Street, 1997, p. 2). What is needed then, is an approach that "rather than conceiving of patients as recipients of and reactors to the message of others, we propose a focus on patients as active interpreters, managers, and creators of the meaning of their health and illness" (Vanderfort *et al.*, 1997, p. 13). Malan states that empowerment results in peoples' direct participation in the decision-making process (1998, p. 69). Furthermore, the acknowledgement and utilization of cultural identity is the central element of true empowerment. Accordingly, "development communication that does not succeed in having the marginalized articulate their own needs, and preferences are doomed to failure in the long term."

The Role of Health Communication

Health Communication can be defined as the art and technique of informing, influencing and motivating institutional and public audiences about important health issues. Its scope includes disease prevention, health promotion, health care policy, business as well as the enhancement of the quality of life and health of individuals within the community (Ratzan, Stearns, Payne, Amato, Liebergott, & Madoff, 1994, p. 362). What is required is an understanding and appreciation of the basic issues underlying health communication. According to Kroger (1994, p. 218) these are *professionalism, systemism* and *consumerism*. Let us discuss each of these.

Professionalism

According to Paisley (1990) social scientists point to three principal avenues for influencing social change: education, engineering and enforcement. Kroger (1994, p. 218) maintains that educator's influence through instruction and persuasion. A trend in professional education has been defining competencies for professional practice of health communication (Maibach, Parrott, Long, & Salmon, 1994, p. 352). A study conducted by Maibach *et al.* (1994, p. 353) lists the competencies required by professional health communicators to include the following:

- ability to apply relevant theories to program and development efforts at both the individual and societal level
- conduct program planning and implementation which requires knowledge of the full range of health communication goals
- good knowledge of the mass media and of its communication tools and
- ability to evaluate at all levels of strategy development and implementation.

Professional health communicators therefore need foundational competencies in order to gain an understanding of a broad base of human behavior. Foundational competencies suggested by Maibach *et al.* (1994, p. 356) include an individual and societal understanding of behavioral theories, functions of the mass media, media production processes and technology, rhetoric and environmental scanning, previous health campaigns, and corporate consumer marketing practices. Appropriate predatory grounds for advanced training as health communication professionals include journalism, health education and public health, psychology, education, public policy, city planning, and marketing communication. Applied competencies are demonstrated in the ability to perform a set of tasks. Individual applied competencies include the ability to collect and interpret formative data, synthesize relevant primary and secondary research findings, and reach action-oriented recommendations. At the societal level applied competencies demonstrate the importance of the health communicator's ability to define public health problems from multiple perspectives and levels of analysis. These perspectives broadly include policymakers, businesses, and the general public. The foundational and applied competencies specified foster reflexive competency.

Reflexive competencies are fostered through providing a full range of understanding and skills required in health communications, thereby enabling professional health communicators to demonstrate and connect health communication outcomes to an understanding of their performance so that actions can be adapted to changes and unforeseen circumstances. In order to equip professional health communicators with these competencies, training institutions must provide graduate-training programs to foster a full range of understanding and skills required in health communication. In terms of development communication, this would involve (Malan, 1998, pp. 73, 76) the recognition, respect for, and utilization of:

- individuals' worldviews and values. This can only be achieved if compassion and empathy are practiced
- local knowledge systems, including traditions, outcomes, beliefs, and symbols and how these influence peoples' view the world
- traditional communication systems - here it is imperative to relate the basic message to the recipients way of life and everyday experiences, so that identification and internalization can occur
- indigenous technologies, and
- oral and nonwritten visual communication especially for the illiterate.

According to Rogers (1994, p. 210) the growth of health communication rests fundamentally on the development of university centers of excellence that engage in scholarly but applied research that trains future generations of health communication experts. The general trend toward prevention in health programs and policies is one reason for the increasing recognition of health communication (Rogers, 1994, p. 211).

Systemism

Kroger (1994, p. 219) contends that a systems approach to disease or disability prevention requires intervention specialists to think holistically. Conscientious health communicators have to examine their roles within a bigger context. Green and Kreuter (1991) have distinguished between interventions in communities versus community interventions. Community interventions call for multiple strategies designed to influence environmental forces and behavioral patterns at several levels within a community. This requires networking and co-operation between all parties involved, not just those within the health system per se. Effective health communication entails being aware of activities on the multiple micro levels of action. The individual is no longer the focus of behavior change strategies, proving that public debate on policy issues is. Health communicators must therefore not only look at developing and deploying messages in a creative manner, but also at issues of distribution. They need to create the message with the correct context-specific cultural discourse.

Consumerism

Consumerism has to do with the notion that a consumer orientation is more productive than a product orientation. This implies that the consumer's wants, needs, perceptions, preferences, and tastes should determine the strategies and execution of the integrated marketing communication aimed at the consumer. Therefore, PHC must fit the requirements of particular local circumstances as well as the development of a customer orientation in the rendering of service. This entails that the community must be recognized as clients and treated as such with regard to the delivery of PHC services. This entails maintaining a clear vision for prioritizing resource allocations and the strengthening of your ability to communicate internally and externally. Community consultation enables the identification of short-term priorities for addressing health care provision problems and on the long term it establishes a reaffirmation of the mandate by conferring public consent. Health-care issues and problems and the size and nature of the community will determine the number and variety of people and associations to consult with. Community consultation is an ongoing process that promotes two-way communication at all times. In essence, PHC represents a broadening of the focus, in that the focus shifts from a curative approval to a preventative one

According to Ratzan (1994, p. 224) the motivation for the shift to preventative medicine has been heightened by the fact that Aids is incurable thus the emphasis has, out of necessity, shifted to preventative medicine. According to Hornik (1996, p. 12) the substantial efforts in public health communication are founded in recognition that much of health status reflects human behavior rather than medical treatment, prevention, and cure. Ratzan *et al.* (1994, p. 363) states that what is required is an understanding and appreciation of both the principles of health and health communication, thus implying that communication competency becomes a central aspect of the health care equation. Hornik (1996, p. 12) postulates that this is why much attention is being focused on understanding why it is that people comply or don't comply with particular behaviors and the development of models of health behavior choice. According to Kreps, O'Hair and Clovers (1994, p. 248) the deployment of increased resources in health care becomes meaningless unless effective communication throughout the health-care delivery process takes place continuously. According to Hornik (1996, p. 11), failure to do this means that the model of influence that comes from a social communication point of view is not respected, thus the quality of communication is not considered.

What is needed is public health communication founded in the recognition of the role of health communication, in affecting secular trends in health behaviors, including both deliberate communication interventions as well as public health communication in general. Only then can public health communication be systematically used to influence secular health behavior, so that there is a change on a scale that can be regarded as meaningful (Hornik, 1996, p. 14).

The challenge is to prevent crises in order to increase the proper management of health services. In line with global trends this entails that the causes of ill health need to be tackled through preventative rather than curative health care.

One way of ensuring this consumercentric approach is to adopt what is referred to as the WIN perspective.

An Outcome Based Model: Workable Integrated Negotiated Health Communication

The basis of the workable integrated negotiated (WIN) perspective is fostering democratic discourse that originates with the initial communication act (Ratzan, 1994, p. 226). Given this perspective, the individual must be empowered to communicate and effectively negotiate to render decisions that affect his/her well-being. According to Ratzan (1994, p. 228) the WIN approach has the potential to significantly affect various levels of education and curriculum of health-care professionals, and to contribute to informed citizenry. Furthermore, WIN can improve the quality and deliveries of health care, as well as broaden the attitudes and beliefs of health-care providers and consumers. In this health communication negotiation model, the individual is the recipient that is targeted to deliberate on the appropriate decision. The result, in part, is dependent on credible agents who make up his/her primary familial group. A secondary, yet important objective is for receivers of such information to become sources in the transactional process to others within the community. In addition to enhancing satisfaction, as well as optimizing successful outcomes, increased patient participation using negotiation concepts in the dyadic health encounter is beneficial for third parties such as insurance companies and other members of the health polity (Ratzan, 1994, p. 233). WIN operates at the individual level and is realized through communication, options, alternatives, standards, and trust (COAST). The promise of implementing WIN within the extrinsic layers of society centers on a parsimonious model for effective decision-making. COAST suggests an active participation by the individual in implementing self-determinism to effect his/her overall health and well being. COAST originates with the initial communication act between individuals, defining interests, establish agendas, identifying cultural nuances, and developing effective listening habits. As the negotiation develops further, options are brainstormed, presented, and discussed along with appropriate alternatives. This important communication act occurs within the context of mutually agreed upon objective standards, thereby imbuing the process with trust. The COAST method inspires and empowers individuals within a similar group to work toward the common interests of quality health, which they collectively define and agree on. The COAST model can be depicted as follows:

Figure 6.1: ***The COAST Negotiation Model***

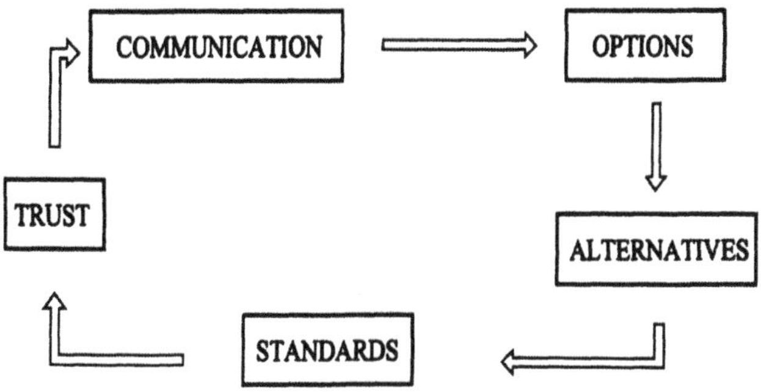

The COAST negotiation approach to the health encounter is communication centered, incorporating essential elements of traditional communication models. COAST points to a dialectical approach with the opportunity to replace unidirectional flow and power relationships between health-care provider and client practiced widely today, with a coactive encounter increasing the clients locus of control, and based on trust and free flow of information. According to Ratzan (1994, p. 230) the key element of this strategy is the development of a dialogue which encourages individuals to select between alternatives. Essential to this approach is trust, the transactional product of open and honest sharing of information and credible feedback among the involved parties. Research reveals that the degree of trust within the health encounter can be positively correlated with the degree of compliance and overall satisfaction of the parties involved. According to Rattan (1994, p. 245) the challenge is to be involved dialectically in the communication process from its inception with in this transactional, holistic approach to health communication.

Patient Centered Care: The Patient as a Central Construct

Gerteis, Edgman, Levitan, Daley, and Delbanco (1993, p. 5) use the term "patient-centered care" to describe an approach that consciously adopts the patient's perspective through a focus on the "patients experience of illness and health care and the systems that work and fail to work, to meet the patients needs, as they define them." According to this definition patient-centered care has seven primary dimensions:

i) respect for patients' values, preferences and needs;
ii) coordination and integration of care;
iii) information, communication and education;
iv) physical comfort;
v) emotional support and alleviation of fear and anxiety;
vi) involvement of family and friends; and
vii) transition and continuity.

Patient-centered care is seen as emerging from an increased focus on the social causes of illness; one that admits the symmetrical influence of social, biological, and psychological forces and acknowledges the integral role of communication. Patient-centered care has, according to Lambert *et al.* (1997, p. 30), emerged from two broad fronts:

1. The notion of wellness has shifted from the health of the body

to the health-related experiences of the patient, reflecting a broader biopsychosocial conception of illness; and

2. An increased acceptance of the patient in care who participates in discussing health issues and therapy.

Vanderford, Jenks, and Sharf (1997, p. 14) identify three key assumptions that underlie the patient-centered approach: patients' experiences matter; identity experience of illness; and patients' experiences must be understood in context. Let us discuss each these assumptions.

Patients' Experiences Matter

According to Vanderford *et al.* (1997, p. 14) the patients' experience with health, illness, and the medical community is crucial to our understanding of health communication. This is especially true as individuals play more active roles in their own medical care and health maintenance skills and experiences, and interpretation of health information become the basis for their ability to make medical decisions. Hines, Babrow, Badzek, and Moss (1997, p. 214) suggest that better understanding of end-of-life decisions and more effective interventions to improve them, require that research focus on the communication process. Such a focus can more clearly identify how doctors and patients negotiate issues that both find problematic and may suggest alternative communication patterns that allow doctors and patients to make health-care decisions in such a way that minimize discomfort while facilitating good long term planning. This entails a focus on events and emotions experienced by the patient, who constructs meaning, devises strategies, and modifies life choices in response to information and changes in and about health. According to Vanderford *et al.* (1997, p. 14) all of these issues require an understanding of the increased importance of patient-centered research, as they become less dependent on the professional sector of health care for determining their medical choices. Medical choices and decisions are made best when patients are well-informed, actively involved in the decision-making process, and not coerced into accepting unwanted treatment (Beauchamp & Childress, 1994).

Identity as a Central Issue

Vanderford *et al.* (1997, p. 15) notes that the patient's experience of health and illness is inherently bound to the individual identity, which emerges and evolves through social interaction with others. Conceptions of health, illness, sickness, and disease relates to each individual's sense of what is normal, what is not, which role behaviors to assume, and what changes are experienced (Vanderford *et al.,* 1997, p. 15). Lambert *et al.* (1997, p. 40) notes that the patient role is a negatively valued role. Entry into the patient or sick role is often a last resort following delays and attempts at self-care. This may be because patienthood can often be dehumanizing and disempowering (Lambert *et al.,* 1997, p. 40).

Ahmed, Kolken, and Coelho (1979, p. 13) note that health should be viewed "not merely as a desirable in itself but as a means toward the fulfillment of strategic role obligations and illness as an obstacle to such fulfillment."

According to Vanderfort *et al.* (1997, p. 15) the patient's role can be both stigmatizing and disempowering. Hellman (1994, p. 82) states "...[they are] stripped of many of the props of social identity and individuality, and clothed in a uniform. There is a loss of control over one's body and over personal space, privacy, behavior, diet, and the use of time."

The use of the term "patient" is problem-laden, according to Sharf and Street (1997, p. 4). It denoted illness of health and recovery, and implies a necessary counterpart relationship with a health-care practitioner. It's Latin root *pati* signifies suffering or enduring, connoting a stance of passivity or helplessness, which is consistent with the patient as a compliant recipient of medical directives and procedures assumed in the biomedical model, rather that proactive behavior.

According to Sharf and Street (1997, p. 4) it is even less appropriate to use the word "patient" to refer to individuals engaged in activities focused on disease prevention, health promotion, and maintenance of physical, emotional, and spiritual well-being.

While the use of the term patient may be inappropriate, Vanderford *et al.* (1997, p. 16) note that recent medical controversies have witnessed a new phenomenon of individuals fighting to obtain their right to be labeled as patients. Sufferers of chronic fatigue syndrome and individuals experiencing multiple chemical sensitivity syndrome are just some of the victims unable to obtain socially sanctioned label of patient bestowed on them by legitimate medical authority. Consequently, these individuals lose social and financial support in the face of illness (Brody, 1987). Vanderfort *et al.* (1997, p. 16) note that the issue of identity is central to patients' experience of illness.

Alternative use of discourse to define the role of the patient has similar problems in deconstruction. Sharf and Street (1997, p. 4) observe that the use of the word "client", which derives from Latin root *klei*, as in being at the call of one's patron, has deeply embedded connotations of dependency. The now popular word "survivor" combats the notions of vulnerability and victimization, but is inherently linked with disease, which is what one survives. Even the use of the terms "health-care consumer," along with its counterpart health-care provider, derives from an expression of health as an economic metaphor. According to Sharf and Street (1997, p. 4) within this framework, health care is reduced to monetarily valued commodities of goods and services, provided by professionals, to be selected, bought and used by the public. Other promising alternatives to "patient," such as "citizen" (Arnston, 1989) and "partner" (Quill, 1983; Roter, 1987) carry less symbolic burdens but have a much broader commonsense context. Sharf and Street (1997, p. 5) contend that "...patient is used in this context in a very broad manner to refer to non-professional participants in medical services and health information, and may include individual families, consumers, and advocacy organizations, or community groups."

Bennett and Irwin (1997, p. 86) recognize the constraint language used to describe the patient-consumer-citizen, and how these serve to describe a variety of constructed identities. The theme of identity and role is therefore connected with its construction. The process of identity construction is sought within the social realm and is interaction-based through the opportunities and constrictions within the family social cultural, community and all other contexts to reconstruct the patient's role.

Patients' Experiences Must be Understood in Context

According to Rimal *et al.* (1997, p. 64) citizens make decisions in a variety of health engendering contexts that can be grouped into three interrelated environments: physical, social, and media. An overall healthy lifestyle is predicated on decision-making competencies in all three environments – all three environments can contribute to the individual's decision-making competencies and to varying degrees. Individuals can shape each of the three environments for their own well-being (Rimal *et al.* 1997, p. 64).

Physical Environment

Rimal *et al.* (1997, p. 65) identify three primary locations in which health-care decisions are made:

i) the household where most day-to-day decisions about life-style factors and health are made, and where individuals spend much of their life
ii) the workplace where many of the positive (e.g. exercise facilities) and negative (e.g. stress) determinants of health reside
iii) health-care institutes where adverse health outcomes are treated and preventative measures prescribed.

The roles of individuals across these settings involve different decision-making scripts and strategies. According to Rimal *et al.* (1997, p. 66) three considerations should be taken into account in understanding how physical environments affect health-related decisions:

1. Each environment imposes its own set of options and restrictions, some of which may be health friendly, whereas others may not be. For example, promoting healthy practices at work may influence employees' health decisions whereas the threat of crime in a neighborhood is a reality that will impinge on individuals' health decisions.

2. Physical environments are closely associated with informational normative cues. Galdin, Reno, and Kallgren (cited in Rimal *et al.* 1997, p. 66) distinguish between descriptive normative cues that provide information on what are normal and injunctive normative clues. Cues received from the environment, which might include the observation of others' behavior, are internalized and used as decision-making tools.

3. Some environments are associated with habitual and routine behavior, whereas others promote conscious decision-making. Knowledge about the nature of behavior (e.g. mindful *vs.* habitual) as a function of the physical environments can provide a deeper understanding of criteria individuals use in making health-related decisions.

Rimal *et al.* (1997, p. 66) point out that physical environments do not completely explain individuals' choices of health practices. How individuals construe their environment and their abilities to overcome existing barriers, to a large extent, shapes their choice of activities, likelihood of persevering in the presence of setbacks, choice of social networks, and attributions for success and failure (Bandura, 1986).

Social Environment

With regard to health decision-making, important social environments are those that either promote or inhibit health outcomes. According to Rimal *et al.* (1997, p. 67) two implications emerge from this understanding:

1. Health promotion efforts must take into account the power of injunctive social clues. Incorporating the individual's social environment as a channel of influence into health promotion, is likely to increase their effectiveness (Aspinwall, Kemeny, Taylor, Schneider, & Dudley, 1991).

2. Reciprocal influences exist between individuals and their social environments. Not only do social environments shape, but they are also shaped by individual behaviors as is revealed by studies that demonstrate the role of minority influence (Kitayama, & Burnstein, 1994) as well as these of opinion leaders (Rogers, 1983) on groups. According to Rimal *et al.* (1997, p. 67) it is the collective behavior of individuals ingroups that shapes culture. These authors also point to the fact that there is now a large body of literature that suggests that the family plays an important role in shaping the individuals health. Furthermore, there is also evidence that suggests that children themselves shape parental attitudes and behaviors (Bell, 1979). According to Rimal *et al.* (1997, p. 68) beyond the school and workplace environments, citizens are also community members with rights and responsibilities. Expanding to a community-oriented model of health communication stresses that the shared experiences of individuals can be a motivating factor for a community group to address common health-related issues through collective action (e.g. Medloff & Sklar, 1994).

Rimal *et al.* (1997, p. 68) contend that health behaviors have to be studied within the context within which health decisions are made, with the realization that the role of the family in shaping those decisions is crucial. Ell and Northern (1990) define this process as a definition of family that includes a collective decision-making process that is rooted in a common purpose for all members – that of maintaining and improving the family's well-being. According to Rimal *et al.* (1997, p. 68) this entails by implication that efforts to enhance the quality of individuals' health have to discover and improve the decision-making processes within which an individual functions.

Media Environment

According to Rimal *et al.* (1997, p. 69) the socializing role of the media has been extensively documented. Although the media are excellent vehicles for propagating messages and enhancing people's awareness of various issues, a number of problems still persist:

1. The mass media have proven to be largely ineffective in motivating people to change their high-risk behavior, especially with regard to AIDS; and

2. The prevalence of unhealthy behaviors depicted in the media (e.g. junk-food consumption and violence) are closely associated with either corresponding practices in real life (Gerbner, Gross, Morgan, & Signorielli, 1981) or, at a minimum, skewed perceptions of reality.

3. There is growing concern in the research community that media-based efforts are not reaching the undeserved population; that the gap between the haves and have-nots impacts on individuals' health practices and are, thus, perpetuating the knowledge gap in society (Freimuth, 1990).

4. Efforts to counter the preponderance of negative media images (e.g. tobacco through sport sponsorship) are severely handicapped by a lack of corresponding public funds, which presents further barriers to setting a healthy media agenda.

According to Rimal *et al.* (1997, p. 71) we need to look at the media's role differently and that emphasis should be placed on educating citizens in a way that improves citizen's decision-making skills about their well-being. The media need to provide models of functional decision-making processes for how people can be healthy, not merely to disseminate health information.

Clearly, health professionals will not only have to provide citizens with the information they need to make functional health-care decisions, it will also be necessary for health professionals to encourage patients to accept responsibility during the encounters, to make decisions about their health; to develop with their patients' decision-making scripts so that their patients can, as citizens make functional health-care decisions in their homes and communities and to prove feedback to patients about the decisions that were made. Decision-making authority for their health needs to be transferred from health officials in a way that creates a sense of self-efficacy. According to Rimal *et al.* (1997, p. 71) citizens' competencies to make individual and collective health-care decisions become the outcome of choice.

Conclusion

It would appear as if the dominant paradigm in health-care delivery in many countries is still the biomedical approach. Consequently, the principles of outcome-based models are excluded from both the education and practice of primary health-care providers. This results in an ability to recognize and acknowledge that health care is culturally bound and impacted by communication, and that the relationships between care providers and recipients depends on the quality of health information rather than the quantity. The new cornerstones of effective health communication are disease prevention, health promotion, and maximizing one's well-being. (Ratzon, 1994, p. 225). However, this entails shifting the paradigm from the traditional unidirectional format in which the physician is the sole focal point of information, toward an outcomes-based approach in which the health-care provider shares in the information flow, leading to decision making between the provider and recipient. This entails a reframing of our understanding of the patient as an active citizen involved in individual and collective decision-making. An understanding of patients' based on unidirectional models of influence from health care providers to recipients is inadequate for a broader conceptualization of health. The new strategy requires an integrative, overarching theory of health built on sound, contemporary theories of communication (Lambert *et al.* 1997, p. 41).

Hence, the implementation of health strategies within a development context is reliant on the following elements (Malan, 1998, p. 63):

- Consultation with relevant parties (participatory communication directed at maintaining basic needs)

- Adaptation and recognition of cultural identity of recipients
  - traditional means of communication should be used when possible, including oral and folk communication
  - acknowledging the wisdom of the recipient
- Mobilization through involvement resulting in self-development and empowerment of the recipient
  - health should not be seen as something that has been determined by the delivery of health services, but by overall development
- Accountability to the recipient
- Dialogic, horizontal and contextual communication that is emancipatory and interactive as health issues is very often characterized by imbalance often minimizing the existence of medical pluralism.

References

Ahmed, P.I., Koker. A., & Coelho, G.V. (1979). Toward a new definition of health: An overview. *Psychosocial dimensions.* New York: Plemum.

Anon, A. (1993). Your patients' expectations. *S.A.. practice management,* 14:2.

Arntson, P. (1989). Improving citizens' health competencies. *Health Communication,* 1;1: 29-34.

Aspinwall, L.G., Kemeny, M.E., Taylor, S.E., Schneider, S.G., & Dudley, J.P. (1991). Psychosocial predictors of gay men's AIDS risk-reduction behavior. *Health Psychology,* 10: 432-444.

Bandura, A. (1986). *Social foundations of thought and action.* Englewood Cliffs, NJ: Prentice Hall.

Beaucham, T.L., & Quill, J.F. (1994). *Principles of biomedical ethics.* (4th ed.). New York: Oxford University Press.

Bell, R.Q. (1979). Parent, child, and reciprocal influences. *American Psychologist,* 34: 821-826.

Bennett, K.C., & Irwin, H. (1997). Shifting the emphasis to "patient as central": Sea of change or ripple on the pond? *Health Communication,* 9:1.

Bidol, H.F. (1997). Effects of expectancies and physician verbal messages on gay/lesbian/bisexual patients' satisfaction. A paper presented at the 47th Annual Conference of the International Communication Association, May 22-26. Montreal, Canada.

Brody, H. (1987). *Stories of sickness.* New Haven: Yale University Press.

Cassata, D.N. (1991). Health communication theory and research: A definitional overview. *Communication Yearbook* 4. New Jersey: Transaction Books.

Downie, R.S. Fyfe, C., & Tannahill, A. (1990). *Health promotion models and values*. Oxford: Oxford University Press.

Ell, K., & Northen, H. (1990). *Families and health care: Psychosocial practice*. New York: Aldine de Gruyter.

Feachem, R.G., Graham, W.J., & Timaeus, I.M. (1989). Identifying health problems and health research priorities in developing countries. *Journal of Tropical Medicine and Hygiene*, 92.

Freimuth, V.S. (1990). The chronically uninformed: Closing the knowledge gap in health. In E.B. Ray & L. Donohew (eds.), *Communication and health: Systems and applications*. Hillsdale, NJ: Lawrence Erlbaum Associates, Inc.

Freimuth, V.S., Edgar, T., & Fitzpatrick, M.A. (1993). The role of communication in health promotion. *Communication Research*, 20;4: 509-516.

Gerbner, G., Gross, L., Morgan, M., & Signorielli, N. (1981). Health and medicine on television. *The New England Journal of Medicine*, 305;15: 901-904.

Gerteis, M., Edgman-Levitan, S., Daley, J., & Delbanco, T.L. (eds.) (1993). *Through the patients' eyes: Understanding and promoting patient centered care*. San Francisco, CA: Jossey-Bass.

Gilman, S.L. (1988). *Disease and representation*. London: Cornell University Press.

Good, B.J., & Good, M.J. (1981). *The meaning of symptoms: A cultural hermeneutic model for clinical practice*. The relevance of social science for medicine. Dordrecht.

Goosen, H. (1988). Primary health care and disease prevention. *South African Panorama*, 33, 7.

Hill, P.S. (1997). African-American women: Conflict in the clinic. A paper presented at the 47th Annual Conference of the International Communication Association. May 22-26. Montreal, Canada.

Hudson, M. (1997). S.A. Gesondheidsdienste erg olik. *Insig*. May.

Himes, S.C., Austin, B.S., Badzek, L., & Moss, A.H. (1997). Communication and problematic integration is end-of-life decisions. *Health Communication*, 9, 1:.

Hyde, M.J. (1990). Experts, rhetoric and the dilemmas of medical technology: Investigating a problem of progressive ideology. In Medhurst, A. *Communication and the culture of technology*. Pullman: Washington State University.

Kaplan, R.M. (1997). Health outcomes and communication research. *Health Communication*, 9, 1:.

Keesing, R.M. (1987). Anthropology as interpretive question. *Current Anthropology*, 28;2: 161-176.

Kim, Y.M., Odallo, D., Thuo, M., & Kols, A. (1997). Client communication and the quality of family planning counseling: Interaction analysis in Kenya. A paper presented at the 47th Annual Conference of the International Communication Association. May 22-26, Montreal, Canada.

Kitayama, S., & Burnstein, E. (1994). Social influence, persuasion, and group decision making. In S. Shavitt & T.C. Brock (eds.) *Persuasion: Psychological insights and perspectives* (pp. 175-193). Needham Height, MA: Allyn & Bacon.

Kleinman, (1980). Culture, health care systems, and clinical reality. *Patients and healers in the context of culture.*

Lambert, R.L., Street, R.L., Cegala, D.J., Smith, D.H,, Kurtz, S., & Schofield, T. (1997). Provider-patient communication, patient-centered care, and the mangle of practice. *Health Communication,* 9;11: 27-43.

Lammers, J.C., & Geist, P. (1997). The transformation of caring in the light and shadow of "Managed care". *Health Communication,* 9,1:.

Lull, J. (1995). *Media, communication, culture.* Oxford: Blackwell Publishers.

Majerovitz, S.B., Greene, M.G., Adelman, R.D., Brody, G.M., Leber, K., & Healy, W. (1997). Older patients' understanding of medical information in the emergency department. *Health Communication,* 9, 3

Malan, C.W. (1998). Development communication as part of culture. *Communicare,* 17, 1:.

Medoff, P., & Skiar, H. (1994). *Streets of hope: The fail and rise of an urban neighborhood.* Boston: South End Press.

Phillips, D.R. (1990). *Health and health care in the Third World.* New York: Longman.

Quill, T.E. (1983). Partnerships in patient care: A contractual approach. *Annals of Internal Medicine,* 98.

Ratzan, S.C. (1994, November). Health communication as negotiation. *American Behavioural Scientist,* 38;20: 224-247.

Rimal, R.N. Ratzan, S.C., Arnston, P., & Freimuth, V. (1997). Reconceptualizing the "patient": Health care promotion as increasing citizens' decision-making competencies. *Health Communication,* 9;1: 61-74.

Rogers. E.M. (1983). *Diffusion of innovations.* New York: Free Press.

Roter, D. (1987). An exploration of health education's responsibility for a partnership model of client-provider relations. *Patient Education and Counseling,* 10.

Sharf, B.F., & Street, R.L. (1997). The patient as a central construct: Shifting the emphasis. *Health Communication,* 9;1: 1-11.

Shaver, L.D. (1997). A taxonomy of the doctor/patient visit. A paper presented at the 47th Annual Conference of the International Communication Association. May 22-26, Montreal, Canada.

Singer, M. (1990). Reinventing medical anthropology: Towards a critical realignment. *Social Science & Medicine,*30, 2:.

Thornton, B.C., & Kreps, G.L. (1993). *Perspectives on health communication.* Prospect Heights, IL: Waveland.

Vanderford, M.L., Jenks, E.B., & Sharf, B.F. (1997). Exploring patients' experiences as a primary source of meaning. *Health Communication,* 9;1: 13-26.

Chapter 7

Health Promotion and the Myth of Community

Gwendolyn J. Lusi
Freddy Batundi
Kigali CBR Program, Congo-Zaire

Failed development projects litter the African landscape. Each one started with a bright idea, bright hopes, new equipment, and generous donations of outside resources. However, few survived to become self-sustaining. They generate a mass of evaluation reports, which conclude mostly around the terms "lack of community ownership," on the assumption that there is a community, that it has a representative voice and that it can own something. The buzzwords of the last two decades - community based health care, and community determined health care - are also dependent on this notion. Certainly, in traditional rural agriculture-based communities, this ideal model, represented by the image of a village meeting under the mango tree, may still exist. Even if the model exists, group dynamics are over-simplified for the convenience of the outsider. The observed realities of the end of the millennium in African communities are very different. We do not claim to present here a sociological analysis of contemporary Africa, but rather present certain features of community, which we have observed in our work in Rwanda, describe the contribution of our community-based rehabilitation (CBR) program in the prevention of disability, and the most appropriate partners we have found for effective community action.

Background to the Program

Our CBR program contributes mainly to secondary arid tertiary prevention of disability; primary prevention is sometimes a spin-off from our activities through clinics, or through home visits, but it is not our main activity. The Kigali CBR program is a local church initiative dating from January, 1997. It is an off-shoot of a ten-year-old program for widows and orphans of AIDS and, since 1994, widows and orphans of the genocide. The widows and orphans program has been a good foundation to build upon: it was never institution-based. It uses the extended family, providing limited, but strategic, financial support to relatives fostering orphaned children, by providing sheltered accommodation for child-headed households or terminally ill widows and their children. The social workers from the church live in the same geographical area as the families they support; they are themselves widows, and their economic situation is in many respects the same as the people they assist.

A visitor to Rwanda will immediately be struck by the difference between the population distribution in Rwanda and in neighboring African countries. There are a few large towns, a few small towns, but villages are rare. This is the most densely populated country in Africa, but people prefer to live on their land and build their house within their plantation, rather than building close to their neighbors. People ask: *"Utuye uhe musozi?"* "Which hill do you come from?" not "Which village do you come from?" Within population centers, the focus of communal activity is the *commune* and the *secteur*, which are structures of local government. The lack of community feeling, trust, and collaboration was both a consequence and a cause of the long-standing divisions in Rwandan society, and is especially evident in the aftermath of the war of 1994.

Within this country the church can play a crucial role in creating community, and it is our choice of foundation for the community-based rehabilitation program. The church is typically a "community of choice." Catherine Lysack uses this very appropriate term to describe what is happening in many societies in the world.

> This loosening of the 'ties that bind' has transformed social groups (communities) based on geography, shared identity, and local culture into communities of choice. We are destined to succumb…to one global culture and an

unending cycle of chosen identities that are discarded when their usefulness is outlived (Lysack, 1998).

What Rwanda has already experienced is likely to become the norm for other African societies in the 21st century. For that reason alone, the programs developed here deserve attention, since they could well become models or warnings for the future. Whether our program is a model or a warning remains to be seen; it is too early to decide. However, the strategies we are using may be of interest to readers who are considering entering the field of rehabilitation in urban centers in Africa.

Why a Community-Based Approach?

The first problem is one of capacity. Rehabilitation institutions in Rwanda cannot offer enough places for the children needing them. Gatagara Center for the physically handicapped and the blind can take 200 children into residence. Butare School for the Deaf, and Nyamirambo School for the Deaf in Kigali can take 100 children each. A very small number of children benefit from the excellent services they offer. The 400 fortunate children are a tiny fraction of the number of children of

Table 7.1: ***School-Aged Disabled Children (6–15 years)***

		Schooling			
Type of Handicap	*Total*	*No*	*%*	*Yes*	*%*
Polio	1,987	1,029	52	958	48
Deformity	1,747	1,109	63	638	37
Deaf	1,411	1,241	88	170	12
Mentally Retarded	728	644	88	84	12
Cerebral Palsy	549	517	94	32	6
Blind	544	378	69	166	31
Psychological Problems	392	293	75	99	25
Amputation	260	118	45	142	55
Hemiplegia	224	170	76	54	24
Scoliosis, Cyphosis	160	92	58	68	43
Elephantiasis	134	96	72	38	28
Spinal Column Truama	111	84	76	27	24
Head Truama	99	54	55	45	45
Myopathology	75	60	80	15	20
Leprosy	61	43	70	18	30
Other	18	13	72	5	28
Total	**8,500**	**5,941**	**70**	**2,559**	**30**

school age with severe physical or sensory handicaps. The national percentage of 15 year olds who have completed primary education was 85 percent for boys and 83 percent for girls in 1992 (Office National, 1994).A nationwide survey of disability carried out by Handicap International in 1995 showed that 70 percent of school-aged disabled children (6–15) had never been to school (Handicap International, 1995). Our own survey, conducted in 1997 and 1998 door-to-door in 12 sectors of the town of Kigali identified the following disabilities among preschool- age children (<1–6 years).

Table 7.2: ***Disabilities Among PreSchool-Age Children (<1–6 years)***

Disability	*No.*
Physical Disability	125
Partial Deafness	111
Eye Problems	93
Deaf and Dumb	46
Epilepsy	41
Cerebral Palsy	39
Mentally Retarded	11
Polio	8
Psychosis	8
Total	**466**

Second, there is a problem of equity: the cost of institutional care is very high, whereas there are no resources and no service at all available for the large majority who need care.

The third problem is one of take-up. Even the places that are available to children in institutions are not always optimally occupied. For example, the school for the blind had 20 empty places in the academic year 1997-98, and some of the children studying there were partially sighted (low vision) and could have benefited from learning to read print with low vision aids in normal schools. The same applies for medical care: the fact that services are available does not mean people in need will use them. Many barriers must be addressed before people come for care: fear; ignorance; prejudice; difficulty of physical access; and lack of financial resources. This is especially true for the disabled person and the family member responsible for that person. These barriers are best addressed in the community.

There are many advantages to a community based approach: the person with a disability can be more easily identified in the community; community-based social workers are able to address all disabilities (physical, sensory, intellectual, social) and are not just limited to medical prevention programs usually associated with "health." Social workers and volunteers with a limited training can inform people of services available to them, persuade them to use the services, and assist them with access. They can be advocates for the needs and rights of the disabled within the community, for example, the right to schooling for the disabled child. Professional services are just one aspect of rehabilitation: if professional advice is not followed and applied day after day in the home, then it will not bear fruit and will cause further discouragement to the family. Most importantly, within the community, it is possible to advance on all fronts together: we aim to draw up rehabilitation plans that address the medical, functional, educational, economic, social and spiritual needs of the person. These plans take into account the resources that are really available: they cannot be theoretical or impractical, or costly.

Strategy

In July and August 1997, we trained 12 workers for four days for the identification of disabilities, and began a house-to-house census in five sectors of the town where the orphans' program was already working. The reaction of the population to the census was frequently hostile: "Another research! Why don't you do something for us instead of just writing down information!" They had been the objects of many research projects. We were pushed faster into interventions than we really wanted to go. We arranged collaborative agreements with some medical specialists and before the end of the first month, we held clinics for epilepsy, eye problems, physical handicap and deaf children.

After the first census, during the last quarter of the year, we retained and trained six social workers from among the 12 researchers; the church employed those chosen. They receive salary assistance from Christoffel Blindenmission, as well as some funds to cope with urgent needs of indigent people. Each month, the team meets together for a training session, for troubleshooting and for planning the month ahead. In July and August 1998, we did a second census in new areas of the city. By this time, volunteers had assumed some of the long term caseload of each social worker, and the system of specialist referrals, day-care centers and follow-up of rehabilitation plans was familiar and easier. We are now able to undertake training for other programs, and accept interns from the university.

Key Partners for Success

After analyzing our brief experience in Rwanda in the changing community context of contemporary Africa, we can suggest to future programs two key partners for community based rehabilitation: the *church* and the *government*. We began our work from a base in a particular church. However, in reaching out to the community over the past 18 months, we have collaborated with many other churches across the ecclesiastical spectrum; we have also worked in close collaboration with other national and international nongovernmental organizations (NGOs) and in some sectors, with the local government. At national level, the ministries have been very helpful, and have fostered this spirit of collaboration among agencies in Rwanda in a way that is not often seen among competitive agencies like NGOs.

Church

The church-based approach has been successful for several reasons. First, the church is the only nationwide grassroots institution with a specific mandate to care for the underprivileged. Jesus requires his followers to engage in social action as a spiritual duty: "As much as you have done this to the least of these children, you have done it to me" (Matthew 25). In a country where 85 percent are practicing Christians, where each local church has a building and a community network, the church is an immense resource, if it can be mobilized effectively.

At the outset, even our own church was hesitant about opening its doors to the disabled. We have used our office at the church as a clinic, for epilepsy consultations, for examining children with running ears, for people lacking limbs, for children with cerebral palsy. There is tremendous social prejudice against receiving such people, and church members are not immune to it. Thanks to the leadership of two church elders, after the program had been running for six months, they began to show interest. Then the interest grew exponentially; we were invited to pastors' training sessions, to church women's groups, to Sunday worship, to explain the program and to recruit volunteers. Then we arranged training and orientation for the volunteers; so far, 20 of the 55 trained have in fact become active volunteers. They are assigned with a social worker to the follow-up of a disabled person close to their own home. Some follow two or three people, some help with identification (census), some help with crowd control on clinic days, and some help in the day-care centers.

In a rural area of Kibungo, after one of the pastors' training sessions, the church decided to call together the disabled who could be identified by the members of the congregation, to find out what their needs are. The church members then decided they would need some financial resources to meet these needs; they located a field, and together cultivated the field so that the produce could be used to help the disabled. This is a rare occurrence in Rwandan society, where there is no tradition of voluntarism or social service.

Day-care centers are the most exciting areas of community involvement in the urban areas, because they develop in unpredictable ways according to the needs of the people who meet together. They are primarily intended for stimulation and therapy for the mentally handicapped and children with cerebral palsy. Local groups of people identified by our social workers meet; they find a time and a place that suits them, for a half day each week. Two groups meet in church halls, one on the verandah of a local doctor; one group meets in the local government hall, another in a school, another two in the homes of one of the children in the group. We have made available a few donated toys, a few mats, and the time of the social worker. The day-care center provides a time to review progress in physical therapy, to share techniques among parents for dealing with the problems of disability, and to give the children an opportunity for social contact. We can bring specialists (physical therapists, educationalists) to consult more effectively during these groups. One group of mothers has begun a small co-operative for purchasing, laundering, and selling secondhand clothes; they have also begun an awareness-raising campaign in other *prefectures*, in collaboration with a sister organization, Handicap International.

National Government

In Rwanda, there is positive and negative aspects to the highly bureaucratized, verticalised government administration. From the minister to the householder, there is a direct line of command and real control which is unprecedented in Africa. The householder is under the supervision of the *nyumba kumi* (supervisor of a group of 10 households); this person is supervised by the *conseiller du secteur*, who answers to the *bourgmestre* of the commune, who is supervised by the *prefet* of one of the 12 prefectures of the country. The country is very small (barely 500 *kms* east to west, north to south), with only 7.5 million people; it has good roads and communications, so control is relatively easy, compared to some of Rwanda's neighbors.

On the negative side, this control enabled the organization of the swiftest and most destructive genocide of human experience; people obey orders from the government, and no one can hide from the authorities. Such authoritarianism works against community initiative.

On the positive side, the government can orient and coordinate the efforts of churches, NGOs and associations on behalf of the disabled. In CBR, we work with the Ministry of Health, the Ministry of Social Affairs and the Ministry of Education. Ministers and service directors within the ministries are accessible, they call together key players in the field, listen to objectives, problems, and strategies. As a result, there is trust, and because of that trust, we can refer cases and specialize. For example, our program has taken a key role in training of new CBR programs; we, in our turn, refer to HealthNet for professional expertise for the physically handicapped, to Handicap International for economic integration for our clients, to the institutions for the disabled for technical resources and assistance in integrated education for the disabled. The ministries can also make available to us the structure of the government administration: the social workers in each commune; the *agents sanitaires* in the health districts; the information channels of official radio and the press.

Conclusion

Any community-based program has to beware of paradigms, the sociologist's illusion; and we are obliged to challenge the myth of the cohesive community working together for its own development. Africa is not immune to the global trend of urbanization and individualism, and it is time for health strategists to bring their thinking up to date. After reviewing the Rwandan experience of CBR, we question the wisdom of community approaches and ask ourselves the questions: Where should we go to look for community in Africa? Is there a place for vertical direction in service provision to the community? Our intent in this paper has been to suggest that communities of choice, such as the church, can fill the gap at grassroots level; and that vertical hierarchy can give validity and strength to community programs in societies that do not resist authority.

References

Lysack, C. (1988). Community: A refuge from global culture. *Asian Pacific Re-*

habilitation Journal, 9;2.
Office National de la Population. (1994). *Rwanda: Enquête démographique et de santé* 1992. Kigali: Office National de la Population.
Handicap International. (1995). *Enquête nationale sur l'ampleur du handicap au Rwanda*. Kigali: Handicap International.

Chapter 8

Health Issues in Africa: The Role of Women

Arglenda Friday
African American Research Library and Cultural Center, Ft. Lauderdale, Florida

This case study is based on research collected during a volunteer effort conducted in Kenya as part of an HIV/AIDS health education campaign in Kendu Bay. The objective of this paper is to assess knowledge, perceptions, and behavioral changes that may be issues for consideration and further investigation in response to the spread of AIDS in a rural community.

The chief goal of the campaign was to distribute condoms to local residents while encouraging safer sex practices and family planning. While engaged in these aspects of the initiative, the volunteers determined there were other more important issues that needed to be factored into the campaign, such as women's concerns and behavior, and cultural practices of the target audience - the Luo people.

The primary emphasis of the initiative soon became centered on the role of women for two key reasons. First, women are much more susceptible to contracting HIV/AIDS from unprotected sex, and secondly, because the culture of the ethnic group limits the major life choices of most Luo women. Major life choices are defined as including property ownership, decision-making as it relates to fertility and childbearing, economic independence and viability, and educational opportunities.

The targeted region of the health education campaign consisted of several tribes and ethnic groups, however, as the majority of the residents were Luo and because a large number of the Luo spoke English, most of our energies were directed toward this group. Within the target audience, energies were soon directed to three subgroups: working women; rural housewives; and commercial sex workers or prostitutes.

Using surveys, workshops, group discussions and community meetings, teams of volunteers went into the community and homes to interact with residents and gauge their knowledge of HIV/AIDS. There were also discussions and sharing of information about family planning and effectiveness of contraceptives being promoted in the region. Depo Provera injections were the most widely used method of birth control.

Based on the findings and results of this study, possible replication in other African and developing countries can be considered with modifications to accommodate religious and cultural differences or issues unique to a particular location.

Following a brief discussion of the demographics, and social mores and customs of the Luo tribe, the report will focus on activities and projects used by the volunteers to address health communication, health promotion, and disease prevention in Kenya.

Demographics

Situated on the eastern coast of Africa, Kenya lies astride the equator. Slightly more than twice the size of Nevada, the republic measures 224,960 square miles and is bounded by the Sudan, Ethiopia, Somalia, Uganda, Tanzania, and Lake Victoria.

Following several decades of high birth rates, Kenya has a population of over 28 million people. It has ethnic and racial diversity, although African peoples indigenous to Kenya now form over 98 percent of the population (Middleton, 1998). They fall into five main clusters or three major cultural and linguistic groups - Bantu, Nilotic, and Cushitic, with Bantu comprising over 70 percent of the population. Major ethnic groups within the three large cultural groups include:

Bantu: Kikuyu (21 percent), Kamba (11 percent), & Luhya (14 percent)
Cushitic: Galla, Somali
Nilotic: Luo (13 percent), Turkana, Maasai, Pokot, Nandi, Kipsigis,

and Tugen
Other: Arab, Swahili (Arab-Africans); Europeans (mostly British)

The pluralistic character of Kenyan society is also reflected in its religious groups. The majority of the population, 66 percent, is Christian (Catholic and traditional Protestant), followed by tribal religionist (19 percent) and Muslims (6 percent) (EIU Country Report, 1995), however, most practice a mixture of traditional beliefs with an intermixing of certain Christian elements (Shipton, 1989).

The country has a literacy rate of 70 percent. Primary education is free although it is not compulsory or universal. Several thousand continue matriculation at the 8 technical training institutes and universities. English is the official language, but Swahili is the national language and several other languages are spoken by over 25 different ethnic groups (Shipton, 1995).

The National Hospital Insurance Fund provides Kenyans with medical care, but the free medical services for children and low contributions to the insurance fund strain the resources of the 324 hospitals and over 5,000 doctors and health care professionals. While life expectancy is about 58 years, Kenya has had one of the highest birthrates in the world. However, recent efforts to promote family planning and smaller families have had some success (Tiffen, 1994). According to U.N. estimates, the population is increasing at about 3 percent annually with almost half of the population under the age of 15 years, and about 75 percent of the population living in rural areas (Kenya Census Bureau of Statistics, 1997).

Social and Cultural Factors

The diversity of ethnic and religious groups is equally reflected in the social, cultural, political, and economic characteristics of the different groups. Many view the nuclear family as the basic social unit of the society, but polygyny, wife's inheritance, and extended families or subclans, are common with many groups. Because most rural women are responsible for crop cultivation, large families and extended relations are even more important.

Economically, tourism is emerging as the principal source of foreign revenues, given Kenya's coasts and beaches on the Indian Ocean, and the country's popular game reserves (Amboseli, Maasai Mara). Manufacturing and service sectors employ large numbers of urban dwellers and immigrants from the countryside. However, for most rural residents, subsistence farming is the main source of work (Downing, 1998).

In 1967, Kenya became the first sub-Saharan African country to launch a national family planning program to address the alarming birth rate. While the campaign promoted family planning, surveys found most women wanted to have large families, preferably around eight. The primary reason given by women wanting large families was that the children constitute an economic asset and are much needed to help the women with agricultural responsibilities (Middleton, 1998) and to assist them in old age.

The Luo People

Having large families is but one of many distinct characteristics of the Luo, our target population. Living on Lake Victoria, the Western Nilotic-speaking Luo is Kenya's second-largest people. Their population is estimated to number about 2.6 million, with over three-fourths of this population living in Nyanza Province, whose largest city is Kisumu. The Luo tribe occupies large areas in three districts around the Lake so most of our outreach effort was to this group with occasional interactions with their neighbors - the Gusii, Nandi, Kuria, and Maasai. DhoLuo is the principal language, but many Luo are proficient in English and Swahili.

Rural dwelling Luo live mainly in scattered multi- or single-house homesteads. Cattle herding and farming are fundamental aspects of their social structure. The majority are farmers but most keep livestock as well for trade and marriage bride wealth (marriage payments from the groom and his kin to the bride's family). Many of the men (about one third) seek work outside the Luo homeland, such as manual labor in the cities, towns and on sugar plantations. Left behind and using mostly hoes and simple farm tools, women do most of the farm and housework while men do more animal tending. Given the proximity to Lake Victoria, many Luo are fishermen (Shipton, 1998).

Homogeneous in language, the Luo are linked by marriage and other kin ties. Their society is well known for large clans and patrilineal descent that extend over generations. Age, wealth, and respect are deeply intertwined such that it is natural for elder men to control family resources and the wealth. Likewise, they control the allocation of the bride wealth cattle, land, and other resources. Elder men receive much public respect; and the land and cattle are inherited patrilineally (although women do most of the farm work).

A third of rural Luo homesteads are polygynous. Patriliny, bride wealth, and polygyny all reinforce each other. Women assume the husband's name and move to his home after marriage. Gender roles are fairly distinct. Women farm and generally keep separate houses, gardens, and storage granaries within the circular homestead or compound of the larger polygynous family (Ocholla-Ayayo, 1980).

Fertility is very important in this society, probably even more for the woman than the man, as reproduction is the value system by which men judge exchanges, be it exchanges of livestock or women. The success of marriages, and wives' social status both depend on their producing children.

In addition, because many cultures, such as the Luo, do not allow women to inherit property, producing large families may be a hedge against homelessness and starvation. Given these social and economic criteria, fertility, family structure (polygyny, levirate or widow inheritance—marriage of a widow by the brother of her deceased husband, and arranged marriages to older men), and cultural beliefs become critical factors for consideration in designing and implementing a health education campaign.

Luo Health Conditions

The Luo people face important health challenges, many of which are influenced by their social structure and practices. Other challenges stem from the environment and lake location to cause seasonal and chronic malnutrition. Common ailments include malaria, marasmus, childhood diarrheal diseases, perinatal gynecological illnesses, schistosomiasis, and in the past two decades, AIDS.

Preliminary research into the social structure of the Luo tribe, our targeted outreach group, and their location (proximity of Lake Victoria), indicated the appearance of a higher incidence in this Kenyan region of persons with HIV (Kenyan Ministry of Health, 1995). In addition, more of them appeared to be succumbing to many of the opportunistic diseases from which persons in the region normally recover - such as malaria, tuberculosis, or typhoid. However, with compromised immune systems, perhaps they were more susceptible to these diseases.

The opportunistic diseases also levied a high toll on children of persons with HIV and AIDS. During several of the home visits, particularly where one parent had died from AIDS-related complications and the other had full-blown AIDS, the children appeared to experience more problems with malaria, diarrhea, malnutrition, and tuberculosis.

It seemed that most of the health conditions of the children were exacerbated by the remote location in the bush, the lack of clean water, and, in some instances, meager or no meals because the sick parent was unable to garden or gather food. In addition, they may have been too far away for neighbors or relatives to be of much assistance.

In spite of all these challenges, Luo continue to address such health problems with a diverse, and flexible combination of Western medicine, religious faith, and traditional healing including witchcraft, herbs, and ritual (Shipton, 1998).

HIV/AIDS Epidemic

According to the U.N. report released at the 12th International AIDS Conference in June (Altman, 1998), countries south of the Sahara account for the world's 21 highest rates of HIV among adults aged 15–49 years. In certain areas of Africa, one in four adults is infected with the virus. The country-by-country analysis of the disease indicates that of the 30 million people infected with HIV, 21 million were in Africa, over 40 percent of whom are women, and most are under the age of 40.

According to the World Health Organization epidemiological reports (1995), Kenya has reported over 75 thousand cases of AIDS since 1986. Prevalence in major urban areas, primarily Nairobi and Mombasa, is over 25 percent among women. In rural areas, HIV prevalence has risen from 1 percent in 1988 to 27 percent in 1995 at many of the 16 surveillance sites. Actual cases of HIV infection and AIDS could actually be much higher than reported given the number of undiagnosed cases.

Other staggering statistics indicate that millions of young African children will be orphaned by the loss of their parents to AIDS, and many of these children will fall victim to opportunistic diseases associated with their compromised immune systems, having contracted the disease at birth from their mothers.

The HIV/AIDS epidemic affects Kenya and other developing countries in many ways. Not only is there loss of life, there are a number of related issues including loss of workers, loss of family support systems, and heightened risk of transmission generated by the increased commercial sexual exploitation of orphans, children, and adults, particularly infected women with no means of economic support. Dr. Peter Piot (1998), head of the United Nations AIDS Program, has done extensive research on transmission of AIDS and sexually transmitted diseases (*http://www.unaids.org,* 1997). He was among the first to document a number of important aspects of the current HIV/AIDS epidemic, such as the existence of AIDS in Central Africa, the heterosexual HIV transmission, the role of sexually transmitted diseases in HIV transmission, the interaction between HIV infection and tuberculosis, and the effect of HIV/AIDS on social and economic development.

Even children who are neither infected with HIV nor orphaned by AIDS are affected by the socioeconomic fallout from the epidemic in hard-hit communities and countries. An AIDSCAP study estimated that, by the year 2005, Kenya's Gross Domestic product (GDP) will be 14.5 percent smaller than it otherwise would have been had AIDS never occurred (*http://www.cdc.gov.nchstp/hiv_aids/stats/hasrlink.htm,* 1997).

Given this setting, any efforts to prevent the spread of the disease require addressing several issues simultaneously. The U.N. AIDS (Altman, 1998) program cited four reasons why the infection rates are so high in Africa:

1. More women of childbearing age are HIV infected in Africa than elsewhere.
2. African women have more children on average than those in other continents. Thus, one infected woman may pass the virus on to a higher average number of children.
3. Nearly all children in Africa are breastfed, which is thought to account for between a third and a half of all HIV transmission from mother to child.
4. New drugs are less readily available than in industrialized world.

Also, other sexually transmitted diseases are known to speed transmission of AIDS and may go untreated in poor countries.

Thus, any disease prevention program must be able to address these issues and offer viable solutions given the cultural and socioeconomic conditions of the country. In addition, given the role and status of women in these societies, solutions must be tailored to meet their needs if health promotion campaigns are to realize any degree of success.

The HIV/AIDS Campaigns

Our HIV/AIDS campaign consisted of a two-pronged approach to disease prevention in rural areas from our base camp at Kendu Bay. Kendu Bay is situated in the hills of the Nyanza Province, on the main road between the city of Kisumu and Lake Victoria. Our group of volunteers were based at Kendu Bay because there is a hospital and large nursing school at the site. Thus, it would be easy to train a larger number of nursing students to be volunteer health care workers for community outreach and training. In addition, because the students came from different tribes, there were more languages from which to select trainers to teach community workers.

The hospital had a few HIV/AIDS patients from whom we could gather additional information about community attitudes and treatment. Further, the location provided opportunities to work with agrarian women, fishermen and young students at a nearby boarding school for boys and a nearby school for children with disabilities. The Luo people became our target group because of their close proximity and because of the social characteristics of the society, which might lead to a higher incidence of HIV/AIDS.

Given these conditions and social issues, our objective was to encourage people to change behavior and beliefs in order to save lives and prevent further transmission of HIV infections and death from illnesses associated with AIDS. The primary objective was to reach a large audience, the plan being to do extensive community outreach in hopes that each informed and properly trained person would spread the word to others. The other component of the health education campaign was to encourage correct and regular usage of properly stored condoms.

A secondary project, family planning, was added to the our campaign platform, because of the similarities of our prevention goals, and because of shared resources with the Family Planning Unit and shared transportation.

To achieve these objectives, the first goal was to educate and train community health workers to work within the villages and local communities to encourage safe sex practices. The second goal was to distribute free condoms and check on the health status of persons infected with HIV or AIDS to help their families cope with the disease while also trying to stop the transmission of the disease to other family members. The third operative or sub-issue with the condom distribution was to encourage family planning.

Given the language differences, we relied rather heavily on the interpreters to translate into DhoLuo and Swahili. Many of them were nursing school students or multilingual members of the community. Social status and protocol dictated that the male team members and interpreters work with male leaders in the community, although women were the primary community health workers.

The timing of workshops and community meetings were also influenced by the economic needs of the community health workers and their work schedules most of the women were busy farming or otherwise caring for their families so they did not have a lot of time to talk about sex.

During the six-week period, the volunteers were engaged in health education activities five days a week and met with over 500 individuals. Most of the activities consisted of conducting workshops and sessions to train community health workers (CHWs) to network with neighbors in their villages and compounds. Literature was distributed and the CHWs were instructed to gather data for record-keeping purposes. Information was to be collected on such items as the number of house calls made, number of condoms dispensed, comments from participants, effectiveness of condom usage and safe sex practices, effectiveness/side effects of contraception, and other relevant issues.

Other projects included assisting the commercial sex workers (CSWs) or prostitutes to encourage their clients to practice safer sex. An unplanned visit for a session on safer sex practices and abstinence was held at a boarding school for young men at the request of the school director. It seems some of the students confessed to visiting local prostitutes when a cache of condoms were found. Despite loud protests of some of the faculty, a condom demonstration session was held and fact tips about HIV transmission and symptoms were warmly received by the young students.

During the course of the campaign, several other issues arose that required agenda modifications. As the health campaign had already been written when the volunteers arrived, there was little room for adjustment. However, interactions with the community suggested there had been little input from the target audience during the planning phase, therefore they were less inclined to buy into the project although their fear of the "hunched-shoulders curse" (the term was used to describe the physical conditions of persons in advanced stages of AIDS) soon outweighed their dissatisfaction with being left out of the planning process.

Another "omission" that soon became apparent was the failure of planners to incorporate tribal beliefs and local custom into the strategy. Many felt that when otherwise healthy persons engaged in normal behavior (marriage, sex within the marriage, and creating a family) become seriously ill from malaria or other common ailments, a spell or bad deed was involved for which the sick person had received a curse. Few would attribute the illness to sexual relations with one's spouse or breastfeeding children.

Finally, while the collaborative learning approach or "each one, reach one" was a good idea, there could have been more insight and local input into the selection of the community health workers expected to do the teaching. The hierarchy within the compounds, and "chief gossips" might have been better vehicles for spreading the word about safe sex. Likewise, some felt uncomfortable talking to strangers about such personal issues as one's sex life.

In spite of the minor glitches, the campaign plan to "promote a healthier life for Kenyans" was adopted. Implemented through the use of health education, family planning, open communication, safe sex practices, and disease prevention, the plan was executed with varying degrees of success.

Health Communication

The form and channels of communicating health issues are important because of the impact they have on listeners and their behavior. Both parties, the teacher and the listener, must be able to communicate and discuss matters openly and have adequate knowledge of the issues to be able to agree upon a plan of action.

The primary goal during our health initiative was to educate and encourage the use of safer sex practices. However, before we could begin to educate the participants, we had to establish open channels of communication whereby individuals would feel free to discuss such personal and sensitive issues as sexual intercourse, or relations with a spouse.

Given the limited time period and the large number of sessions we were trying to convene, trust had to be established quickly and effectively. Our group split into teams of two to three persons and went to different groups almost daily. House calls were needed occasionally to follow up on diagnoses and treatment programs but the bulk of the effort was concentrated on the outreach effort.

Several of our workshops were in mixed groups consisting of both men and women. The meetings with women-only tended to be more productive, thus leading to the thesis that the role of women is critical to the HIV/AIDS prevention. Their discussions tended to generate more realistic and difficult questions perhaps because the patrilineal structure of the society gave them fewer options and less control over their lives. However, visits with the women may have been more open and honest simply because the team consisted of two young African-American females with whom they could relate.

Sessions with mixed groups generally centered around the mechanics of proper storage and usage of the condom. All too frequently male participants would then try to steer the discussion away from safer sex to political arguments about the origin of AIDS and whether the lubricant in the condoms was actually a source of germ warfare used by capitalist countries to annihilate Africans and take control of the large wealth of natural resources.

Instead of trying to curtail these discussions, we used these issues as springboards from which to encourage safer sex so that Kenyans would be healthy and alive to defend the country from the capitalists. We then encouraged them to stay healthy by limiting relationships to as few individuals as possible (in other words, eliminate extramarital affairs), and by getting tested regularly for early detection and treatment.

Communication with the females was more challenging. In the group settings, they usually allowed the males to dominate the conversation while they focused on the mechanics of correct condom storage and usage, massive distribution of the free condoms, and taking advantage of the meeting and the break from work to visit with friends and neighbors.

Workshops with women-only were productive because we were able to address serious issues and listen to their fears and concerns. In most cases, the Luo women were married to men that worked away from the homestead. Many saw their husbands infrequently because of the distance from Nairobi and Mombasa where many of the men worked. Most expressed concerns that their spouses might be interacting with prostitutes in the city, thus exposing the wives to HIV or other sexually transmitted diseases.

Infidelity was not a matter for discussion, especially when the husband was home so infrequently and when there were so many other pressing issues the couple may need to discuss. Besides, if the wife suspected infidelity and attempted to leave, there were few options available - where would she go with no money or skills, and children to feed. There was also Luo societal constraints that strongly discouraged or even prohibited divorce.

Many women indicated that sexuality was not an issue they discussed in marriage. Rather, a wife's duty was to please her husband and be fertile in order to produce many healthy children. Further, if she became troublesome, the husband might also have grounds for physically abusing her and taking on another wife that was more compliant, supportive, and appreciative of his labor (Goody, 1997). In fact, one of the participants was beaten by her husband for attending a session and treated at the hospital.

In spite of these obstacles, our team was able to encourage the women to focus on eating nutritiously and staying healthy so that if they should become infected from spousal infidelity, they might be able to live longer and healthier lives, even with HIV, to care for their children. We also encouraged them to explore more nonphysical intimacy with their spouses in hopes that the men may have less desire to visit prostitutes and may, instead, try to come home more often for sex and intimacy with their wives.

Polygyny and widow inheritance posed additional challenges for our workshop presentations. While widow inheritance is more common in Ghana and West Africa, our hospital cohorts felt some parties were engaged in the practice and encouraged us to address the issue in the sessions. Also, as many of the elder Luo men have multiple young wives, they were less inclined to allow them to attend the workshops for fear we would be corrupting the women. In these instances, we were obliged to rely more on the community workers to communicate with the wives.

Our objective in these situations was to encourage the wives to share information with each other and to attempt to keep the circle of sex partners within the marriage to a minimum. If one wife contracted a sexually transmitted disease, she was encouraged to confer with the other wives in order that they might all be treated and cured.

Levirate or widow inheritance was another critical issue. With this particular social structure, the brothers of the deceased male inherit his wives. If the decedent died of AIDS, and his brother inherited an infected wife, the brother assumes the risk of becoming infected by the new wife and of transmitting the disease to his own wives. There was considerable discussion about the need to use "symbolism" to indicate inheritance. In other words, the safer interpretation of "widow inheritance" might dictate that the brother simply hang his coat in the widow's house to show that he has accepted responsibility for her and the family, rather than have a physical relationship with her. Whether this position gains popularity and acceptance remains to be seen.

By far the most interesting workshop was held with a group of commercial sex workers or prostitutes. Here, the objective was to help them generate ways to convince their customers to use condoms. Lively discussion ranged from using full body massages and foreplay to surreptitiously put a condom on the partner to simple refusal of services for men unwilling to cooperate. However, most of the sessions were devoted to identifying and detecting symptoms, and types of treatment for STDs and HIV.

Another engaging aspect of the communication platform of the campaign was the "buzz outside the hospital and workshops." The hospital staff forewarned us that while our efforts to educate and communicate were admirable, participants in our workshops were more inclined to accept the advice and information of a neighbor or friend with whom she has a close social relationship, particularly if the friend has personal knowledge of the health concern whether it involve family planning, STDs or HIV infection. This position has been supported by other researchers and written with anecdotal evidence presented in an article by Naomi Rutenberg and Susan Watts (1997) entitled, "The Buzz Outside the Clinics: Conversations and Contraception in Nyanza Province, Kenya."

The gist of their research was that if nurses and health care professionals give good information about family planning, why do the women go outside and talk with other women? They surveyed Luo women in villages and community-based distribution programs (CBDs) near Kendu Bay, the site of our workshop, and found that a great deal of social interaction takes place between women in the compounds or as they walk together to the lake or village. The women share information and compare notes, particularly about the side effects or symptoms. The women were also inclined to blame the contraceptives or medical treatment for birth defects or other health problems, irrespective of the true cause of the problem.

Our volunteers had the same experience. For example, we were told most persons with AIDS were "killed" when they came to the hospital, therefore, persons with "the curse" should not go to the hospital because they will surely die. In reality, the patients generally came to the hospital when they had exhausted all home and traditional remedies and died from serious complications of the disease, rather than from any treatment at the hospital.

Our recommendations for coping with the "outside experts" mirrored those of Rutenberg and Watkins. First, for there to be effective communication with the target group and for the program to succeed in promoting behavioral and attitudinal changes, the informal gossip networks needed to be an integral part of the program and structure. In fact, women from these informal social networks should have been co-opted into the planning process and the program, and encouraged to become the community health workers.

Second, the concerns of the women about the cultural and moral issues, or the side effects of family planning and repercussions from family members opposed to protected sex practices were quite valid. These issues should have been fundamental to open communication to help the program planners find solutions to the HIV transmission crisis.

Health Promotion

There are cultural taboos, moral matters regarding infidelity, economic variables, and other issues to consider when promoting condom use and open discussion with sexual partners about safe sex. In addition to literature and condom distribution, we found a combination of short lectures, group discussion with assigned questions, role-playing, and demonstrations to be most effective. Games and prizes also heightened their interest and increased participation. Likewise, a short series of two to three sessions were better than all-day workshops that were too time consuming for most attendees. Use of visual aids - placards, dildos for practice with condoms were equally well received.

An introduction with a few statistics and an overview of what was to be covered in the workshop was followed by the distribution of blank sheets of paper upon which attendees could take notes and write down questions. Everyone was instructed to write down one or more questions about HIV/AIDS for general discussion at the end of the session. The primary reason for requiring questions from everyone was to prevent embarrassment, especially if only one or two persons had questions.

Following the overview, a short lecture was used to present the facts about HIV and AIDS. The facts were covered in broad generalities to make certain everyone understood the vocabulary and primary issues:

- Terminology and key words
- Transmission of HIV/AIDS and STDs
- Symptoms
- Prevention and Treatment

Handouts and fact sheets were distributed so attendees could follow the lecture and use them in the exercises.

The next segment of the workshop was the scripted "Question and Answer" team approach to reinforce the lecture. Depending on the size of the group, teams of two to four participants were paired off to analyze questions and respond to situations. Scripts varied according to the audience. After each script or question, a brief discussion ensued to consider how the situation might be "improved" or handled differently to guarantee the safety or minimize the risk of infection for the participants, particularly for the prostitutes or women with unfaithful spouses.

Games and prizes were warmly received and made participants more responsive and enthusiastic. The game approach was good because the instructor could ask hard questions in the form of hypothetical to make everyone feel at ease with the discussion. For example, in one game the women were paired off and given three cards saying "no risk, low risk, high risk." The instructor then read or showed placards about various types of sexual behavior. Each duet discussed the issue then raised a card identifying the risk factor. After all cards were raised, the correct answer was given along with an explanation as to why or how the risk was assessed. The top three pairs of women getting the highest number of correct responses won prizes.

In addition to lectures and games, it was important to make certain participants knew how to correctly use condoms for disease prevention. To break the ice and engage participants, the instructor put on a condom-rolling it down to the elbow and saying–"if any man tells you a condom is 'too small for him,' do what I have just done. For indeed, if his penis is longer than the length of your forearm, you probably need to avoid him anyhow." Following embarrass laughter, they paid close attention to the next segment of the workshop - condom demonstration. Dildos were used to make certain condoms were being used correctly.

Other classes were held to discuss the care and treatment, and social issues such as stigma, ignorance, and fear, related to living with persons who have HIV infection and AIDS. Again, to keep communications open and to minimize embarrassment, emphasis was placed on promoting proper nutrition and healthy environments rather than on individual cases. Fact sheets on "low risk" interaction with AIDS persons were distributed. They listed activities, such as hugging and massaging the body as ways of comforting the patient and minimizing exposure. Lists of nutritious foods to combat malnutrition and diarrhea; and reminders about sterilizing water, shared utensils; and general good hygiene were also promoted. Combating myths about curses was challenging but the informed team found ways to encourage early testing so that persons could make certain the illness was a "treatable" curse.

Disease Prevention

The third segment of the health education campaign focused on disease prevention. The primary way to prevent transmitting HIV and other sexually transmitted diseases is through education and the promotion of safer sex practices. Dissemination of current information is needed to keep health care professionals abreast of new treatments and therapy for HIV/AIDS. While there is a growing number of websites *(http://*

www.nih.gov; http://ww.unaids/document/epidemio/june98/factpercent 5Fsheets/pdfs/Kenya.pdf) and publications available with information and statistics on AIDS in the international arena, our remote site lacked access to such technology. However, when team members went to Nairobi on business, we gathered current data and information to share with hospital staff and health educators. Collaboration with regional hospitals and clinics and other social service agencies was another important component of a successful disease prevention effort in Kenya and other African countries (Brooten, et al., 1997).

On the local site in Kendu Bay, most emphasis was placed on promoting proper nutrition and sanitation as part of general good health practices. While there was limited access to drugs and medication at the local hospital, few women could afford the drugs or had time to leave their families for hospitalization.

Breastfeeding and pregnancy posed other challenging dilemmas. The social culture encourages large families and breastfeeding - two ways HIV can be spread to children. In fact, in most developing countries, almost one-half of all HIV infections in young children are acquired through breast milk (U.N. AIDS, 1998). To compound matters, many HIV-positive women in Kenya have no idea they are infected. Therefore they do not receive treatment during pregnancy that might prevent HIV transmission to the fetus.

Further, the stigma attached to HIV, similar to Ebola, may cause friends and family to avoid the victim. So many women who know or may suspect they are HIV-positive prefer to behave normally to avoid being ostracized.

In spite of the costs of treatment and the need for more testing and early detection, emphasis on disease prevention would definitely be a worthwhile investment as social costs to Kenya and its Gross Domestic Product are high.

Conclusion

This effort by volunteers was short in duration and plagued with a host of unanticipated challenges. However, the end results were that hundreds of people in the province were trained and/or presented with HIV/AIDS information, and that hundreds of condoms, fact sheets, and literature were distributed. Whether there will be behavioral and attitudinal changes in the Luo people toward health promotion, education and disease prevention will require follow-up studies and further investigation.

The HIV/AIDS program under which the volunteers were working has since lost its funding, but preliminary results indicate more people in the rural areas have knowledge about HIV/AIDS including transmission, symptoms, and prevention. Changes in the social and cultural structure of Luo society, particularly polygyny and levirate, may also need to be addressed if disease prevention efforts are to be successful. Likewise, power as determined by gender in relationships will need to be incorporated into health campaigns in developing countries such as Africa (Mafethe, 1995). When health initiatives promote condom usage within marriages, health care professionals need to be cognizant of the options - such as beatings or other adverse consequences for women. Finally, with increased global travel and migration, there needs to be considerably more research and resource sharing among developed and developing countries if diseases are to prevented.

References

Altman, L. (1998). Parts of Africa showing HIV in 1 in 4 Adults. *New York Times*. Retrieved June 24, 1998 from *http://www.nih.gov/od/98nihplan.pdf*, FY 1998 NIH Plan for HIV-Related Research.

Brooten, D., Thompson, J., Makoza, J., Kaponda, C., Mede, E., Kachapila, L., & Phoya, A. (1997). Collaborating for international research development in Malawi, Africa. *Image: Journal of Nursing Scholarship*, 29(4), 369-373.

Center for Disease Control: HIV/AIDS Prevention Division. *www.cdc.gov/nchstp/hiv_aids/*

Downing, T (1997). Kenya. In *Encyclopedia of Africa South of the Sahara*, Vol. 2, pp. 425-429. New York: Simon and Schuster Macmillan.

Goody, J. (1997). Kinship and Marriage. In *Encyclopedia of Africa South of the Sahara*, Vol.2, pp. 456-465. New York: Simon and Schuster Macmillan.

HIV/AIDS Surveillance Report. (1998). *http://www.cdc.gov/nchstp/ hiv_aids/stats/hasrlink.htm.*

HIV/AIDS Publications. (1998). *http://www.cdc.gov/nchstp/ hiv_aids/pubs.htm.*

Kenya. (1995). *Worldmark: Encyclopedia of the Nations*. (8th ed.). pp. 197-208. New York: Gale Research, Inc.

Lagarde, E., Pison, G. & Enel, C. (1997). Improvement in AIDS knowledge, perceptions and risk behaviors over a short period in a rural community in Senegal. *International Journal of STDs and AIDS*, 8(11), 681-7.

Mafethe, I. (1995). Africa: Perspectives on gender, culture and power in community health. *Nursing and Health Care: Perspectives on Community*, 16(4), 217-220.

Middleton, J. (1997). Kenya: Peoples and cultures. In *Encyclopedia of Africa South of the Sahara*, Vol. 2, pp. 432-435. New York: Simon and Schuster

Macmillan.

Middleton, J. & Rassam, A. (1991). Marriage. In *Encyclopedia of World Cultures: Africa and the Middle East*, Vol. IX, pp. xxx-xxxi, Boston, MA: G.K. Hall & Co. Macmillan.

National Council for Population and Development (NCPD), Central Bureau of Statistics (CBS) (Office of the Vice President and Ministry for Planning and Development [Kenya]), and Macro International (MI). (1994). *Kenya demographic and health survey, 1993*. Calverton, MD: NCPD, CBS, and MI.

Ocholla-Ayayo, A. (1980). *The Luo culture: A reconstruction of a traditional African Society*. Wiesbaden: Steiner.

Rutenberg, N. & Watkins, S. (1997). Conversations and contraception in Kenya. *Studies in Family Planning*, 28 (4), 290-307.

Shipton, P. (1989). Bitter money: Cultural economy and some African meaning of forbidden commodities. *American Ethnological Society Monograph Series*, No. 1, Washington, D.C.

Shipton, P. (1997). Luo. In *Encyclopedia of Africa South of the Sahara*, Vol. 3, pp. 63-65. New York: Simon and Schuster Macmillan.

Turner, B. (Ed.) (1998). *Statesmen's yearbook*. New York: St. Martin's Press.

UNAIDS/WHO Working Group on Global HIV/AIDS and STD Surveillance. (1998). *http://www.unaids.org/unaids/document/*.

World Health Organization. (1998). *Kenya: Epidemiological fact sheet on HIV/AIDS and sexually transmitted diseases*. Geneva: United Nations AIDS.

Chapter 9

Traditional Medicine and Biopsychosocial Fulfillment in African Health

E. S. Ataudo
University of Calabar, Nigeria

Every society has its own method of managing illness and of controlling its environment. Illness management is a process that evolves from generation to generation. The technique of healing has been with human societies from time immemorial and has formed a network of social structure and social relationships. Each society functions within the constraint of its own unique system of social structure, language and communication, belief and customs, attitude, behavior and 'cultural facts'. These taken together form the 'social web'–a binding force, of any society. Thus, each society is unique. Traditional medicine is an established part of culture; and in African societies, traditional medicine remains the major way of coping with illness, especially in rural communities where modern medical services are inaccessible.[1–4] "It seems paradoxical that at a time when modern scientific medicine appears to be making such giant strides and enjoying unparalleled prestige, so much interest should be taken in traditional medicine, in both developed and developing countries alike."[4]

The long affinity of traditional medical practices is identified with African 'cultural fuels' (such as ways of behavior, belief system, customs, attitudes, values). My thesis is that as a society would not negotiate its sociocultural imperatives for a borrowed culture or rid itself of the traditional culture in the present age of cultural revival, it becomes imperative for society to contain its major 'cultural idioms' such as traditional medicine.

Traditional societies regard health as a state of balance or equilibrium, both internal and external, and they believe in the efficacy of traditional medicine to achieve this balance.[4] This encompasses the physical, mental, social, moral and spiritual well-being of an individual. It means, therefore, that traditional medicine is in the domain of 'biopsychosocial health' because it treats the whole person. The concept of biopsychosocial health reflects the definition of health by the World Health Organization which states the "health is a state of complete physical, mental and social well-being and not merely the absence of disease or infirmity."[5]

A healthy body is a healthy mind and lives in, and enjoys the comfort of, a healthy social environment. "In our concept of biopsychosocial health, as a component of biosocial development, we believe that health care is not a matter solely to be evaluated by physicians alone, but as good health concerns all in society, laymen, as well as physicians, each person is better to be taught to conserve his own health (self-health) as a fundamental direction of biopsychosocial care."[6] However, the question that often comes to mind is whether or not traditional African medicine promotes or encourages biopsychosocial fulfillment? To attempt a brief answer it is necessary to define the concept of traditional medicine, and of modern medicine, and to show the extent to which traditional medicine promotes the biopsychosocial fulfillment in African societies. This chapter defines biopsychosocial health and briefly discusses its relationship with traditional medicine. Here, 'traditional medicine' is used inter-changeably with 'native African medicine'.

The Meaning of Traditional Medicine

Traditional medicine is the medicine of the people by the people and for the people that has been practiced and handed down from generation to generation. It is the 'first contact medicine'. This practice reflects the sociocultural imperatives of the people who practice it (culture, customs, belief, behavior, economic system, political system, etc.). Different authors have different meanings for traditional medicine. Some of these are: traditional medicine refers to those beliefs and practices founded in tradition and which are generally accepted uncritically by the people. Such practices are continued from one generation to another largely because "things have always been done this way" and because the people have faith in the effectiveness of the beliefs. These beliefs and practices are often associated with the supernatural which lends a moral credence, or more strongly, a moral imperative to their appropriateness.[7, 8]

Traditional systems of medical care in Africa reflect the perceived taxonomy of disease causation.[9] Traditional medicine is regarded in the rural communities as an alternative to Primary Health Care.[7, 10, 11] Traditional medicine is regarded by patients who have faith in its healing power as a 'psychological opium that helps to alleviate pain and suffering by recreating a sense of belongingness and awareness of self in the midst of fear and death. In this way the sufferer has regained his/her sense of touch with realities in the brotherhood of relatives and friends, traditional medical doctors, and the community at large who are wholeheartedly involved in life-and-death crusade. Here a biopsychosocial situation is involved in which the biophysiological, the spiritual and the social vacuum created by the ailment is consciously taken care of by these 'life-crusaders'. Traditional medicine is a form of domestic health care, based on general medical knowledge, and practiced within the family. This includes the area of self-treatment. It is also known as folk medicine or indigenous medicine. Traditional medicine represents a structured system of ordering, classifying, and explaining illnesses, comprising equally elaborated concepts of treatment.[11] Traditional African medicine is the totality of all knowledge and practices, whether explicable or not, used in diagnosing preventing or eliminating a physical, mental or social disequilibrium and which rely exclusively on past experience and observation handed down from generation to generation, verbally or in writing.[7] The importance of traditional medicine in African societies cannot be over-emphasized. This is because it is to the traditional healers that the great majority of the people of the developing countries turn in times of sickness. For 80 percent of the population 'primary health care' is synonymous with traditional medicine. For this reason alone, it is essential for health professionals to be fully aware of the work of these traditional practitioners and of their place in society.[1, 7-9] For centuries, the peoples of Africa, like those of other continents, speculated on the enigma of life and death. Most tribes and kingdoms failed to see any reason why life should not last eternally. They accordingly made use of practices thought likely to perpetuate the individual's life. These practices have now become an integral part of their cultural heritage. There is no break of continuity between the world of the living and the world of the dead. Ancestors live on in their descendants and act on their lives, and certain religious faiths entertain the idea of communication between the two worlds.[7] This, in essence, is the concept of traditional medicine in African health.

Biopsychosocial Health

Biopsychosocial health, as its name implies, views the health of any population in its physical, mental and social environment. "Increasingly over several years, in the matter of health care, it has become clear that quality of life is more and more a function of the biosocial development of the society. Good health is a function of good health communication, and good health is not only good clinical health but also good social health."[12] And again, the concept of biopsychosocial health, as a component of biosocial development, "health care is not a matter solely to be evaluated by physicians, but as good health concerns all in society, laymen as well as physicians, each person is better to be taught to conserve his own health, (self health), as a fundamental direction of biopsychosocial care."[13] "We ought to remember however that fundamental medicine has always been biopsychosocial. Evidence for this is forthcoming in the Vedas and Upanishads of ancient India, in the psychology of the shaman, in the metaphysic of the hakim, and in the expression of contemporary healers. Including modern sophisticated medicine, all such concepts in effect integrate good health from cultural, social, biologic and economic perspectives."[14] Thus we see biopsychosocial health is viewed in the context of the definition of health by the World Health Organization (WHO), health as "a state of complete physical, mental, and social well-being and not merely the absence of disease or infirmity."[5] The relationship of this definition with the concept and practice of traditional medicine together with the concept of biopsychosocial health is illustrated in Figure 9.1.

Characteristics and Philosophy of Traditional Medicine Which Have Made It a Socio-Cultural Force in the Treatment of Ailments

It should be noted that traditional health care delivery is inter-twined with the Nigerian sociocultural models and any attempt by the social system to disengage it, will cause a dysfunctioning effect. This is because traditional medicine has formed a part of the people's way of life as far as coping with any ailment is concerned. It is part of the socio-religious structure of indigenous societies. Values, attitudes, behavior, beliefs in

Figure 9.1: *The Relationship Between Biopsychosocial Health, WHO Concept of Health and the Practice of Traditional Medicine*

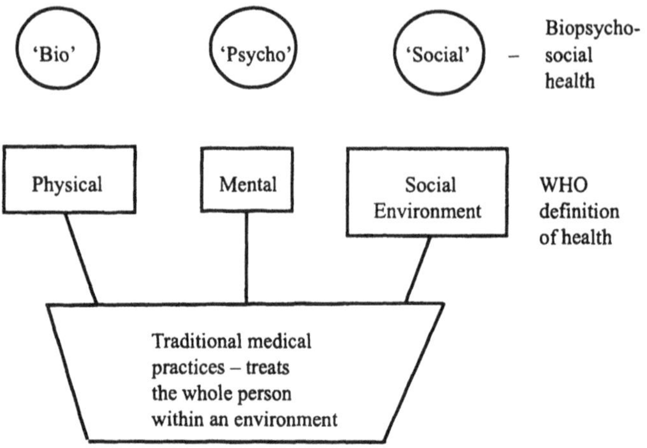

respect of health and illness were developed within these socio-religious and cultural foundations. The role of traditional medicine can also be seen on occasions when the traditional doctors would use musipsycho-sound and pleasing voice, with or without moaning or chanting, or the use of imagery as a form of meditation to get a positive or desired result, or the call-and-response form of interaction between the traditional doctors and their clients where the clients or their families talk back to the doctors during a healing episode.[15] The power of traditional medicine can also be seen in its 'placebo effect' where the client's faith in the healing art of the traditional doctor induces him/her to believe that whatever the traditional doctor does to counteract the evil plans of the enemy or of the spirits or the offended ancestor will surely work. A case in point is the result of a psychiatric treatment of a foreign student in London by Lambo. The student had believed that his rivals had invoked some evil powers to worry him. As a result of this, his dead father appeared to him several times in the dream and wanted him to make some sacrifices to him in order that all those things might go away from him. Simple advice brought the student back to normal mental state.[16] As part of African philosophy the traditional doctor represents the interpreter of the unknown, the supernatural of wrong, and the one individual who cares and who is involved in the problems of his/her clients, and who teaches his clients to believe in the one 'Supreme Being' who Controls heaven and earth.[17] There are many other characteristics and philosophy of traditional medicine not mentioned here because of time and space, However, those mentioned above appeal to the patients' 'biopsychosocial touch' and milieu which in turn treats the 'whole person' and helps to bring about the fulfillment of biopsychosocial needs in African Health. There are a number of reasons for the persistence of traditional medical practices in Africa in general and in Nigeria in particular, among which are Traditional Medical practices built from simple home remedies with which the people are familiar to what they have learned during the process of their socialization into their respective societies; it serves as a basis for primary health care, especially to those who have no access to modern medical services, thus, it fills a health vacuum; it is part of a larger culture of the society, it has been practiced from generation to generation; it has been internationally recognized by the World Health Organization (WHO); it exists side by side with modern medical systems; traditional doctors play important roles in the management of the patient, and contact between the patient and the traditional doctor is much closer than between the patient and the modern medical doctors. The traditional doctor is a down-to-earth-doctor and "is a far better *health communicator* than his sophisticated technologically educated medical brother."[13]

It can reasonably be concluded from the above discussions that traditional medicine promotes the fulfillment of biopsychosocial needs in West African health.

Endnotes

[1]Bannerman, R. N. Traditional medicine in modern health care.
3, 8–26, 1983.

[2]Pifferling, J. H. Some issues in the consideration of non-western and western folk practices as epidemiologic data. *Social Science & Medicine*, 9, 655–658, 1975.

[3]Bonsi, S. I. Traditional medicine in modern Ghana. Unpublished Ph.D. dissertation, University of Missouri, Columbia, 1973.

[4]World Health Organization (WHO). Health manpower development: Training and utilization of traditional healers and their collaboration with health care delivery system. Unpublished WHO document No. EB 57/2:Add. 2, WHO, Geneva, 1975, p. 4.

[5]World Health Organization. The constitution of the world. *World Health Or-*

ganization Chronicle 1, 29, 1947.

[6]Day, S. B. *Health Communications,* p. v. The International Foundation for Biopsychosocial Development and Human Health, New York, 1978.

[7]Ampofo, O., & Johnson, Romauld, F. O. Traditional medicine and its role in the development of health services in Africa. WHO Africa Technical Papers No. 12 (37-63), Regional Office Africa (Afro), Brazzaville, 1978.

[8]Bhatia, I. C. *et al.* Traditional healer and modern medicine, *Social Science & Medicine* 9, 15–21, 1975.

[9]Bichman, W. Primary health care and traditional medicine: Considering the background of changing health care concepts in Africa. *Social Science & Medicine.* 13B, 175–182, 1979. Imperato, P. J. *African Folk Medicine: Practices and Beliefs of the Bambara and Other Peoples,* p. 54. York Press, Baltimore, 1977.

[10]Ampofo, O. Health manpower development: Training, and utilization of traditional healers and their collaboration with health care delivery system. In *Sociology and Medicine* (Edited by Coe, R. M.). McGraw–Hill, New York, 1970.

[11]Zeller, D. Traditional and Western medicine in Buganda: Coexistence and complement. *Rural Africa* 26, 91–103, 1975.

[12]Day, S. B. Editorial. *Biopsychosocial Health,* Vol. 3. Foundation One, The International Foundation for Biosocial Development and Human Health. The American Biopsychosocial Health Association, 1981.

[13]Day, S. B. *Nigeria 2000: The Biopsychosocial Way.* Calabar, 1982.

[14]Day, S. B. *Biopsychosocial Health.* A Monograph Publication in Health Communications and Biopsychosocial Health. Biosocial Development and Human Health, New York, 1980.

[15]Staples, R. *Introduction* to *Black Sociology,* pp. 150–180. McGraw-Hill, New York, 1976.

[16]Lambo, T. A. *African Traditional Belief: Concept of Health and Medical Practice.* Ibadan University Press, Ibadan, 1963.

[17]Mbiti, J. S. *African Religions and Philosophy.* Morrison & Gibb, London, 1980.

Chapter 10

Psychology and Health in Africa

Bernice N. Ezeilo
University of Nigeria, Nsukka, Nigeria

Any health care program aims to alleviate the sufferings of its clients and restore this client as a holistic entity to a state of health that enables the client to function at an optimum level. The health care programs in Africa have for long focused attention on health problems as caused by environmental factors and pathogenic organisms. A great deal of diseases are labeled idiopathic or of unknown origin. Some of these idiopathic conditions may be psychogenic as implied in the several publications relating psychological variables to physiopathology.[1] The experience of the present author[2] and other practicing Nigerian clinical psychologists suggest that Nigerian clients with idiopathic conditions readily respond to psychological intervention.

There is a worldwide recognition of the fact that much human organic pathology contains significant psychological origins and correlates, and have psychological consequences. Besides, over 60 percent of persons reporting physical ailments have mostly psychological problems. For example, Ezeilo's study at Enugu[3], Nigeria showed that 65.15 percent of undergraduate out-patients showed no organic pathology following medical and laboratory examinations, but reported symptoms of psychological distress on a Symptoms Inventory.

This implies that the people who sought medical attention would benefit from psychotherapeutic rather than chemotherapeutic attention. The current increase in the rate at which patients leave the hospital system and seek help from prayer houses, religious 'healers' and traditional healers for their health problems, which had not been dealt with within the health care delivery system, suggested that something is missing in this system. Some patients patronize traditional and religious healers while undergoing medical treatment.[4]

Clinical psychological experience in Nigeria suggests that many of those patients who patronize these healers often become worse before coming to the attention of the psychologist, but recover following psychotherapeutic intervention. There is clearly a need for full integration of psychological services into the health care delivery system in order to enhance patient care. This may avert the exodus of patients from this system in search of the services of those who may further destroy them physically and emotionally. Such an integration has already been effected in the United States of America, Britain, Europe, and also Cuba where public health psychology forms part of the public health programme.[5]

To emphasize the relevance of psychology to health, special journal issues[1, 6–10] have been devoted to works relating psychology to health issues in developed and developing countries. The book edited by Dasen *et al.*[7] emanated from two workshops sponsored by the World Health Organization (WHO) which examined the application of cross-cultural psychology to health care delivery. As far back as the early 1970s, the WHO had recognized the importance of behavior in health work.[7] Many African countries are yet to integrate psychological services into their health care programmes at the primary, secondary and tertiary levels.
ntries are yet to integrate psychological services into their health care programmes at the primary, secondary and tertiary levels.

The Nigerian Experience

For a decade now Nigerian psychologists have been advocating the inclusion of psychological services in health care programmes. Uzoka and colleagues[11] evaluated the need for the discipline of psychology to be encouraged to play its role in various areas including health care delivery. They proposed firstly, that national policy makers must recognize the growing international advocacy for both preventive and curative programs "which include proper nutrition, proper water supply, proper environments (social and physical) and the availability of good health care facilities" (p. 7). These authors then urged that "psychology must insist on a broad appraisal of its functions which encompass the whole range of health care whether psychiatric or otherwise". It was emphasized that even in general hospitals, psychologists have a role to play in patient appraisal, interviewing and counseling. In respect of psychiatric care, the authors advocated the immediate decentralization of the psychiatric hospitals so as to ensure that our people receive attention closer to their homes; and that staffing of the proposed centers should involve a team concept in which psychiatrists, clinical psychologists and psychiatric social workers/nurses as well as traditional healers would participate in the healing process. A further advocacy by the authors was for a comprehensive health insurance program and the development of viable day care centers. The authors finally argued that "psychologists should be seen as collaborating professionals in the training of medical and paramedical personnel" (p. 8), and should be properly represented on the training staff of medical schools, nursing schools and psychiatric establishments. Other Nigerian psychologists and medical doctors have also contributed to the issue of psychology and health through their empirical studies, keynote lectures and theoretical papers. Some of the areas addressed include psychological correlates of health problems, symptom presentation, psychological treatment and the role of changing culture and lifestyles.

Some Psychological Correlates of Health Problems in Nigeria

One variable studied by Nigerian psychologists is the self concept.[12–15] Using various self concept measures, these workers found negative and low self concepts to be related to sickle cell disease[12], various organic illnesses in an out-patient sample[14], and some psychiatric diagnoses.[15]

Johnson and Dada[16] conducted an attitudinal survey, in Lagos, of psychological reactions to cancer, using both cancer patients and "normal" individuals. They found the cancer patients significantly more angry, depressed and frightened than normal subjects. Onwuzurike[17] found need satisfaction to be related to beer drinking among a sample of Nigerian university students, while Shindi[18] draws attention to the role of meaninglessness in the aetiology of neurosis in a rapidly changing African society like Nigeria. Ezeilo[19] compared fertile and infertile literate Igbo women using scores from Beck's Depression Inventory (BDI), an alienation scale and Rotter Locus of Control scale. The infertile women were found to feel more depressed and alienated than the fertile women. Both groups were equally externally oriented. This confirms clinical observations that important correlates of infertility in the Nigerian woman include depression and feeling of alienation.

Symptom Presentation

Various researchers have shown that African clients tend to present psychological distress through somatic symptoms.[3, 20–24] These symptoms like heat in the body, body pains, insomnia, crawling sensations all over the body show no organic basis. Known psychosomatic symptoms with obvious organic concomitant like hypertension, asthma, peptic ulcers sometimes reach the attention of the clinical psychologists, but their psychogenic factors are yet to be empirically documented.

Psychological Therapies

Nigerian clinical psychologists are involved in treatment in the general and psychiatric hospitals, psychological clinics attached to departments of psychology, and in their private practice. There are then a few reports on therapy using mostly models developed in Western countries which are sometimes modified to suit the peculiar needs of the individual client. Ezeilo[19, 25] described the treatment of stuttering and functional infertility respectively, using an eclectic approach that incorporated procedures tailored to the clients' needs. The management package for stuttering, for example, include detailed clinical interviews and assessment to determine the aetiological factors and encourage carthasis. In the course of this, Azrin and Nunn's[26] habit reversal procedure was introduced, followed by a stress management training program. The management of functional infertility follow the same pattern but clinical assessment precedes appropriate behavioral techniques (e.g. progressive relaxation and assertive training) and marital and sex therapy. Success is determined by reduction in frequency and eventual elimination of stuttering, and conception following treatment of the infertility.

Awa[27] reported the use of hypnobehavioral techniques as an adjunct to drugs in the treatment of essential hypertension. Nigerian clients also respond to the use of psychological treatment techniques in the management of functional impotence[28], brain fag syndrome[29], enuresis[30], psychosomatic symptoms in a couple.[31] The techniques, mainly behavioral, include relaxation procedures, assertive training, biofeedback[32], and conjoint marital therapy.

The effect of hospitalization is not left out. Omoluabi[33] studied the effect of long term hospitalization on cognitive and affective functioning of orthopaedic patients and found this to be adverse.

Cultural Changes, Changing Lifestyle and Health

Some Nigerian workers have drawn attention to the changing disease patterns following changing behavior patterns of the "modern" Nigerian. In his review of stress and illness research. Nweze[34] discuss the "big man" diseases like stroke, hypertension and in fact sudden death now on the increase in Nigeria. He suggested that these might result from the stressful effects of social and cultural changes which "are far more exceedine the coping and adjustment resources of average Nigerians". He reported that 30 percent of obituaries in newspapers are in the 30–65 age group, being people who occupied high positions in society who died suddenly.

Following a comprehensive literature review, Oshuntokun[35] observed the epidemiological transition taking place in developing countries with increasing frequency of non-communicable diseases associated with economic development, industrialization and psychosocial maladaptation. His paper dealt with hypertension, coronary artery diseases, diabetes mellitus, obesity, cerebrovascular accidents, some types of cancer, dental caries, traffic accidents and violence, multiple sclerosis, Alzheimer disease, epilepsy and other neuropsychiatric diseases. He drew attention to the increasing incidence of these diseases in African countries among both urban and rural dwellers. He also drew attention to the importance of changing lifestyles and behaviour patterns in the aetiology and maintenance of these diseases.

The Nigerian experience has highlighted the fact that the health status of the Nigerian today, in fact the African, depends to a great extent on psychological variables. The behavior of the African may determine his or her health status. Recognition of this fact has led Nigerian clinical psychologists and medical doctors to advocate for some time now the incorporation of psychological services into the health care delivery system.

When Dean of Faculty of Medicine at the University of Nigeria Teaching Hospital, Enugu Nwokolo[36] included a one year compulsory course in general psychology in the curriculum of premedical students in that institution. When he left the issue lapsed.

In 1988, he reiterated the call to include behavoural sciences in the medical curriculum.[37] In evaluating the role of psychology in personal and national survival Onuigbo[38] advocated the exposure of medical students and nurses to psychological knowledge with a view to enhancing the way doctors and trained nurses relate to patients. He also examined the contributions of psychology in different facets of medical care and urged the Nigerian Psychological Association to work towards making such contributions in the Nigerian context. Enekwechi[39] in the same vein, after reviewing the work on the integration of psychology and medicine in developed countries argued for the need for Nigerian authorities to incorporate the skills and services of clinical psychologists into the health care scheme to improve the welfare of the Nigerian patient.

After reviewing the areas of health care delivery in which the clinical psychologist can contribute to patient management, Ezeilo[40] recommended that a full department of clinical psychology be established at the onset of a new Nigerian college of Medicine, with particular reference to the new Anambra State University of Technology College of Medicine at Nnewi. These envisaged areas of contribution will be examined shortly.

The Present State of Affairs

The positive responses of the Nigerian authorities have been most encouraging. Following these calls, the Nigerian Association of Clinical Psychologists initiated some dialogue with the Minister of Health in 1986. In 1989 a Nigerian clinical psychologist - Professor A. F. Uzoka - was included in the committee to develop a mental health policy for the country. The committee's report included a recommendation for full integration of psychological services in the mental health program.[41] Some state governments in Nigeria have recently advertized for clinical psychologists to be recruited to work in the general hospital.

The new University Teaching Hospital of Anambra State University of Technology has incorporated from the onset a plan for full department of clinical psychology with out-patient facilities, consulting rooms and a 10-bed ward for in-patient behavior therapy. Provision is made in this department for clinical psychologists, a psychological technician and administrative staff.[2]

It is encouraging to note that some state ministries of health have started recruiting clinical psychologists for their general hospitals and health centers (Anambra State Civil Service Commission, January 1990).

Contributions of Psychology to Health-Care in Africa

What contributions can psychologists make in promoting the health of the African? About a decade of clinical psychological experience with Nigerian clients – males and females, children, youths and adults, literate and non literate, from urban and rural communities – has convinced me that the health status of the African will be greatly enhanced if psychological services are incorporated into all facets of health care delivery system.

The role of the psychologist in health care in Africa, like hisher counterpart elsewhere, should include service to the patient and the community at large. the teaching of medical personnel, supervision and training of some specialists and finally research. These will now be further examined.

Service to Patients

Long close contact with patients both within the hospital setting as a registered nurse, and nurse tutor; and outside it as a clinical psychologist, has left me in no doubt that there is no clinical department in the health care system in Africa that does not benefit from the services provided by clinical psychologists for enhanced patient management.

Medicine

Many medical problems are either psychosomatic in nature; or have psychological consequences which may influence the rate of recovery.

Psychosomatic illness are organic pathologies known to result from continuously high autonomic arousal due to prolonged stress. These include for example hypertension peptic ulcer, asthma and others.[35] It is sometimes stated that all non-pathogenic organic pathologies are psychosomatic. The African is not immune to such diseases. It is our belief that psychosomatic illnesses cannot be effectively treated without psychological intervention.

In Nigeria many patients, communicate their psychological distress through somatic complaints like internal heat, pain all over the body and "oria ime ahu" that is "ailments deep in the body". These symptoms do not respond to drug treatment but readily subside with psychological therapy.

Sick role inclination and health seeking behavior are important psychological variables which determine the course and outcome of medical intervention. The necessity for medical attention and hospitalization does have negative psychosocial consequences which may be related to relapse leading to readmission or the patient seeking other sources of help. The conscious terminal patient also benefits from psychological attention in terms of helping him/her better cope with impending death.

Surgery

Some of the issues raised above also apply to the surgical patient, namely: psychosomatic problems, sick role inclination and health seeking behaviour and the effect of hospitalization.

Surgical conditions are associated not only with physical trauma but with such emotional trauma may influence the recovery process. Pre-operative anxiety is a common feature owing to fear of anaesthesia, and fear of surgery itself. Sometimes doctors and nurses talk of reassuring the patient or prescribing anxiolytic drugs. Mere reassurance, especially if attempted by an unskilled person, may not reduce anxiety. The effect of anxiolytic drugs are usually transient, and temporary. Pre-operative psychological intervention may greatly facilitate the patient's response to surgical procedures.[42]

Paediatrics

Several problems of childhood, e.g. enuresis, stuttering, epilepsy, asthma and non-organic mental retardation are known to be related to pathogenic family relationships, which the clinical psychologist deals with in marital and family therapy. Even nutritional disorders, non-compliance with drugs and many other paediatric problems related to economic hardship may result, for example, from the inability of the alcoholic breadwinner to provide the money for proper feeding, purchase of drugs and general maintenance of the child. The behavioral management of mental retardation, whether organic or not, is within the domain of clinical psychology. It is our conviction that the management of every paediatric problem must incorporate psychological treatment either of the child or the family.

Obstetric and Gynaecology

A look at the aetiology and correlates of many obstetric and gynaecological problems do reveal the presence of psychological factors. Such problems include infertility, sexual dysfunctions, repeated abortions and preeclampsia. Fortunately such patients do benefit from psychotherapeutic intervention.[2] Besides, psychoprophylactic procedures enable women to go through pregnancy and labor without much pain.

Psychiatry

There is no psychiatric condition that has no psychological base or consequence. Clinical psychologists have long been associated with psychiatric departments and hospitals in Nigeria but their services are yet to be fully utilized in many cases. We believe that clinical psychological intervention must be an adjunct to drug or electro-shock therapy to increase cure rate and reduce relapse. Absence of such an intervention in the psychiatric setting has greatly contributed to patients patronizing the prayer houses and religious crusaders instead of the health system.

Community Medicine

Psychological services are of even greater relevance in the primary health care program. Every illness originates in the community. Illness may be due to ignorance of health promoting behaviors, e.g. essential hypertension may result from faulty stress coping behaviors, or to faulty beliefs – cows urine poisoning following treatment of convulsion with concoctions containing cows urine; another due to superstition when several school children at Enugu were wounded and some died following the belief that mermaids had visited the school, or the anxiety that grip some "religious" persons who believe that the demon is actively visiting homes and destroying them.

Knowledge of psychological factors in the aetiologies of both physical illness and psychopathologies enables the health psychologist to plan preventive programs for the community he/she covers. With the presence of health psychologists at health centers and polyclinics, many illnesses can be nipped in the bud through early detection and treatment, and by psychoeducational programs. Such programs include teaching the community healthy attitudes, beliefs, behaviors and prevention of many illnesses.

Besides patients and members of the public, hospital staff and students can benefit from psychological services. To function efficiently in their work situation, there is need for the staff to be healthy. It is well known that emotional stress lowers productivity. Provision of psychological services to staff would improve their functional efficiency and hence their productivity in the health care system. Besides, the need for healthy interpersonal relationship among staff cannot be overemphasized. Training in healthy interpersonal behaviors is part of the psychological services to hospital staff and students.

Teaching and Training

This is a second function for the psychologist in the health care delivery system. For any medical programme to be complete the student should be exposed to courses in psychology. Recognizing this the Nigerian Medical Council[43] has included an introductory psychology course in their medical training curriculum. This introductory course which is offered to premedical students should include information on determinants of behavior. More advanced psychology courses in the clinical years should include psychodiagnosis and behavioral medicine. This would prepare the future doctor to recognize the problems that require specialist psychological attention. It would also enable the doctor who finds himself or herself alone to handle simple problems of psychological origin.

Others who benefit from psychology courses are nurses, midwives, graduate students in clinical psychology, psychiatry, social work and health assistants.

Psychologists in the health system also supervise the training of interns/residents in specialist subjects like psychiatry.

Research

The last but not the least of the roles of the psychologist in the health care delivery system is research. Such research may be in innovative and culturally relevant techniques in psychodiagnosis, psychotherapy, prevention and psychoeducation. It may be research in interpersonal communication among health personnel and between health personnel and patients, or in the area related to compliance.

Conclusion

The Nigerian experience has shown that the African patient can benefit from psychological attention. To improve the health and general well being of the African whether literate or non-literate, rural or urban, there is need to integrate psychological services in the health care programs at the primary, secondary and tertiary levels.

It is necessary to note that integrating psychology into the health care programmes will make demands on the available psychological manpower. Pupil clinical psychologists (with B.Sc.) and trained clinical, health and medical psychologists with M.Sc. and Ph.D. will be needed. There is need for existing departments of psychology in Africa to step up their graduate programs in these areas, in terms of quality and quantity. Those universities that do not have departments of psychology should strive to establish them in order to help train psychologists for health care programs. Important bodies like the World Health Organization, UNESCO and African Medical and Research Foundations as well as African governments will be of great help in terms of providing funds for training psychologists and research related to psychology and health in Africa.

Endnotes

[1]Gentry, W.D. (Ed.) *Handbook of behavioural medicine.* London: The Guilford Press, 1984.

[2]Ezeilo, G.C. *A brief on the upgrading of Nnewi General Hospital into the University Teaching Hospital, ASUTECH. Nnewi.* An invited working document submitted to Anambra State (Nigeria) Ministry of Health, 1989.

[3]Ezeilo, B.N. Somatization of psychological distress among Nigerian undergraduate medical outpatients. *Psychopath. Africaine* xviii, 363-372, 1982.

[4]Goke-Panola, M.A. Psychological management of infertile women, in *Psychology and Society,* Wilson, E.B., (ed.). Nigerian Psychological Association, 1986.

[5]Averasturi, L.G. Psychosocial factors and health: The cuban model. In *Health and cross-cultural psychology: Toward application,* Dasen, P.R., Berry, J.W., & Sartorius, N., (eds.), Newbury Park, CA: Sage, 1988.

[6]*British Journal of Clinical Psychology,* December 1982.

[7]Dasen, P.R., Berry, J.W., & Sarsonus, N. (Eds.) *Health and cross-cultural psychology: Toward applications.* Newbury Park, CA: Sage, 1988.

[8]Broome, A.K. *Health psychology processes and application.* London: Chapman & Hall, 1989.

[9]*Journal of Behavioral Medicine.*

[9a]*J. Consult. Clin. Psychology,* December 1982.

[10]*Journal of Health Psychology.*

[11]Uzoka A.F., Eyo, I.S., Obi-Keguna, H.U., Ikeagwu, E.K., Okpara, E., Ibeh, O.A., Iwuh, I.I., & Ozioko, J.O.C. Nigerian psychology and public policy: A working paper presented at the *Annual Conference of the Nigerian Psychological Society* held at the University of Lagos, 6-9 February, 1980.

[12]Pela, O.A., & Okafor, I.A. Self concepts in Sickle cell disease. *IRCS Medical Science Journal,* 10: 178-179, 1982.

[13]Ezeilo, B.N. Self concepts in medical outpatient and normal Nigerian undergraduates. *Social Science & Medicine,* 17: 1309-1313, 1983a.

[14]Ezeilo, B.N. Psychological distress and self concepts in a sample of Nigerian undergraduates. *IRCS Medical Science Journal,* 11: 61, 1983b.

[15]Ezeilo, B.N., & Onyeama, W.P.J.C. Self concepts and psychiatric diagnosis. *Psychopath. Africaine,* xxi, 103-114, 1986/87.

[16]Johnson, B.C.A., & Dada, I.O.I. An attitudinal survey of the psychological reactions to cancer. *Nigerian Journal of Clinical Psychology,* 3: 29-38, 1984.

[17]Onwuzurike, C.A. Need satisfaction and beer drinking among university students in Nigeria. See Reference #27.

[18]Shindi, J. Meaninglessness: the noogenic neurosis of our time–Challenges for Nigerian psychology. *Nigerian Journal of Basic Applied Psychology,* 1: 152-164, 1988.

[19]Ezeilo, B.N. Some psychological factors in infertility among Nigerian women. A paper presented at the *International Canference on Health Psychology* held at University Hall, Cardiff. Wales. 18–22 September, 1989.

[20]Okhimina, F.O.A., & Ebie, J.C. Heat in the head as a psychiatric symptom. Paper presented at the *4th Pan African Workshop,* Accra, Ghana, 1973.

[21]Binitie, A. A factor-analytical study of depression across culture (African and European). *British Journal of Psychiatrics,* 127: 559-563, 1975.

[22]Anah, C.C. Treatment of patients with the complaint of heat in the body. *African Journal of Psychiatrics,* 3: 177-182, 1977.

[23]Ayorinde, A. Heat in the head: A semantic confusion? *African Journal of Psychiatrics,* 1: 59-63, 1977.

[24]Nweze, A. Emotional stress and psychoneurotic symptom expression among undergraduate students. See Reference #27.

[25]Ezeilo, B.N. The treatment of stuttering: The need for an eclectic approach *Nigerian Journal of Clinical Psychology,* 3: 41-47, 1984.

[25a]Ezeilo, B.N. Psychological treatment of functional infertility. Nigerian Journal of Psychology (In press).

[26]Azrin, N.H., & Nunn, R.G. A rapid method of eliminating stuttering by a regulated breathing approach. *Behavioral Research Therapy,* 12: 279-286, 1974.

[27]Awa, A.E. Hypno-behavioural approach: An adjunct to medication in the treatment of essential hypertension. In *Clinical psychology and The Nigerian Society,* Enekwechi, E., & Onwuzurike, C.A. (eds.), pp. 372-389. Nigerian Association of Clinical Psychologists, 1984.

[28]Awaritefe, A. The treatment of functional importance. *Nigerian Journal of Clinical Psychology,* 5: 157-161, 1986.

[29]Omoluabi, P.F. Psychological treatment of brain fag syndrome. *Nigerian Journal of Psychology,* 5: 23-34, 1986b.

[30]Shindi, J.A. Enuresis: A review of therapeutic efforts. *Nigerian Journal of Psychology,* 5: 75-86, 1986.

[31]Uzoka, A.F. Treatment of osychosomatic symptoms in a couple through assertiveness training and conjoint marital therapy. *Nigerian Journal of Clinical Psychology,* 5: 73-83, 1986.

[32]Omoluabi, P.F. Biofeedback therapy: Appraisal and demonstration. In *Psychology and society,* Wilson, E.B. (ed.), Nigerian Psychological Association, 1986a.

[33]Omoluabi, P.F. Does long-term hospitalization affect psychological function. See Reference # 27.

[34]Nweze, A. Current developments in stress and illness research: A selected review in medicine and psychology, *Nigerian Journal of Clinical Psychology,* 3: 1-9, 1984.

[35]Oshuntokun, B.O. Life styles and changes in patterns of non-communicable diseases in developing countries. *Nigerian Journal of Basic Applied Psychology,* 1: 165-181, June 1988.

[36]Nwokolo, C. Personal Communication. 1975.

[37]Nwokolo, C. Some current insights into tomorrows medical curriculum. Text of the second Professor Okoronkwo Ogan Memorial Lecture held at Hotel Presidential Enugu, 14 April, 1988.

[38]Onuigbo, W.B. The role of psychology in personal and national survival. Keynote Address delivered at the *Annual Convention of the Nigerian Psychological Association,* held at the Univerity of Nigeria, Nsukka, 24 April, 1986.

[39]Enekwechi, E. The role of psychology in health care delivery system in Nigeria. Unpublished manuscript. Department of Psychology, University of Nigeria, Nsukka, 1986.

[40]Ezeilo, B.N. The need for a department of clinical psychology in a Nigerian College of Medicine. Unpublished manuscript. Department of Psychology, University of Nigeria, Nsukka, 1987.

[41]Uzoka, A. F. Personal Communication, 1990.

[42]Kayode, C.M. Psychology in aid of health effects of psychotherapy on surgical pain. Paper presented at the *Conference of Nigerian Association of Clinical Psychologists* held at the Aro Neuro-Psychiatric Hospital, Abeokuta, 21-24 February, 1989.

[43]Medical Council of Nigeria. *Guidelines on Minimum Standards of Medical Education in Nigeria.* Harrison Pnnting Press, Lagos, 1984.

Chapter 11

A Sociological Contribution to the New Public Health in South Africa: Why and How?

Leah Gilbert
University of Witwatersrand, South Africa

> Health is a crossroads: It is where biological and social factors, the individual and the community, and social and economic policy all meet. In addition to having its own intrinsic value, health is a means toward personal and collective realization; it is therefore also an index of the success achieved by a society and its government institutions in the search for well-being, which, after all, is the ultimate goal of development (Frenk, 1994, p. 68).

Against this background, this paper aims to explore the dimensions of the "New Public Health" and to examine sociology'*s* role in general and in the South African context in particular.

Societies differ in their definitions of health problems, as well as in their ways of seeking explanations and organizing them, and these differences are shaped by social factors as well as historical development. The evolution of public health has been associated with these factors. It is for this reason that an historical perspective of the relevant developments has been applied throughout this chapter.

Firstly, the changes that have occurred in society, health and medicine linked to the need for a sociological understanding for health professionals, will be examined. Within this framework, the socio-environmental model of health and disease, which is the outcome of the new understanding, is presented. This is followed by a discussion of the development of public health and primary health care with its links to sociology. Finally the "New Public Health in South Africa" and the potential role sociology can play in its research, practice and education are dealt with.

Shifts in Society in Relation to Health and Disease

"Sociology is a relatively recent addition to the syllabuses of health care professionals: yet the interrelationship between sociology and health is not new. Indeed the very early social surveys by Rowntree (1901) and Booth (1892, 1894) showed that ill health was related to poverty and one of the early classic works in sociology took suicide as its subject (Durkeim, 1897)" (Bond & Bond, 1986, p. 1).

Thirty or even twenty years ago, it was uncommon for students preparing themselves for a career in health to study topics drawn from the social and behavioral sciences. Today, however, the curriculum for the training of all health professionals includes a considerable amount of sociological input. At the same time, there is a growing amount of social research in the health field.

It is clear that those in charge of the planning of training programs for health professionals have realized that the knowledge and skills required for their successful practice need to be extended to include the social and behavioral sciences. It is important, therefore, to examine the developments that have created the need for an additional, different perspective in "health practice".

The following section explores the major shifts that have occurred in society in relation to health and disease, which are responsible for the changes in the curriculum and increased focus on social aspects in health research.

Changing Patterns of Disease

The 20th century has seen what has been termed "the conquest of epidemic disease" in the western world. Although this term was coined before the outbreak of the AIDS pandemic, its implications for the issues discussed here remain valid. In most of the developed world, the pattern of causes of death has shifted dramatically from the predominance of infectious diseases in the nineteenth century to that of chronic diseases today. What it means to the practice of health professionals is that since most of the conditions people suffer from today are long term, chronic, degenerative ones, there is a need for a continuous encounter with different health professionals. In addition, most of these conditions are incurable, and health professionals merely play a role in assisting the person in the "management of the disease" so they continue to live as normal a life as possible for as long as is medically possible. They do not *cure* the disease but take *care* of the patient. This brings with it a range of psychological and sociological issues that health professionals need to have some understanding of in order to be able to help patients react to and cope with their conditions.

Causation of Disease

The shift in patterns of disease discussed earlier is linked to a change in the concept of causation of disease. The "doctrine of specific aetiology" or monocausal model of disease which was associated with the germ theory, has been replaced by a *multi-causal model* or *multi-factorial* approach. According to the new approach, the great majority of diseases today are caused by a multiplicity of factors and complex interrelationships between them. Therefore the way to examine disease and disability is to take into consideration all the variables and contributing factors as well as the interdependence between them. This approach is the cornerstone in current epidemiology and is well illustrated in the models presented by Kark (1974). It suggests that the physical and biological causes of disease often work in relationship with a variety of other causes, including psychological, social and environmental factors, rather than a specific disease being the product of a single risk factor. This approach brings the social and behavioral sciences into the picture and creates the need for its contribution.

Comprehensive Care–Multi-Disciplinary Approach–Team Work

The understanding of the complexity of factors involved in the disease process, calls for *comprehensive care* integrating the patient's physical, psychological as well as social well-being. Since this kind of care could not be provided by a single health profession, it has brought with it the need for a multi-disciplinary approach based on *team* work. In the ideal situation, the different disciplines contribute additional dimensions towards the well being of the patient or to the health system as a whole. Working with other members of the team and interacting with various disciplines requires insight into and understanding of social behavior.

Sociological Factors in the Aetiology, Development and Treatment of Disease

In light of the developments discussed above, it is clear that there is a greater awareness of the importance of psychological and sociological factors and the role they play in the different stages of the disease process, from its aetiology, development and treatment to its outcome.

The recognition of the pervasive effects of social and psychological factors on health and disease has resulted in attempts to explain the differential distribution of disease in the population, or why certain groups are more susceptible to disease. This development shifted the emphasis to an examination of related lifestyles and behaviors and has in turn given rise to a wide range of conditions that contribute to the inequalities in health and disease of various social groups.

Demographic Change

Infant mortality rates (IMR), which are generally regarded as sensitive indicators of a country's level of health, have been declining in all Western countries, though disadvantaged groups always have the highest IMR. This, coupled with the development of public health measures, has led to an increase in life expectancy. The result is a general increase in the population of the elderly, and due to lower birth rates, their relative proportion in the total population. This phenomenon has been termed the "Ageing of the population". Big groups of older people in the population bring with them a host of psychological and sociological problems and needs. Quite often these are the people in need of health care, suffering mostly from degenerative conditions.

Health Promotion and Disease Prevention

The realization that some of the major diseases of our times are incurable, coupled with the increasing cost of medical care, has shifted the emphasis towards the prevention of disease. The latter part of the twentieth century is characterized by the growing health promotion movement and the emphasis on "health and maintenance rather than disease and treatment". Numerous health professionals spend a substantial proportion of their time focusing on the preventive and promotion side of their practice. Health promotion and disease prevention rely on peoples' attitudes and behaviors, and as such are mainly in the domain of expertise unique to the social and behavioral sciences.

The Emergence of Health Care Organizations

The provision of health care has developed into complicated organizational structures. Most health professionals operate within the structures of big and growing medical organizations, such as clinics and hospitals. Their activities are greatly influenced by overall governmental policies with regard to health care and its means of financing it in particular. This necessitates a basic understanding of the workings of bureaucracies and organizational structures, which form one of the areas of concern of sociology.

The Bio-Medical and Psycho-Socio-Environmental Models of Health and Disease

Some of the 'shifts' or 'changes' discussed in this context represent components of a more general shift in the dominant framework or 'paradigm' of thinking in medicine, namely, the shift from the sole emphasis on the so called "bio-medical model" to the inclusion of a more comprehensive "psycho-socio-environmental model" of health and disease.

Bio-Medical Model

This term was given to the scientific paradigm in medicine. The basic assumptions underlying this way of thinking are:

- The nature and causes of health and disease - all diseases can be traced to a specific aetiology (or origin) such as virus, parasite or bacterium.
- The patient - the treatment focuses on the patient's body, and the assumption that it can be treated like a machine in that it is passive during treatment.
- The nature of the intervention - focuses on treatment and the belief that medical knowledge and skills ('engineering') is sufficient to 'make the patient's body better'.

- The role of medicine - medical care with its technology and chemical intervention is perceived to have played a major role in the eradication of infectious and parasitic diseases as well as in lowering IMR.

These assumptions created the link between health and the medical care system, and maintained the powerful image of the role of medicine in improving health. However, the real result is an emphasis on treatment of disease (rather than health), based on technological! chemical means, organized around medical specialties. This emphasis is reflected in the education of health care professionals as well.

In essence, the bio-medical model views health and disease through the 'microscope' and offers technical solutions to what are to a large extent social problems (Harding, Nettleton and Taylor, 1990).

Psycho-Socio-Environmental Model

This represents a shift in the thinking mode about health, disease and the role of medicine in improving and maintaining health. While the bio-medical model focuses on the impact of medicine in the elimination of disease, the psycho-socio-environmental model focuses on the promotion and maintenance of health through socio-environmental and behavioral changes. It emphasizes the role of peoples' behavior, what work they do and how and where they live their lives, in determining their health status. There is recognition of the fact that the above factors are not less significant than the biological ones considered by the bio-medical model. Prevention, management of illness and comprehensive rehabilitation are, therefore, more appropriate than intervention.

According to this, people are no longer seen as passive victims of disease, but can themselves participate in their recovery as well as in the production of good health. More than that, changes in society and the environment are perceived to greatly contribute to disease management, prevention as well as health promotion. Thus social solutions are being sought to the problems of health and disease in society.

The bio-medical model keeps health in the biological context, while the psycho-socio-environmental model puts it in the social context, and as such offers a broader perspective, or a macroscope view.

The two models represent different 'paradigms' of thinking, and emphasize different aspects of health and disease. Although the adoption of the "psycho-socio-environmental model" by all health professions who adhere to the "bio-medical model" is encouraged, it needs to be said that the two models provide complementary explanations rather than alternative or competing ones. As such, they broaden our understanding of health and disease in society and the role of health professionals in it.

The Development of Public Health

Societies differ in their definitions of health problems, ways of seeking explanations and organizing them, and these differences are shaped by social factors as well as historical development. In a similar manner, the public health field, which has been developing since the Industrial Revolution, has been subjected to these influences and has undergone reconstitutions that have reflected new relationships between society and state "particularly in their ways of reacting to health problems of individuals and populations." (Paim, 1992, p. 136)

The public health movement of nineteenth-century England and America was stimulated by unhealthy social conditions in both industrialized urban and rural areas (Feinberg et al, 1994). It emerged as "social action" to combat the spread of infectious diseases (Afifi & Breslow, 1994).

In tandem with the developments discussed earlier, various interventions were initiated by the medical profession. These varied initiatives have been alternatively named as, public health, community health, social, community or public medicine.

It is significant to note that the common denominator is a 'group' - community or public - and the distinguishing feature is the use of the word 'health' or 'medicine': it is not just a semantic difference, but illustrates the confusion and inconsistencies within the different approaches.

The impetus to all these interventions and more recently the 'new public health' movement was the inadequacy of the 'bio-medical model' to explain disease patterns and the realization that health of an individual includes the family, work environment, community and society at large (Tarlov, 1992).

The term "public health" is charged with ambiguous meanings. One particular problematic connotation equates the adjective "public" with government or "non-personal" health services. This has been addressed in the more recent comprehensive conception of public health.

A search for a definition of 'public health' produces a variety of interpretations, of which only a small sample will be introduced here: "Public health is one of the efforts organized by society to protect, promote, and restore the people's health. It is the combination of science, skills and beliefs that are directed to the maintenance and improvement of the health of all the people through collective or social actions. The programs, services, and institutions involved emphasize the prevention of disease and the health needs of the populations as a whole. Public health activities change with changing technology and social values, but the goals remain the same: to reduce the amount of disease, premature death, and disease produced discomfort and disability in the population. Public health is thus a social institution, a discipline and a practice" (Last, 1988, p. 107); "Public health is conceived of as the effort (organized or unorganized) of a society stemming from its commitment to meet and attain its health ideals." (PAHO, 1992, p. 4)

In an attempt to come to grips with public health and what it is, Menendez (1992, p. 93) states that "[public health may be defined or regarded as a science, as a set of disciplines, as a series of techniques, as a political/technical sector of the state, as a social phenomenon that is managed by part of civilian society and so forth."

According to the Pan American Health Organization (PAHO, 1992), the most important elements in public health are:

- strategy of population based intervention
- health promotion
- multisectoral activities
- the role of the family and
- the mobilizing capacity of values inherent in such concepts as quality of life, social participation, citizenship and social control.

A comprehensive outline of the public health approach is presented by Feinberg et al (1994) and includes the following elements:

- Understanding of health problems in the context of defined populations.
- Recognition that many problems of public health are deeply rooted in the behavior of individuals and their social context.
- The public health problems of the late twentieth century are rooted in the technologies of economic development: industrialization, super-urbanization, agricultural mechanization, rapid and mass transportation, communication and information management and massive exploitation of natural resources.

- Public health problems continue to require the engagement of the body politic, in the form of government participation, for their solution.

Considering the various presentations, it is vital to remember that the "revolution of the health-related knowledge, attitudes, traditions and practices of each individual society is causally related to specifics of that society's economic, political and social context" (PAHO, 1992, p. 4).

This is particularly relevant to the South African context, where the history of public health is linked to the social and political structure, as will be demonstrated later.

The Primary Health Care Approach

At the International Conference of Alma-Ata in September 1978, the countries of the world unanimously declared that primary health care was the key strategy for attaining the societal goal of "health for all by the year 2000" (WHO-UNICEF, 1978). It is important to note that this goal was established as a collective decision to direct health-related efforts in a common direction. The countries were well aware that this is a social and political response to a social and political problem – a problem of global proportions but one that was clearly most severe in the developing countries (De Rivero, 1992). The social and political problem refers to the inequities among different population groups as far as their health status is concerned, as well as to the distribution of resources allocated to health.

The conference in Alma Ata and the declaration that followed (WHO, 1978) are seen as milestones in consolidating thinking and practice in public health (WHO-UNICEF, 1978).

That public health sees itself as a multidisciplinary entity became evident in the 1970s in the forging of the concepts and strategies of primary care, which seek to globalize the approach to health problems from a new 'medicine-community relationship and multisectoral action to change living conditions in which disease is generated (Orellana, 1992).

The most significant contribution to the development of the Primary Health Care Approach (PHCA) are the main principles it is based on, which distinguish it from the dominant paradigm in the traditional curative medical care services. These principles consist of equitable distribution, community involvement, focus on prevention, appropriate technology and a multi-sectoral approach. Primary health care starts with people and recognizes the major role they play in solving multi-faceted health problems.

Some of the sources of the ideas that led to the development of the Primary Health Care Approach which are significant in the context of this paper, were:

- Changing theories of development, which helped to link health to other sectors and emphasized the need for an integrated, intersectoral approach that stresses equity.
- Disenchantment with a technological approach to diseases and medical services, which did not sufficiently consider social, economic and political aspects of life. It was argued that health care had to be more appropriate to the situation in developing countries (Walt & Vaughan, 1981).

These ideas put sociology in the forefront as a discipline that has contributed to the developments so far, as well as a major potential discipline required in the realization of some of the above principles.

Although nearly 20 years have passed since the Alma-Ata meeting, and although attempts to implement the PHCA all over the world have not met with great success (De Rivero, 1992), it remains the most significant approach that has been guiding health developments all over the world. In fact, sociological theories and concepts have been used and need to be further applied in order to analyze some of the failures in implementing the PHCA.

The History of Public Health in South Africa

There is no comprehensive document that gives a thorough account of the history of 'public health' in South Africa, and it is not the intention of this paper to produce one. However, mention will be made of the most significant developments in South Africa, which ironically influenced the development of public health elsewhere, but not in South Africa.

Although the principles of Primary Health Care and its associated outcomes were officially embraced by the World Health Organization only in 1978, there were significant innovations in this area in South Africa in the 1940s, which were later adapted to address relevant problems in highly developed nations in several instances in the 1960s (Geiger, 1993).

In 1940, two young South African Physicians, Drs. Sidney and Emily

Kark, opened a health Centre in Pholela, Zululand, Natal. Without going into a detailed account of their activities it is meaningful to refer, in this context, to the main principles that guided their operation as well as some of the outcomes.

Some of the main components of the activities in Pholela included a "community diagnosis" in order to define the population and its broad characteristics. This involved epidemiological and environmental surveys to assess health status and other relevant problems. The work was carried out in multi-disciplinary teams, which included physicians, nurses, midwives and laboratory personnel. More importantly, health workers from the community were recruited and trained to act as health educators. Their main focus was the community rather than the individual, and Primary Care was regarded as the basis for targeting additional medical interventions. Incorporated in the activities was a process of ongoing surveillance and evaluation, which included quantitative as well as qualitative research methods, to measure impact and identify new problems as they arose.

The Pholela model was so successful that it became a model for a network of some 40 health centers, established by 1948, predominantly in black communities (Geiger, 1993), and by 1954 it had its educational counterpart: the Department of Social, Family and Preventive Medicine at the University of Natal Medical School, the first black medical school in South Africa. Although the work at Pholela and other centers was published in the South African Medical Journal (Kark & Cassel, 1952) and international health journals, "it remained virtually unknown–or, at best ignored as irrelevant–in the United States" (Geiger, 1993, p. 101).

Yach & Tollman (1993) present a detailed account of "Public Health Initiatives in South Africa". Although it is not the intention of this paper to go into the details, it is important to mention John Casel's name as Kark's collaborator in Pholela, as well as the work done by Mervyn Susser and Zena Stein in Alexandra Health Centre and University Clinic in the mid-1950 during a period when apartheid policies were being intensified. Harry Phillips and Eva Slaber were a third husband-and-wife team, who contributed in this area by focusing on social aspects of child health problems in Cape Town (Yach & Tollman, 1993).

The Gluckman Commission with Kark as its technical advisor and the report (1945) that followed served as a blueprint for the development of the health centers with the support of the ministry of health with Gluckman as health minister, and can therefore be considered as one of the major landmarks in the evolution of public health in South Africa.

According to Geiger (1993) and Tollman (1991), the work carried out in South Africa laid the foundations for the formation of the core elements that came to be defined later as Community Oriented Primary Care (COPC). Directly and indirectly, this influenced the development of Primary Health Care and Public Health in the USA and Israel (Tollman, 1991; Geiger, 1993; Yach & Tollman, 1993).

From the historical/sociological point of view, the key to the development of these health centers in South Africa "was the early realization of the need to focus on broad aspects of health" (Yach and Toilman, 1993, p. 1046). They adopted the 'Psych-socio-environmental model' in their approach before the 'model' had been constructed as such. Factors such as family structure, culture, urbanization and the migrant labor system were identified and considered in their association with disease patterns.

The irony of this early example is that the very same forces these pioneers took into account in their understanding of health and disease, namely wider societal influence, were responsible for their collapse, as put by Yach & Tollman (1993, p. 1047): "the disjunction between the social philosophy and community development objectives of community-oriented primary care, together with the White supremacist ideology of the governing National Party, led to the movement's demise and the departure of its leading proponents."[1]

During this period the contribution of sociology to 'public health' was mainly as a source of knowledge with regard to the social aspects of health and disease and the implication thereof in the planning of comprehensive health programs as well as in training of health professionals.

In the years that followed there was very little or no formal consideration given to the development of 'public health' as was understood by most of the world. The results were and still are apparent in the existing health services, with their fragmentation, emphasis on curative services, characterized by gross maldistribution of resources between the private/public sector, different racial groups, urban and rural areas and the corresponding disparities in the health levels of the people (ANC, 1994).

Presently, there are no schools of Public Health in South Africa. The training in "community health" is available to doctors and nurses in a limited intra-professional capacity only (Ijsselmuiden, 1993). Some of the existing departments of community health, however, offer training towards a "Diploma in Public Health". Additional training in the form of short courses is offered on an ad-hoc basis by the new "public health" initiatives.

Since the dominant ideology during the apartheid era did not encourage the study of the links between society and health, most of the 'sociological' contribution was in the way of sporadic research that critiqued the features of existing structures (Westcott & Wilson, 1980; De Beer, 1984) and the nature of training health professionals (Rudolph et al, 1985).

In the early eighties, some collaborative efforts were made in departments of Community Health and Dentistry where research and teaching included some sociological elements and students became familiar with the terminology and philosophy of the Primary Health Care Approach (Hammond, 1984; Gilbert, 1985).[2]

Against the background of the government's unwillingness to address the health problems of the majority of the people, voluntary organizations and resource groups have responded to the health needs of communities in many different ways, resulting in some "community based health projects" that came into being on this basis (Zwi, 1986).

The publication of *Critical Health* by an editorial collective on a voluntary basis and the articles published in it, can be seen, to a large extent, as reflecting the efforts of people in South Africa who were concerned with the outcomes of an unjust social system on the health of its people (Buch, 1987).

The creation of the National Medical and Dental Association (NAMDA) and the conferences that followed produced additional material that can be classified under the umbrella of public health (Owen, 1987).

In light of the wide definition of public health, as discussed earlier in the paper, all the developments mentioned above can be seen as contributing to 'public health' in this country and to the understanding of the links between society and the health of its people. In a review of De Beer's book, Jacklyn Cock states: "This book makes a valuable contribution toward exposing the relationship between social injustice and ill health in South Africa" (Cock, 1984, p. 69).

The establishment of the Progressive Primary Health Care Network and other progressive organizations as well as their later amalgamation were signs of a growing movement pushing for the transformation of existing health structures. Even the 'old' government in 1991 began talking about Primary Health Care and familiarized itself with the appropriate terminology; however, there were no substantial outcomes.

With the political transformation, which took place after the election in 1994, the scene has been set for the metamorphosis of thinking paradigms and structures in health as well.

The ANC National Health Plan (1994) in combination with the Reconstruction and Development Programme, which can be considered as the guiding documents for the new government, places great importance on Primary Health Care. It seems that despite the difficulties, the new government is committed to the principles of the Primary Health Care Approach and their practical implementation, and the new National Health System presented by the Minister confirms this.

In line with the above it strongly supports the current initiatives to establish schools of Public Health: Thusano School of Public Health, Western Cape Public Health Programme and the Natal Institute For Community Health Education (Ijsselmuiden, 1993).

What emerges is that there is a great need for the establishment of a strong public health movement based on the Primary Health Care Approach, integrating training, research and service.

The New Public Health: Concepts and Critique

The reason why the term "new" public health has been introduced in this paper is that it is a term that has surfaced in the literature during the past few years. Although based on the analysis so far, it should be obvious what is meant by 'public health', it seems necessary to redefine it in terms of "new" as opposed to something different or something in a process of change.

According to some (Editorial, 1991, p. 1381-1382), "public health has been enjoying a renaissance". The definition adopted by the Acheson Inquiry refers to public health as "the science and art of preventing disease, prolonging life and promoting health through the organized efforts of society" (Department of Health, 1988).

Based on the above the British experience of this "new" public health has two elements:

1. development of the multisectoral and multidisciplinary new public health movement; and
2. shaping of the new public health doctor and the newly styled specialty of "public health medicine".

According to Frenk (1992, p. 70), "the essence of public health is that it adopts a perspective based on groups of people or populations. This populational perspective inspires its two applications, as a field of knowledge and as a sphere of action."

As a multidisciplinary field of research, the 'new' public health can be defined according to Frenk (1992, p. 70) "as the application of the biological, social and behavioral sciences to the study of health phenomena in human populations."

The reality that health problems emerge mainly in response to conditions of life, requires that public health remain highly adaptive, especially when living conditions are changing rapidly (Afifi & Breslow, 1994). Therefore one of the main features of public health in the past and today in particular is its dynamic nature. Its core disciplines must always remain "on the ready" (Afifi & Breslow, 1994, p. 224).

Sociology as a discipline in the center of the study of society and change is therefore well situated to contribute to this necessary feature of constant adjustability and adaptability to changing circumstances. This is particularly relevant to South Africa as a society in transition. The HSRC's national research program on "Global Change & Social Transformation", or on a smaller scale, the research program in the Sociology department, University of the Witwatersrand, Johannesburg, with "Southern Africa in Transition" as its main theme can be seen as examples of such a response.

It is of significance to note that although the understanding is that the 'new' public health has developed to meet a whole new set of diseases (as discussed earlier)–those associated with increasing longevity and overpopulation, with industrialization, with inequalities in health, environmental damage and ecological imbalance during a re-evaluation of the effectiveness of therapeutic medicine–it is perceived as a specialization of "medicine" and remains in that realm, dominated by the medical profession.

Menendez (1992, p. 94) maintains that "public health, both as knowledge and as a political and technical sector, was and continues to be in the hands of either physicians or technicians from other disciplines who have adopted the medical perspective". According to Menendez (1992), this is the key to understanding not only the orientations that have been imposed on public health but also the errors of interpretation that have been made.

It seems that the relative power of medicine in relation to other disciplines is a central "bone of contention" within the public health movement. The continuing struggle over the relationship of public health to medicine explains why so many terms have been used in the field, either to define public health or to indicate the specific contributions of the medical profession.

An additional point of critique relates to the rendition of the population model, which is a major component of public health. One interpretation of this model is that "the 'patient' is a population, that is, a group of people...with certain characteristics in common" (Ijsselmuiden, 1995). Without underplaying the importance of the population model as a component in public health, this kind of interpretation merely demonstrates the emulation of the medical model by public health experts, in their use of terminology, reasoning and understanding of health and disease.

The new public health movement seeks the active participation of individuals and communities in decisions that affect their health and in taking the action required to make them healthier.[3] If one adopts this premise, public health action will be based on the population model and its active participation in the intervention. However, often, even the language used defies the declaration. One talks about 'population-based control strategies'. An example given by Ijsselmuiden (1995, p. 98-99) is typical of this misconception: "A good example of the relevance of these last two factors (democracy and population model) is the continuing tuberculosis epidemic in South Africa. More than sufficient knowledge on tuberculosis exists, and adequate treatment has also been available for over 40 years. The tuberculosis epidemic in South Africa, however, is out of control, with at least 75,000 new cases annually – and the numbers are still rising. Only through adequate application of population-based control strategies and the equitable distribution of expertise and resources, may we hope to start making an impact on this epidemic."

Here lies the explanation to the failure to 'control' the epidemic. TB is a disease firmly rooted in the cultural and social structure, in addition to poor nutrition and living conditions which contribute to its rapid spread, the beliefs associated with the understanding of the disease and the way to treat it are embedded in the culture of the people and peoples' responses to attempts by 'public health officials' to control the epidemic are shaped by these beliefs.[4] A complicating factor is the fact that in the South African setting, the 'controlling' body was/is mainly white and most of the 'population' in whom TB was/is to be controlled is black – so the issue acquires a racial angle as well. All this means is that in reality, people affected by TB in South Africa had little or no say in the way TB should be controlled, and were definitely not reached on the level of social understanding of the meaning of the disease; solutions therefore were, and continue to be, unsuccessful. Early attempts by the government to control the spread of HIV were fraught with similar problems. Cases like these present an example and offer opportunities where sociology could make a real contribution to public health.

As referred to earlier, although public health challenges the bio-medical model, it is in a strange way trying to emulate it in reasoning and structure in order to gain acceptance among the very people or propagators of the philosophies it criticizes.

Najera (1992, pp. 113-114) talks about "[t]he difficult and lopsided marriage spoken of by Fee (1987) between the rich and powerful medicine and the weaker public health...public health has been relegated to the less dominant role in an unequal marriage within a macho society." Fee (1987) states more accurately that "public health is struggling for autonomy and independence, while at the same time wishing to have status of her stronger companion, as well as his[5] protection."

Najera (1992) takes the argument further by suggesting that some of the schools and practices of public health have assumed the role of the "submissive wife" without expressing the crisis openly. He further proposes some crucial questions for public health to think of:

- Might it not be thought necessary to begin a conceptual search for new ways of thinking about health?
- Could we come to believe that, although it has been in many senses ultimately an abortive process, the gestation of public health over the past 80 years is finally making us - however recently and timidly - begin to think about health?
- Could we promote a process of change and a true rebuilding of our thinking about health, totally liberating health from medicine if medicine continues to be totally dependent on, and revolve around, disease?
- Shall we work to generate a new theory? (Najera, 1992, p. 114)

Interdisciplinary thinking and intersectoral collaboration is forging the path towards a theory of health.

Feinberg et al (1994, p. 255) maintain that "the field of public health has never attained the status of a recognized, single independent profession and thus endures an ongoing crisis of identity."

Training For Public Health

The debate about what constitutes public health is reflected in the various approaches to training in public health. In the USA (Fee & Acheson, 1991, p. 161), "[o]ne option was to regard public health as a unique amalgam of the biomedical, engineering, and social sciences, requiring specialized training in each of these fields. Some suggested that public health be treated as a combination of sanitary engineering and bacteriology, so that the contribution of engineers and physicians could both be honored. Others regarded public health as mainly a problem of social reform and social organization, in which social and political scientists should take a leading role. Yet others thought that public health should be a specialized branch of medicine, drawing on physicians' knowledge of disease processes, diagnosis and therapy."

As can be seen from the analysis thus far, the major tensions are between public health and clinical medicine and between the social and biological approaches to health, and these feature widely in the debates about the nature of training in public health.

Basic questions about the form of education for public health center around "who should be trained?" "What should be taught in what proportions and who should do the teaching?" "What is the appropriate mix of disciplines and the balance between theory and practice?" "What is the proper role of physicians, nurses, engineers, statisticians, sociologists, economists etc. and how should these different professional groups relate to each other within the larger endeavor of public health?" (Fee & Acheson, 1991).

The answers to these questions are as varied and complex as the definitions and interpretations of 'public health' in different and changing social contexts. They are shaped by the same forces and accompany the historical changes. This is linked to the dynamic nature of public health.

In addition to constant changes in the training, the multidisciplinarity of public health ensures that the material is presented from different perspectives and this changes according to the nature of the problem under consideration.

In an attack on public health, Vandenbroucke (1994, p. 994) states: "There is a discipline in medicine that over the past 200 years has been known by various names: sanitary medicine, public hygiene, public health, social medicine and community medicine. Its newest incarnation proudly calls itself 'the new public health' ... In each new generation of doctors, however, this branch of medicine attracts not only analytical minds but also people who feel a strong personal vocation to improve health in society by attacking plain injustice" (1994, p. 225).

A similar sentiment is echoed by Fee and Rosenkrantz, where they present the declining numbers of physicians in schools of public as a problem and state that "[t]hose attracted to the field will continue to share with their non-medical colleagues a social commitment that often conflicts with the dominant priorities of the medical system and that transcends the care of the individual patient to focus on the health of populations" (1991, p. 271).

Sociology and Public Health

The purpose of this paper has been to examine the links between sociology and public health in general, focusing on the South African context in particular. It is conspicuous that sociology can and has been making a contribution to public health. It is also important, however, to point out some of the many ways in which sociology can benefit substantively, theoretically and methodologically from collaboration with the field of public health.

Riley (1994) mentions two of the ways in which social science efforts to understand and to improve health have benefited from interchanges with the field of public health:

1. in demonstrating how people's lives are influenced by changes in social structures and environments; and
2. in defining goals for structural interventions that could enhance people's lives in the future.

It has further been argued that "[t]he large number of congruent or complementary theoretical and methodological approaches shared by the two fields has made the development of working relationships in research, teaching and service areas mutually profitable" (Suchman, 1963, p. 9).

Sociologists working in public health need to be problem-orientated, not discipline-orientated. This applies to all disciplines involved; however, it should not be confused with forfeiting the unique contribution a discipline like sociology can make to solving health problems through multi-disciplinary efforts.

Health, illness and health care constitute significant areas of sociological concern. The development of the 'sociology of health' is confirmation of the above. In addition to advancing sociological knowledge, research in the field of public health offers a number of opportunities for methodological progress. The growing concern of public health with international health programs offers fertile ground for the development of comparative or cross-cultural research. In fact, the methodology adopted for public health research is, to a large extent, the methodology of social research.

The close affinity between sociology and public health is in terms of unit of study, theory and method. They share a common concern with populations of individuals, a theoretical orientation toward abstract generalizations and a similar methodological approach. They also share a 'problem' focus. To a large extent public health problems are social problems. The social forces that determine whether a health condition will be viewed as a public health problem are similar to those that define a social problem in general.

Suchman (1963) goes so far as to say that it is not incorrect to attribute much of the origin of public health movement to early attempts of social reformers to meet social problems created by the industrial revolution and the rise of urban slum. As Dubos states, "out of the reform efforts of the nineteenth century, there emerged our modern concepts of sanitation and public health." (Dubos, 1960, p. 168).

There is no doubt as to the necessity of sociology's participation in public health. However, there is a need to point out some of the potential dangers, one of which is the danger of sociology being 'taken over' by health professionals as another one of their contributing disciplines. Notwithstanding the fact that the inclusion of sociology in public health is of utmost importance, one needs to maintain the independent perspective of the discipline in order to be able to study health in the social context and public health as a social phenomenon.

One should not confuse the contribution of the discipline of sociology to public health with the adoption of public health as a sociological approach to health. Sociological contribution to public health is beyond its influence on the performance of medical practitioners in clinical work or health service administration (Jefferys, 1991).

Additional tensions of collaboration can be attributed to:

- ordinary problems related to the interdisciplinary nature of the collaboration between people with different 'scientific' paradigms of thinking and operating;
- strain associated with practitioner – researcher relationship;
- different cultural backgrounds;
- low status within a rigid status-conscious institutional setting; and
- differing conceptions of self and expectations of others.

In summary, the areas where sociology can contribute include:

- social factors as determinants of the distribution of disease;
- social factors in the aetiology of disease;
- definition of a public health problem in sociological terms;
- social factors as responsible for society's responses to illness influencing reactions to public health programs; and
- basic social research.

This can be used in training public health workers in order to equip them with the necessary background knowledge. On a more instrumental level sociology can contribute by providing useful knowledge with regard to the social factors that need to be taken into consideration in planning, development and operation of public health programs, in particular with regard to community participation, support and action. As such sociologists can contribute to teaching, research and practice in public health.

The very definition of public health research involves an effort to achieve interdisciplinary integration. As stated by Frenk (1992, p. 72), "[c]learly all human populations are organized into societies. Therefore, the social sciences are indispensable for fully understanding health in populations - that is public health."

Public health as an institution provides sociology with an opportunity to explore its structure, key role players and the associated tensions, goals and objectives, and interrelations with other 'agencies' in the community.

Since the current development of public health in South Africa is only beginning, it is vital to identify the areas where mutual contributions can be made. It seems that there are six major questions that need to be answered.

Although the full answers to these questions as set out by Suchman (1963) are beyond the scope of this paper, it is hoped that the paper provides the background to start thinking about the following questions:

1. What are the current needs in public health that sociology is attempting to meet, and how did these develop?
2. What is the nature of the relationship of sociology to public health? What forces lead to convergence or divergence of the two fields?
3. What contribution does sociology have to make to public health in the understanding of health problems?
4. What contribution does sociology have to make to public health in the study and organization of public health structures and

personnel?
5. What activities do sociologists in public health engage in; where, how and with what results?
6. What problems of collaboration exist between sociologists and public health workers and how are these being met?

Any social science program in public health must accept the responsibility of working on problems that are meaningful and useful to public health. A social science program to be meaningful must be free to develop an inherently social science approach to public health problems.

Conclusion

Although there is great variety in the understanding and implementation of public health, there is wide agreement that the challenges to public health today are as serious, if not more so, than those at the end of the nineteenth century (Jefferys & Lashof, 1991). This is probably more poignant in the South African context.

In the latest South African interpretation of public health, Carel Ijsselmuiden, as chairman of the "Transvaal School of Public Health" initiative, made the following statement: "Public Health is a social movement which was started in the middle of the 19th century around issues of hygiene, sanitation and occupational health, and which focuses now on equity in health and in access to health care, and on the balance between development, health and well-being. By definition, therefore, Public Health is not the property of a specific profession, nor of professionals in general, but both as a practice and a social movement it belongs to all. As a discipline, Public Health is the academic or scientific expression of the people's right to optimal health and to a fair distribution of disease interventions and health care" (Ijsselmuiden, 1993, p. 67).

Since sociology in South Africa has the potential to make a valuable contribution in the training, research and practice of Public Health, it should seize this opportunity and work towards the development of a force in Public Health, where its guiding philosophy and principles do not remain meaningless declarations of intent, but are mirrored in its reality. By doing so, it will support the following plea made by Yach & Tollman (1993, p. 1049):

> The work in public and community health in South Africa during the 1940s and 1950s represent extraordinary coherent and comprehensive integration

of teaching, service and research dimensions of public health practice...Having made this original contribution, it is time for South Africans to reclaim this experience and apply its profoundly contemporary lessons to the current reality.

Endnotes

[1]Cassel was recruited as professor and chair of epidemiology at the University of North Carolina at Chapel Hill in 1960. Kark left to found the Department of Social Medicine and Health Cantre at the Hebrew University in Jerusalem.

[2]This chapter does not attempt to give a full review of the above activities, and therefore these are just a few examples of outcomes; there are probably many more which have not been mentioned.

[3]Alma-Alta and subsequent direction provided by the WHO "Health for All by The Year 2000" strategy (European Office of the World Health Organization, 1985, Targets in Support of health for all by the year 2000 in the European region. Copenhagen: WHOEURO).

[4]This was acknowledged by Kark and his team in their work in Pholela in the 1940s.

[5]The notion of differential power structure is carried further with the use of gender allocation.

References

Afifi A. A., & Breslow, L. (1994). The maturing paradigm of public health. *Annual Review of Public Health*, 15: 223-235.

ANC (1994). *A National Health Plan for South Africa.*

Bond, J., & Bond , S. (1986). Sociology and health care. New York: Churchil Livingstone.

Booth, C. (1892). Pauperism: a picture and the endowment of old age, and 1894, The aged poor in England and Wales, cited in: Bond J. & Bond, S., 1986, *Sociology and health care*, New York: Churchil Livingstone

Buch B. (1987). The struggle for health. *Critical Health*, 21: 4-10.

Cock J. (1984). Book Review, The politics of genocide - by De Beer C. *Critical Health*, 11: 69-73.

De Beer C. (1984). The South African disease: Apartheid health and health services, Southern African Research Service, Johannesburg.

Declaration of Alma-Ata (1978). WHO-UNICEF.

De Rivero D. T. (1992). Public health and primary health care: A critical evaluation. In Pan American Health Organization (PAHO), *The crisis of public health: Reflections for the Debate* (pp. 155-165). Washington, D.C.: World Health Organization.

Department of Health (1988). *Public health in England (The Acheson report).* London: HM Stationery Office.

Dubos, R. J. (1960). Beyond traditional medicine: The crisis in American medicine. A special supplement to *Harper's* magazine.

Durkeim, E. (1897). Suicide: A Study in sociology. Cited in Bond, J. & Bond, S., 1986, *Sociology and health care.* New York: Churchil Livingstone.

Editorial (1991). What's new in public health? *The Lancet*, 337: 1381-1383.

Fee, E., & Acheson, R. M. (1991). *A history of education in public health.* Oxford: Oxford University Press.

Fee, E., & Rosenkrantz, B. (1991). Professional education for public health in the United States. In Fee, E., & Acheson, R. M., 1991, *A history of education in public health* (pp. 230-271). Oxford: Oxford University Press, Oxford.

Fineberg, H. V., Green, G. M., Ware, J. H., & Anderson, B. L. (1994). Changing public health training needs: Professional education and the paradigm of public health. *Annual Review of Public Health*, 15: 237-257.

Frenk, J. (1992). The new public health. In Pan American Health Organization (PAHO), The crisis of public health: Reflections for the debate (pp. 68-84). Washington, D.C.: World Health Organization.

Geiger, H. J. (1993). Community-Orientated primary health care. In Morgan, R. E., & Rau, B. (eds.), Global leaming for health (pp. 99-106), Washington, D.C.: National Council for International Health.

Giddens, A. (1989). *Sociology, polity press.* Cambridge.

Gilbert. L., & Rudolph, M. (1986). Oral health status - A comprehensive approach. *Journal of The Dental Association of South Africa*, 41: 9-11.

Gluckman Report (1945). *Report of the National Health Services Commission on the Provision of an Organised National Health Service for All Sections of the People of the Union of South Africa 1942-1944.* Cape Town, RSA: South African Government Printer.

Hammond, M. (1984). An alternative analysis of health care in South Africa. *Critical Health*, 10: 4-13.

Harding, G., Nettleton, S., & Taylor, K. (1990). *Sociology for pharmacists: An introduction.* London: Macmillan Academic and Professional.

Ijsselmuiden, C. (1993). The Transvaal School of Public Health: Towards education for health. *CHASA Journal*, 4: 67-71.

Ijsselmuiden, C. (1995). Sociology and its relevance to the New Public Health. In Allais, C. (ed), *Sociology of health and illness* (pp. 93-106). Isando: Lexicon Publishers.

Jefferys, M. (1991). Medical sociology and public health: Interdisciplinary relationships 1950-1990. *Public Health*, 105: 15-21.

Jefferys, M., & Lashof, J. (1991). Preparation for public health practice: Into the twenty-first century. In Fee, B., & Acheson, R. M., 1991 (pp. 314-335), *A history of education in public health.* Oxford: Oxford University Press.

Kark, S. L., & Cassel, J. (1952). The Polela Health Centre: A progress report. *South African Medical Journal*, 26: 101-104; 131-136.

Kark, S. L. (1974). *Epidemiology and community medicine.* New York: Appleton-

Century-Crofts.
Last, J. M. (1988). *A dictionary of epidemiology*, 2nd edition. New York: Oxford University Press.
MacLeod, S. M., & McCulllough, H. N. (1994). Social science education as a component of medical training. *Social Science & Medicine*, 39: 1367-1373.
Menendez, E. L. (1992). Public Health: State sector, applied science or ideology of the Possible. In Pan American Health Organization (PAHO), *The crisis of public health: Reflections for the debate* (pp. 92-110). Washington, D.C.: World Health Organization.
Morgan, R.E., & Rau, B. (eds) (1993). *Global learning for health*. Washington, D.C.: National Council for International Health.
Najera, E. (1992). Public health, a theory aimed at a practice: Is a reconstruction needed? In Pan American Health Organization (PAHO),), *The crisis of public health: Reflections for the debate* (pp. 111-120). Washington, D.C.: World Health Organization.
Orellana, H. S. (1992). Public health situation and trends In Pan American Health Organization (PAHO), *The crisis of public health: Reflections for the debate* (pp. 151-154). Washington, D.C.: World Health Organization.
Owen, C. P. (ed.) (1987). *Towards a national health service. Proceedings of the NAMDA Annual Conference*, University of The Western Cape, Cape Town.
Page, S. L. (1994). A new mandate for public health. *Public Health Reports*, 109: 469-471.
Paim, J. S. (1992). Collective health and the challenges of practice. In Pan American Health Organization (PAHO), *The crisis of public health: Reflections for the debate* (pp. 136-150). Washington, D.C.: World Health Organization.
Pan American Health Organization (PAHO) (1992). *The crisis of public health: Reflections for the debate*. Washington, D.C.: World Health Organization.
Rosenberg, C., Medicine and Society 1993-1994, Department of Social Medicine, The University of North Carolina at Chapel Hill.
Rowntree, B. S. (1901) Poverty: A study of town life. Cited in Bond, J., & Bond, S., 1986, *Sociology and health care*. New York: Churchil Livingstone.
Rudolph, M. J., & Brand, A. A., Gilbert, L., & Van Zyl S. (1985). Dentistry and the community. *Journal of the Dental Association of South Africa*, 40: 761-764.
Suchman, E. A. (1963). *Sociology and the field of public health*. New York: Russell Sage Foundation.
Tarlov, A. R. (1992). The coming influence of a social science perspective on medical education. *Academic Medicine*, 67: 724-731.
The Alma-Alta Conference on Primary Health Care (1978). *WHO Chronicle*, 32: 409-430.
Tollman, S. (1991). Community oriented primary care: Origins, evolution, applications. *Social Science & Medicine*, 32: 633-642.
Vandenbroucke, J. P. (1994). New public health and old rhetoric. *British Medical Journal*, 308: 994-995.
Walt, G. & Vaughan, P. (1981). An introduction to the primary health care ap-

proach in developing countries. *Ross Institute of Tropical Hygiene Publication No.13*, London School of Hygiene and Tropical Medicine.

Westcott, & Wilson (ed) (1980). *Perspectives on the health system: Hunger, work and health*. Johannesburg, South Africa: Ravan Press.

White, R. M. (1994). Changing lives and social structures: Common concerns of social science and public health. *American Journal of Public Health*, 84: 1214-1217.

Yach, D., & Tollman, S. M. (1993). Public health initiatives in South Africa in the 1940s and 1950s: Lessons for a post-Apartheid era. *American Journal of Public Health*, 83: 1043-1050.

Zwi, A. (1986). Health services provided by voluntary organization. *Critical Health*, 16 & 17: 4-47.

Chapter 12

Influence of Interpersonal Communication and Social Support on Health Decisions in an African Context

Andy O. Alali
California State University, Bakersfield

The literature suggests a link between interpersonal communication, social support, and the health decisions people make (Rimon & Zimmerman, 1987; Ezeh, 1993; Kuseka & Silberman, 1990; Piotrow et al., 1997). This appears to support the notion that interpersonal communication, social support and health decisions are contextually bound, especially when examined with the perspective that self-disclosing communication in social support networks may be intrinsically gratifying to members of that group. It also follows the school of thought that the intent or willingness to disclose and the amount and veracity of information disclosed result from the affirmative support received from the social network. The expectation is that the interaction that takes place within social support networks and between those with affirming relationships is likely to produce optimal results, with implication on individual health decisions and the overall health promotion objectives of the responsible health agency. And, in critical health contexts where culture and tradition collide with public health objectives, it becomes crucial that we fully understand the dynamics of interpersonal communication and the intricacies of social support networks that interact with individual health decisions. In this respect, one would expect that social support networks play a crucial role in individual health decisions because of the ability to provide a supportive communication environment, "by offering tangible assistance, expressing acceptance, and listening as recipients 'vent' their feelings" (Cline & Boyd, 1993, p. 131).

Analysis of research evidence suggests direct impact on family planning contexts, as it appears that most people "talk with their spouses or partner, friends, and others to seek information, confirmation, or emotional support" before they consult with their service providers (Piotrow et al., 1997, p. 163). Clearly, other research findings are supportive of the notion that the "talk" which takes place in support networks may, in fact, impact on observable health behavior. For example, in the African countries of Egypt, Ghana, and Zimbabwe, researchers found that communication between spouses about family planning predicts high levels of contraceptive use (Rimon & Zimmerman, 1987; Ezeh, 1993; Kuseka & Silberman, 1990). Similarly, as the interpersonal contacts and social support networks increase, they appear to significantly impact on individual decisions to engage in family planning (Kim, Marangwanda & Kols, 1996).

The evidence from the research on family planning and social support networks serve as the backdrop for the analysis in this chapter. An equally important consideration here is the notion of self-disclosure, which features prominently within the circle of those in a supportive interpersonal context. It is necessary to determine the extent to which self-disclosure impacts on health decisions because of the support networks' ability to guard or publicize personal health information. Clearly, the actions of a recipient of personal health information can influence the discloser's health decisions. Therefore, this chapter examines the role and influence of interpersonal communication and social support networks in health decisions. The analysis is based on data collected by the author in Zimbabwe.

The Zimbabwe Case Study

The research sought to determine four key issues: how interpersonal communication about health is initiated and terminated; the social networks often used for discussions about health; the types of health issues discussed within the social networks; and the influence of interpersonal communication and social support on health decisions.

The focus on women, in this chapter, is intentional because they are often overlooked in most African health contexts and research endeavors. In light of this concern, the author interviewed 350 females from a sprawling high-density suburb of Harare, Zimbabwe. Each was asked to complete a four-part survey comprising 10 items; participation was voluntary. Apart from soliciting basic demographic information from the sample, participants were asked to identify the social support networks with whom they disclosed their health status in the six months prior to the survey; to identify or specify the health issue(s) they discussed with their social support networks within the same six-month period; and to list specific reason(s) why they discussed their health status with the social support networks they identified. The study yielded the following findings:

Demography

The sample was representative of several age groups. A few of the sample (3.7 percent) reported they were between the ages of 15 and 18, while 47.1 percent of the sample comprised those within the 19–29 age group. Those who identified their ages as between 30 and 39 comprised 24.5 percent of the sample; 9.4 percent were 40 to 49 years of age. Only 3.7 percent were 50 years of age or older. Some participants (11.3 percent) did not identify their age.

As with the sample's age, their marital status also varied. A majority of the respondents were married (58.4 percent), with only 39.6 percent identifying themselves as single. A few of the sample, or 1.8 percent, said they were divorced.

Social Support Networks

There were three types of social support networks to whom participants said they self-disclosed their health status in the six months before the survey. In most of the cases, respondents (44.8 percent) said they disclosed their health status more often to members of their family than to their primary-care providers (34.9 percent). A few of the respondents (18.2 percent), however, self-disclosed personal health information to their friends and peers; only 2.1 percent said they use other social support networks that include traditional healers, or "medicine men."

Health Issues

There was an exhaustive list of health issues participants say they self-disclosed in the six months prior the study. All were collapsed into five health categories. A majority of the respondents (66.1 percent) say they discussed "Basic health issues" with their social support networks. Other health issues were: "Gynecological/Reproductive health" (15.3 percent); "HIV/AIDS" (8.8 percent); "Contagious diseases" (2.9 percent); and "Cardiovascular ailments" (6.9 percent).

Reasons for Self-Disclosure

An important component of the study was to determine the reasons why participants disclose personal health information to their social networks. When asked to give reasons why they self-disclosed specific health issues to their social support networks, 25.7 percent said they wanted "To seek help." An equally significant number (22.9 percent) indicated they intended "To share information," while 17.9 percent cited "To get information" as their reason for self-disclosure. Other reasons given were: "To give information" (11.4 percent); "To clarify information" (8.6 percent); "To confide in the person" (6.4 percent); "For satisfaction" (4.3 percent); "I was asked to" (1.4 percent); and a few of the sample (1.4 percent) did not specify their reasons for self-disclosure.

Implication for Health Communication and Campaigns

This Zimbabwe study is an attempt to begin the long road of assessing the roles interpersonal communication and social support networks play in self-disclosure and decision-making within the African health context. Equally important is how affiliative groups can be integrated in public health campaigns so as to encourage healthy lifestyles and achieve health behavioral objectives. We see this as crucial to campaign success because we believe the theory of disease prevention and the practice of health promotion cannot be divorced from the interpersonal relativism that enhance campaigns or, for that matter, render health promotion objectives ineffective. Therefore, it is imperative that communications scholars interested in health campaigns and disease prevention efforts study social support networks to determine the extent to which the health exchanges that take place enable or disable health-realted behavior. The results of such inquiry would help health educators to determine how an existing social relationship and the interaction that takes place within that relationship can be merged and ethically manipulated to achieve health promotion objectives.

The findings in this chapter affirm the perspective that most of health information acquisition is conditioned by the affirming or non-affirming relationships that take place between individuals and their support networks of family, peers and social groups. In this context, it is not unreasonable to expect that the affiliative relationship may, in fact, influence information acquisition since most Africans tend to confide in those they trust and, in times of crisis, turn to them for advice about their health as well as for assistance. The evidence in this study is supportive of the perspective that "people in crisis, particularly those with serious illness, rely on social support as a preventive agent" (Cline & Boyd, 1993, p. 131).

While this study yields a relative picture of what people might do in time of crisis, it does not tell us if they seek accurate information from their social networks. Therefore, we must find ways to plan more effective campaigns that assist individuals in seeking reliable and accurate health information from informed sources. The one way we can achieve the goal of a healthy society is to recognize that health promotion is transactional. The transactional nature of health promotion requires us to understand the rules that govern a communication environment and the cultural variables that impede health promotion objectives. In the process, we can design pre-campaign research that seeks to determine whether there are similarities and/or differences in self-disclosure among peoples of the different African cultures. Clearly, the issue of gender differences in self-disclosure about health is equally a significant issue.

In conclusion, it is important to note that this study is not without limitations. First, the results and conclusions are based on a relatively small sample that may not necessarily be representative of all females in Zimbabwe. Second, it must be noted that this study is retrospective in that respondents were asked to recall or identify their social support networks, and the health issues they discussed in the six months prior to the survey. It is possible that their responses may be based on their best memory of what might have occurred in the six months before the survey; we must give room for lapse in memory. Yet, these limitations do not diminish the importance of the study and, hopefully, its intended contribution to the role social support networks play in self-disclosure and how they impact on health information acquisition, all of which would add to the literature on health communication in Africa.

It is imperative that a more expansive research, comprising a larger sample, should be conducted in the immediate future. Equally important is the need for researchers to explore the role of social pressure in seeking social support. Other research activities should seek to examine the external experiences individuals and members of their social group bring to the network, and the extent to which such experiences impact on group interaction. We see all of these as enabling factors in fully understanding: social support groups; the motivation for joining support groups; the extent to which social support groups impact on decisions; the degree (high–low) of dependence to social support groups; and whether the influence is one- or two-way. As we identify and analyze some of these issues, it is possible to meet the health promotion objective of finding ways to bridge the health information and knowledge gap that currently exists between the informed and the chronically uninformed. Perhaps, the results of these research efforts would serve as the basis for which a healthy African society can be achieved.

References

Cline, R. J. W., & Boyd, M. F. (1993). Communication as threat and therapy: Stigma, social support, and coping with HIV infection. In E. B. Ray (ed.), Case studies in health communication (pp. 131-147). Hillsdale, NJ: Lawrence Erlbaum Associates, Publishers.

Ezeh, A. C. (1993). The influence of spouses over each other's contraceptive attitudes in Ghana. Studies in Family Planning, 24, 163-174.

Kim, Y. M., Marangwanda, A. C., & Kols, A. (1996). Involving men in family planning: The Zimbabwe male motivation and family planning method expansion project, 1993-1994, IEC Field Report No. 3. Baltimore, MD: Johns Hopkins Center for Communication Programs.

Kuseka, I., & Silberman, T. (1990). The Zimbabwe male motivation impact evaluation survey. Evaluation report by the Zimbabwe National Family Planning Council Evaluation and Research Unit, Harare, Zimbabwe.

Piotrow, P. T., Kincaid, D. L., Rimon, J. G., & Rhinehart, W. (1997). Health communication: Lessons from family planning and reproductive health. Westport, CT: Praeger.

Rimon, J. G., & Zimmerman, M. (1987). Print materials review and IEC needs assessment of four Egyptian agencies. Trip Report, October 4–2, 1987. Baltimore, MD: Johns Hopkins Center for Communication Programs.

Part IV

Health Communication in Contexts

Chapter 13

AIDS Communication in Africa: Towards a Practical Framework

Carol A. Okigbo
Minnesota State University, USA

Charles C. Okigbo
North Dakota State University, USA

Susanne Williams
Minnesota State University, USA

The most sobering facts about HIV/AIDS are also the most humbling and most perplexing. At the beginning of the 21st century, more than 36 million people are living with HIV/AIDS; the total number of deaths since the beginning of the epidemic is 21.8 million; and the number of AIDS deaths in 2000 alone was 3 million. Africa alone accounts for 25.3 million cases. It is perplexing that though there is abundant information about how to contract (and also how to prevent) AIDS, yet 5.3 million people were infected in 2000 alone. The global situation is getting out of hand and is far more dangerous than what was projected a decade ago. UNAIDS/WHO (2000, p. 4) found that the "the number of people living with HIV/AIDS at the end of 2000...is more than 50 percent higher than what WHO's

Global Programme on AIDS projected in 1991 on the basis of the data then available." African American communities in the United States and sub-Saharan African countries present the worst scenarios now.

Among African Americans, gay men are at greatest risk. Recent studies show that whereas as many as one in 50 black men in the United States is infected with the virus, among gay men, the rate of infection is as high as 33 percent (CDC, 2000; Carey, 2001). Most of the new infections in 2000 were in Sub-Saharan Africa and among African American communities in the United States (UNAIDS, 2001; CDC, 2001). The situation in Africa is so depressing that DeCock, director of programs for the Center for Disease Control in Kenya, avers that it is the continent's greatest catastrophe since slavery (Carey, 2001).

The HIV/AIDS epidemic has taken many African countries by storm, since the first few cases were reported in the early 1980s, and it has continued to pose a veritable threat to the sustainable development of the continent. Starting with the first reported cases in Zaire in 1981, it spread like wild fire all across the continent, leaving no country untouched and many devastated in the extent of its pervasive prevalence. Even without HIV/AIDS, socio-economic development in Africa was a precarious prospect, as many economies faced (and still have to contend with) declining economic fortunes, internal political instability, inter-ethnic strife, very low per capita incomes, high incidence of diseases, and ever-worsening terms of trade.

The seriousness of these threats lead some to see only negative prospects for the continent's development, and thus to become thoroughly pessimistic about the prospects for positive change. According to UNAIDS/WHO (2000) the epidemic is projected to reduce South African economic growth annually resulting in a gross domestic product which will be 17 percent lower in 2010 than it would have been without AIDS. In diamond-rich Botswana, which has the highest per capita GDP in Africa, in the next 10 years, AIDS will slice 20 percent off the government budget, erode development gains, and bring about a 13 percent reduction in the income of the poorest households.

The HIV/AIDS situation has compounded the economic development problems of the continent, and poses the greatest threat to Africa today. Unless it is checked immediately, there can be no viable options for survival. Life expectancy has regressed to the rates in the 1950s in some countries (UNAIDS, 1998). As recent data on infection rates show, Africa is the worst affected region, with the highest rates of infection. With 25.3 million total cases, Africa has more than all the other regions put together. In some African countries, the rate of infection has continued unabated in the face of initially uncoordinated responses. There are both national and regional variations, which are still changing, and thus show a picture of an evolving phenomenon (Cohen & Trussell, 1996; UNAIDS, 1998). AIDS is ever changing and thus has defied not only a cure but also a vaccine, leading many to characterize it as diabolical (Carey, 2001).

The various African governments have responded differently to the epidemic. While Uganda was quick to accept the situation, and ask for international support in controlling it, Kenya started out denying it (Forsythe & Rau, 1996). In some West African countries today (e.g. Nigeria and Ghana), there is rampant confusion among policy makers on how to deal with the situation. Regardless of how government and public policy makers react to the situation, it is becoming clear that the best approach is to recognize the seriousness of the epidemic, and also design vigorous communication and education strategies to contain it and bring about appropriate changes in behavior.

Persuasive communication and education are still the best AIDS interventions. In analyzing the situation in the United States, Reaves (2001) concluded that the task is to convince at-risk populations that there is no cure. Reports about the promise of new treatment regimens and cocktail of medicines create a false sense of security. The undeniable reality is that prevention is the best intervention. The best prevention is achieved through communication and education campaigns that employ a multiplicity of strategic packages. Information and education are so critical that even empirical mathematical estimations of HIV/AIDS infections using probability models (Hudgens et al., 2001) have to incorporate exposure to and consumption of information and communication. The African epidemic presents a challenge to information management, persuasive communication, and utilitarian education. The most fundamental ingredient is communication, which is the fulcrum around which the other factors revolve.

Communication in Africa

AIDS prevention and control must necessarily involve communication, especially in the contexts of behavior changes. As Lin (1971, p. 178) has noted, "it is human communication (then) that provides the moving force in changing human behavior." However, communication in Africa is more than just messages and media. This quality of African communication can easily elude people who are not deeply steeped in the African view of communication. Communication in Africa has its unique characteristics, some of which have been captured by various scholars (see Doob, 1961; Hachten, 1971; Ugboajah, 1978; Ziegler & Asante, 1993; Oreh, 1978; Bourgault, 1995).

In one of the earliest studies of communication in Africa, Doob (1961, p. 17) noted the futility in trying to see African communication through Western lenses. If an African responds positively to a (Western) communication stimulus (e.g. adoption of a new habit), there are no doubt a "thousand and one communications during the past fifty years which really enabled the present communication as the last in the long series to be successful." Even with the pervasive presence of the modern mass media in Africa today, the individual African is still surrounded by the more enduring traditional media, which Ugboajah (1986) called "oramedia." Moemeka (1998) identified community feelings and communitarianism as important features of African society. These have not been systematically examined by studies of development and health communication, nor have behavior change programmers employed them adequately. In developing the African AIDS communication framework, UNAIDS/PennState paid considerable attention to the unique nature of communication within African communities. Health and wellness have cultural roots, and effective health communication is facilitated by close attention to culture (Airhihenbuwa, 1995).

An analysis of the evolution and uses of both the traditional and modern mass media in Africa shows that they were used more for bringing about change than for frivolous entertainment. Even African talking drums which the uninitiated thought of as just musical instruments provided instruction, rebuke, praise, or some other form of intelligent counsel (albeit in a playful mode). The so-called new creative strategies of edutainment or infotainment have been part of traditional communication in Africa from antiquity. The failure of the early scholars of development communication to recognize African traditional communication and make it a vital part of social change strategies is another evidence that oramedia were grossly misunderstood.

Development Communication: Paradigm Shifts

Modern health communication in Africa is partly an offshoot of the tradition of development communication, which has experienced significant shifts in paradigms, starting from the debunking of the dominant paradigm (direct effects model) of the 1950s and 1960s (Lerner, 1958;

Schramm, 1978). The dependency paradigm, which came next, had a limited acceptability, and was replaced by participatory model, which in turn is now being displaced by strategic planning (Adhikarya, 1995), empowerment (Melkote, 1999), and newer models. These models embody significant promise for the use of communication in preventing and controlling HIV/AIDS. In the case of Africa, the necessity to involve local peoples and also use traditional communication (oramedia) cannot be over-emphasized. Schramm (1979, p. 9) had argued for such local involvement in these words:

> ...the center of development strategy, as far as feasible, will be the local areas, local activities, and as far as possible, local decision making will become central in development planning; two-way, not one-way communication will be emphasized, and horizontal communication will emphasized at the expense of vertical communication.

AIDS Communication: A New Paradigm

The HIV/AIDS epidemic has presented a good testing ground for many of the principles of development and social change communication. The new paradigms of development communication (especially the participatory and strategic planning models) portend great significance for their application in creating awareness, changing attitudes, and ultimately influencing the behaviors of people who are at risk of contracting HIV. The UNAIDS/PennState Framework recognizes that prevention is the best cost-effective strategy to reduce worldwide HIV infection rates.

The HIV/AIDS situation is more serious in developing countries where worsening economic fortunes make it unrealistic to entertain any hopes of the people benefiting from the new drugs that can delay the onset of AIDS from HIV infections. But for prevention campaigns to be successful, they must involve communication and education efforts that are properly planned and implemented with the peculiarities of the target audience in view. Sexual behaviors are cultural manifestations. They are also reflective of sub-cultures and idiosyncratic behaviors. Thus they are not easily identifiable, nor is changing them necessarily similar to changing consumer behavior. This partially accounts for the widely acknowledged gap between knowledge of HIV/AIDS and continuing engagement in risky sexual behavior.

If we accept that communication is a key component in interventions for HIV/AIDS prevention and care, then we should identify the best means of employing the wide range of communication factors to achieve the most desirable results. This was the task of the UNAIDS/PennState initiative. Employing a multi-stage research and consultative process, UNAIDS/PennState health communication specialists identified five common domains of context that characterize universal factors in HIV/AIDS preventive health behavior. The five factors, which are operational in all world regions, are: *government policy, socio-economic status, culture, gender*, and *spirituality*. These can be referred to as pan-regional factors, as they apply to all world regions, regardless of their levels of development. Here is how each of them is explained in the framework:

Government policy. Official government policies and laws play important roles in prescribing the boundaries for public health, and education programs, many of which are directly related to AIDS prevention.

Socio-economic status. People's economic and social statuses have direct relationships to their knowledge, attitude, and behaviors in many important areas, not least of which is health.

Culture. If it is true that we are who we are because of our culture, it is even truer that our state of health is implicated in our cultural beliefs and activities.

Gender relations. Many societies have various ways of expressing the biological fact that people are primarily "gendered" (as male or female) before they become sexually relevant. In many societies, our perceptions of gender roles have important implications in our health-related activities and wellness.

Spirituality. The African world is dominated by benevolent and malevolent spirits that are believed (even by some of the most educated Africans) to have direct effects on peoples' daily activities. Generally, our religious and spiritual values have some relationships with our health and wellness beliefs and activities.

In addition to the five universal factors that operate in all world regions, two other factors apply to each of the major geographical regions. In Africa, the two peculiar factors are *community-based approaches* and *regional integration.*

Community-based approach. The community is vital, and often assumes a super-natural role in African societies. Many African societies are com munity oriented and have less regard for individualism.

Regional cooperation. HIV can travel very fast, and is known to be highly associated with trans-national highways, truck drivers, and sex workers who operate at truck stops.

Thus, the seven elements adjudged to be the most critical factors in African AIDS Communication planning and implementation are: *government policy, socioeconomic status, culture, gender relations, spirituality, community approach,* and *regional cooperation*. Though the last two factors (*community approach* and *regional cooperation*) are peculiar to Africa, they "may also be applicable to other regions" (UNAIDS/PennState, 1999, p. 52).

Though the above seven factors make sense to many people who are familiar with public communication campaigns in Africa, it is apposite to subject them to some form of validation exercise. We have done this here by comparing these factors to the results from two separate empirical studies of communication and AIDS in Africa. The two studies are the UNFPA-Kenya Survey of Kenyan Adolescents (1998), and the AIDS Communication Survey of Kenyan NGOs (Okigbo, 2000).

The First Study: Survey of Kenyan Adolescents

As part of its training program on audience research and segmentation for Population IEC, the UNFPA Training Program for Anglophone Africa, based at the Kenya Institute of Mass Communication, Nairobi undertook a survey of 351 Kenyan adolescents (aged 15 to 19) in Mombasa, Kenya. The sample was drawn from residential areas and high schools, using random selection procedures. A seven-page questionnaire that had 43 open- and close-ended questions and statements was used to elicit various kinds of information on vital aspects of population communication from the respondents. Many of the questions required respondents to indicate what they knew, felt, or did about teenage pregnancy, contraceptive methods, and similar aspects of population communication. They were also asked what they felt were the major health problems in their communities.

Other questions addressed sources of information on health-related issues. A battery of Likert-structured statements required them to indicate how much they agreed or disagreed with representative views on premarital sex, availability of contraceptives, teenage pregnancies, and sex education in school, among other. In addition to the survey part of the study, six focus group discussion groups were constituted to discuss six related themes of adolescent reproductive health, contraceptive use, family life education, family communication patterns, peer pressure, and access to health facilities and to health-related information. The full report was produced by the United Nations Population Fund, Kenya (1994), and parts of it have been published separately (Pratt et al., 2000).

The results showed that HIV/AIDS and STDs were reported to be the most serious health problems that confronted their communities. There were 126 respondents (35.9 percent) that felt this way. Teenage pregnancy was common, as 295 respondents (84 percent) said they knew girls (aged between 15 and 19) who had become pregnant. A large number of the respondents (215 people or 61 percent) reported that such pregnant teenagers usually resorted to abortion. More than three-quarters of the respondents (277 teenagers or 78.9 percent) reported that teenage pregnancy was common.

Regarding knowledge of contraceptives, more than half the respondents said they knew the common contraceptive methods, with the condom and the pill being the most well known methods. The sources for information on reproductive health issues ranged from institutional (hospitals, media and schools) to personal (parents, counselors, friends) channels. The most frequently cited sources were hospitals, clinics, and the Ministry of Health, followed by the mass media, and teachers in school. Personal sources were reportedly less important. This is the expected pattern in African communities where sex talk or reproductive education is not common at the personal level.

TABLE 13.1: ***Frequency of Major Health Problems***

Health Problems	Frequency	%
HIV/AIDS/STDS	126	35.9
Malaria	117	33.3
Dietary	76	21.7
Drugs	25	7.1

TABLE 13.2: ***Frequency for Teenage Pregnancy***

Statement on Teenage Pregnancy	n	%
Know pregnant girls aged 15–19	295	84
Pregnant girls aborted	215	61.3
Teenage pregnancy is common	277	78.9

TABLE 13.3: ***Frequency for Main Sources of Information***

Sources of Information	n	%
Hosp ital/Clinics/Ministry Health	122	34.8
Media	82	23.4
Teacher/School	73	20.8
Parents/Home	47	13.4
Guidance and Counseling	38	10.8
Friends	28	8

Factor Analysis. We subjected the 19 statements on various aspects of teenage sexuality to factor analysis to achieve a parsimonious reduction

TABLE 13.4: ***Factor Analysis Result – Rotated Factor Matrix***

Dimension	Variable Description/Index	Factor 1	Factor 2	Factor 3	Factor 4	Factor 5
	Pregnancy is Common	- 52892	23739	- 04553	23830	31340
	No Pregnancy at First Sex	66998	02815	2828	02377	10357
Cognition	Ignorance of Contraceptive	77672	28753	- 24692	16747	- 03939
	Unavailability of Contraceptive	44067	- 19467	- 23502	06790	- 11578
	Contraceptive Affordability	54980	03884	46611	04428	- 30281
	Parents Discuss Sex	- 01278	43598	04820	10611	- 11481
Protection	Contraceptive Failure	28186	- 83568	08418	00707	11469
	Contraceptive Use	26117	78529	24501	04648	09755
	Contraceptive Availability	25180	43654	42695	47049	11174
	Some Teenage Girls Abort	- 09226	01560	76144	02812	- 21784
Abortion	Boys Impregnate Teenage Girls	- 14237	11595	76579	12914	08131
	Contraceptives Affordability	54980	03884	46611	04428	- 30281
	Contraceptives Availability	25180	43654	42695	47049	11174
	Contraceptive encourages sex	03324	- 00824	15995	80898	- 00574
Emotion	Contraceptive Availability	25180	43654	42695	47049	11174
	Availability encourages Sex	- 01146	07961	- 0594	84654	- 06694
Sexual	Older Men Impregnate	24983	36471	37395	18438	- 51434
Activity	Sex Education	05019	- 28539	00699	11342	69145
	Premarital Sex	05640	15947	- 08053	10011	081151

of the data set. A verimax rotated factor analysis of the Likert statements isolated five factors, which account for 61 percent of the variance. The scree test was the primary criterion for deciding on the number of factors.

TABLE 13.5: *Factor Analysis Factor Transformation Matrix*

Factors	Eigenvalues	% of Variable	Cumulative %
1	3 088	19 3	19 3
2	2 119	13 2	32 5
3	1 555	9 7	42 3
4	1 505	9 4	51 7
5	1 434	9 0	60 7

The first factor (cognition) had five variables that referred to knowledge of teenage pregnancy, contraceptive availability, affordability, and use. The second factor (protection) had four variables that reflected parental discussion and preventing pregnancies with contraceptives. The third factor (abortion) had four variables that suggested boys make girls pregnant, and the latter seek abortion. The fourth factor (emotion) had three variables that referred to contraceptives making young people want to have sex; while the fifth factor (sexual activity) had three variables that measured views on pre-marital sex, sex education, and teenagers being impregnated by older men. The most notable result is the value of knowledge (the cognition factor) in teenage sexuality. This result is consistent with much of the experience of AIDS communication and education, where knowledge is the basic building block without which appropriate behavior will depend on chance. However, knowledge by itself is not sufficient, though its necessity is not arguable.

Focus Group Discussion. The results of the focus group discussions revealed the adolescents' views on the need for sex education in school, further education at home, and more instructional programs within the community. One female respondent said that lessons on AIDS prevention should be "taught by parents, teachers, and elders." There were some indications that the mass media might be sources of negative influence, as one respondent noted, "you watch a movie, and just because you see it (sex) being done, you decide to do it."

The respondents were consistent in reporting their high regard they have for communication and education as the necessary foundation stones for desirable sexual behavior. They also acknowledged the importance of peers and peer pressure, as well as the need for attention to community social values.

Though this study was undertaken before the formulation of the UNAIDS/PennState Framework, some of the results are consonant with some aspects of the framework. The reported high rate of teenage pregnancy implies that these teenagers were engaging in risky sex behavior, and thus would need HIV/AIDS prevention efforts directed at them. The high incidence of abortion can be attributed to the policies of the Kenyan Government, which (at the time of the study) required that pregnant students be expelled from school, without hope of re-admission after delivery. In terms of socio-economic status, the respondents were mostly of middle-class status, and thus had access to both formal education and the mass media, unlike their lower status counterparts. This is useful knowledge in designing appropriate media strategies for them. With regard to culture, it bears pointing out that though the respondents were urban-based, they were not completely isolated from indigenous Kenyan culture.

On gender relations, the respondents saw themselves correctly as boys or girls, and obviously knew there were different role expectations for each group. One of the girls said during the focus group discussions that "boys don't care about prevention; they want enjoyment." As for spirituality, some respondents seemed to be torn between the teachings of their religion and their feelings. The community-based approach was felt to be important and worthwhile. This was borne out in the examination of the sources for health-related information, which showed the dominance of institutional and personal channels. The use of regional cooperation did not feature, even remotely, because it was not addressed at all. The factor analysis results showed that there were clear dimensions on knowledge, protection or prevention, abortion or treatment, emotions, and sexual activity. Such a trajectory is discernible in HIV/AIDS communication, where following the UNAIDS/PennState Framework, the emphasis could be on using the key factors to address issues of knowledge, protection or prevention, treatment, emotions, and non-risk behavior. The next section describes the second study, which was a survey of AIDS communication agencies and AIDS program beneficiaries.

The Second Study: Survey Kenyan AIDS NGOs

The second study was undertaken to determine how selected AIDS prevention agencies in Kenya used various communication approaches (Okigbo, 2000). The quantitative data were collected through two surveys of 72 program officers and 146 program beneficiaries. The program officers completed a nine-page questionnaire that elicited information on various aspects of AIDS communication campaign management. Program beneficiaries responded to various questions on their involvement in AIDS communication programming, perceived impact of the programs, and their knowledge of AIDS. Ten agency managers who did not participate in the quantitative survey were selected for in-depth personal interviews, the results of which complemented the findings from the surveys.

The results showed, among other things, that the agency managers reportedly used strategic planning, which involved pre-search, needs assessment, clear objectives, pre-testing of materials, and evaluation. The program officers and mangers reported extensive use of social marketing. This often involved teaching program beneficiaries new skills relating to AIDS prevention. Among the major communication strategies used were workshops, seminars, and training. Others were posters, drama, and group work. In a list of 10 such strategies and channels, the mass media were the least favored, and came after personal and community (group) methods. The responses from the in-depth personal interviews showed that many managers preferred to adopt multi-media approaches and integrated marketing methods. The four major areas of AIDS communication programming were: awareness creation, risk behavior modification, skills acquisition, and behavior reinforcement.

The respondents had clear notions about the factors that facilitated greater achievement of their organizational goals. Among these were: clear understanding of their target audiences, designing messages with clear calls for action, and focusing on determinants of behavior. One of the most important results was the significant association between beneficiaries' participation in AIDS programming and their level of knowledge. Knowledge of AIDS was assessed through a batch of 16 questions on various aspects of AIDS, and responses were scored to achieve a value that reflected the proportion of correct answers. The range of achieved scores reflected levels of knowledge that ranged from low to high. The beneficiaries who had participated in AIDS programs organized by AIDS prevention agencies tended to know more about two aspects of AIDS: means of contracting, and methods of preventing it.

TABLE 13.6: ***Cross-tabulation of Knowledge of Possible Ways of Contracting AIDS and Participation in Programming***

Participation	No Knowledge	Average Knowledge	High Knowledge	Total
Not Participated	1 0.68	7 4.79	3 21.92	40 27.4
Participated	0 0.0	8 5.48	98 67.12	106 72.6
Total	1 0.68	15 10.27	130 89.04	146 100.00

Chi-square = 5.96, df= 2; Prob < 0.05

TABLE 13.7: ***Cross-tabulation of Knowledge of AIDS Prevention and Participation***

Participation	Average Knowledge	High Knowledge	Total
Not Participated	7 4.79	33 22.60	40 27.4
Participated	2 1.37	104 71.23	106 72.6
Total	9 6.16	137 93.84	146 100.00

Chi-Square= 12.24; df= 1; Prob < 0.001

These results support some of the factors in the UNAIDS/PennState AIDS Communication Framework for Africa. The role of government policies was not specifically examined in the surveys, but in the in-depth interviews, many program mangers averred that advocacy and getting the support of vital publics (including public officers) were important ingredients for success. Socio-economic status and culture were perceived as important, and implied in the attention to audiences, messages, action, and behavior.

Because different ethnic groups in Kenya have different cultural practices relating to sexual conduct (e.g. wife inheritance and virgin marriages), the program officers and managers recognized that their AIDS programming must be culture-sensitive. Again, gender relations was not specifically addressed in the surveys, but the strong endorsement for participatory planning and involvement of beneficiaries would seem to provide sufficient cover for accommodating men-women differences and peculiarities. The spiritual dimension in AIDS communication in Kenya is becoming more conspicuous as the epidemic spreads to the rural areas (where superstitious beliefs are more rampant). Many program managers reported that they often had to contend with uneducated people who associated AIDS with witchcraft and/or sinful behavior.

On the two factors that UNAIDS/PennState adjudged to be peculiar to Africa (i.e. community-based approach and regional cooperation), the community-based approach was more widely endorsed by the respondents. This was evident in the reportedly pervasive involvement of beneficiaries in all aspects of programming. About two-thirds of the program officers reported that their organizations had built-in mechanisms for getting feedback from their beneficiaries. During in-depth interviews, many program managers reported that their work would be impossible without vigorous but well thought out plans for community involvement. This is not surprising, for as Moyo (1992, p. 223) noted of African societies, "life can be meaningful only in community, not in isolation." This is what Moemeka (1998, p. 125) referred to as African communalism – the social order where "the immediate and ultimate goal is not the protection of the rights of the individual or of the goals of groups within the community, but the maintenance of the supremacy of the community as an entity and the safeguard of its welfare."

Regional cooperation was evidently recognized as vital in the successful implementation of many AIDS programs in Kenya. Many of the agencies were part of regional or global networks on HIV/AIDS, and thus already benefited from positive developments in other countries or regions. Program managers reported that though the various governments in Eastern Africa did not appear to cooperate closely in the design of AIDS interventions, the individual health agencies within the region were forging ahead in many collaborative ventures. This was made easier by regional organizations such as UNICEF-East and Southern Africa Regional Office in Kenya, UNESCO Regional Office in Kenya, and funding organizations that are located in one country, but have programming responsibilities for the entire region.

Conclusions from the Results

Though the UNAIDS/PennState Framework was developed after these two studies had been conducted, the research results provide collaborative evidence for the meritorious value of the framework. Both the survey of Kenyan adolescents, with its focus on teenage reproductive health, and the study of Kenyan AIDS program officers and beneficiaries showed the relevance of each of the five universal and two regional factors (proposed by UNAIDS/PennState) in HIV/AIDS communication in Africa. Recent experience (e.g. Uganda and Kenya) has shown that public policy and governments' response to the epidemic are some of the most critical factors in successful program management. Socio-economic status, culture, gender relations and spirituality are also important; so are community-based approaches and regional cooperation. The two studies suggest two areas of interest which the UNAIDS/PennState Framework has not addressed clearly, and which might deserve further attention in future

research. The study of adolescents showed the relative importance of institutional and personal sources of information. The mass media were reported to be less important than personal sources. This was supported by the study of Kenyan AIDS NGOs, where the program officers reported that the mass media paled in importance (to workshops, posters, drama, and group work), as strategies or channels for AIDS communication and education. This is an affirmation of the primacy of personal relationships and an endorsement of the validity of community approaches.

The second area is greater appreciation of the value of African traditional forms of communication. As HIV/AIDS spreads more into the rural areas, where the mass media (already shown to be less influential than personal sources) are even less visible, the need for using traditional forms of communication becomes more urgent. AIDS program officers reportedly used drama, which is often a hybrid between traditional performances and modern theatrical structures. But the wide range of truly indigenous means of conversation, training, socialization, village consultative meetings, and behavior control are largely left out of many contemporary AIDS communication campaigns. These two areas (emphasis on personal influence and greater recognition of traditional communication) deserve more research attention to see if they can fit in this evolving AIDS communication framework for Africa. Future research in Africa should also include the other factors that UNAIDS/PennState (1999) has isolated for the other world regions.

Beyond an African Framework

The development of the UNAIDS/PennState Framework has come at a most auspicious moment in the continuing evolution of both health communication and development communication in Africa. This framework has the potential to rekindle interest in the field of applied communication because of its (framework's) promise of theoretical relevance and practical significance. By reviewing and building on existing models, the framework has avoided some of the pitfalls of the traditional development communication paradigms. But ironically, in this strength also lies its major weakness. By successfully guarding against ethnocentrism, it can easily fall victim to cultural relativism.

The most recommendable feature of the framework is the provision of five common factors that (are expected to) apply in different cultures. These can provide the core and foundation for all AIDS communication programming, regardless of geographical location. One of the weak points is the lack of justification for proposing that the regional factors cannot be common or universal factors too. For instance, the two Asian factors (communication context and epidemic context) may obtain in Africa or Latin America. Similarly, the Latin American factors of advocacy and involvement of HIV+ people may apply to African and Asian situations. The two African factors (community-based approaches and regional cooperation) may apply to Asia and Latin America, as well. UNAIDS/PennState recognizes the need to subject the framework to rigorous scrutiny and validation exercises to refine it further; hence this is called a "framework" to show it is only work in progress. There is no doubt we here have the seeds of a possible new theory of health and development communication. What we need are cross-sectional, longitudinal and cross-cultural quantitative and qualitative studies (involving academics and practitioners) to refine the framework further, and determine the validity of the five common and six regional factors.

The Global Communications Framework for HIV/AIDS

The five common domains that apply to all world regions are:

- Government policy
- Socio-economic status

Figure 13.1: ***Global Communications Framework for HIV/AIDS***

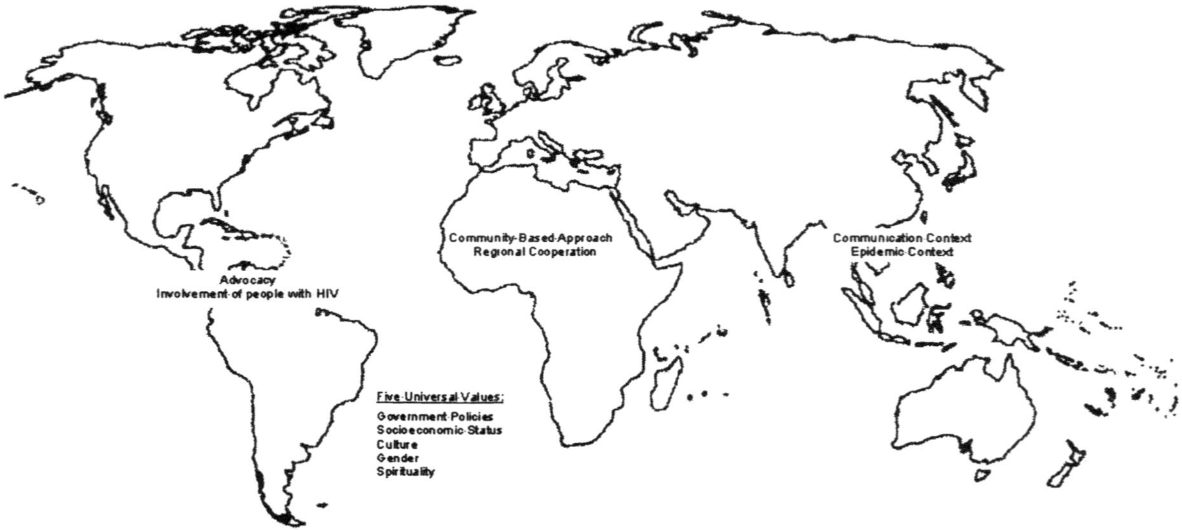

- Culture
- Gender relations
- Spirituality

The two domains that apply to Africa are:

- Community-based approach
- Regional cooperation

The two domains that apply to Asia are:

- Communication context
- The epidemic situation

The two domains of Latin American and Caribbean countries are:

- Advocacy
- Involvement of positive persons in communication programs

References

Adhikarya, R. (1994). *Strategic Extension Campaign. A Participatory-oriented method of agricultural extension.* Rome: FAO.

Airhihenbuwa, C.O. (1995). *Health and culture. Beyond the western paradigm.* Thousand Oaks and London: Sage.

Bourgault, L. (1995). *Mass media in sub-Saharan Africa.* Bloomington: Indiana University Press.

Carey, J. (2001, February 7). A sad truth about AIDS. *BusinessWeek On Line.*

CDC (2000, December 6). *HIV/AIDS Surveillance Report,* 12:1.

CDC (2001). HIV/AIDS Updates. <*www.cdc.gov/hiv/stats*>

Cohen, B., & Trussell, J. (1996). (Eds.) *Preventing and mitigating AIDS in sub-Saharan Africa.* Washington D.C.: National Academy Press.

Doob, L.W. (1961). *Communication in Africa: A search for boundaries.* New Haven: Yale University Press.

Forsythe, S., & Rau, B. (eds.) (1996). *AIDS in Kenya.* Nairobi: FHI/AIDSCAP.

Hachten, W. (1971). *Muffled drums: The news media in Africa.* Ames: Iowa State University.

Hudgens, M.G., Longini, I.M., Halloran, M.E., Choopanya, K., Vanichseni, S., Kitayaporn, D., Mastro, T.D., & Mock, P.A. (2001). Estimating the transmission probability of human immunodeficiency virus in injecting drug users in Thailand. *Applied Statistics,* 50; 1:1-14.

Lerner, D. (1958). *The passing of traditional society.* Glencoe, Il.: Free Press.

Lin, L. (1971). *The study of human communication.* New York: Bobb-Merrill Company.

MAP. (1998). *The status and trends in the HIV/AIDS epidemics in the world.* Geneva: MAP.

Melkote, S. (1999, May 10). Reinventing development support communication to account for power and control in development: Toward a conceptual framework. Presentation made at North Dakota State University.

Moemeka, A.A. (1998). Communalism as a fundamental dimension of culture. *Journal of Communication*, Autumn, 48; 4: 118-141.

Moyo, A. (1992). Religion in Africa. In Gordon, A.A., & Gordon, D.L. (eds.), *Understanding contemporary Africa*, Boulder, CO.: Lynne Rienner.

Norussis, M.J. (1994). *SPSS professional statistics.* Chicago: SPSS Inc.

Okigbo, C.A. (2001). Communication for behavior change: A study of HIV/AIDS prevention programs in Kenya. Unpublished Master's Degree The sis, Department of Communication, Daystar University, Nairobi, Kenya.

Oreh, O.O. (1978). Modes of communication. In Kalu, O.U. (ed.), *Readings in African humanities: African cultural development.* Enugu: Fourth Dimension.

Pratt, C., Obeng-Quaidoo, I., Okigbo, C., & James, E.L. (2000, Fall). Health information sources for Kenyan adolescents: Implications for continuing HIV/AIDS control and prevention in sub-Saharan Africa. *The Western Journal of Black Studies*, 24; 3.

Reaves, J. (2001, February 24). AIDS: The dangers of letting down your guard. *Time.com*

Schramm, W. (1978). End of an old paradigm? In Schramm, W., & Lerner, D. (eds.), *Communication and change. The last ten years – and the next.* Honolulu: The University Press of Hawaii.

Schramm, W. (1979). *Mass media and national development.* Paris: UNESCO, International Commission for the Study of Communication Problems.

UNAIDS. (1998). *Progress Report 1998.* Geneva: UNAIDS/WHO.

UNAIDS/PennState. (1999) *Communications framework for HIV/AIDS: A new direction.* Geneva: UNAIDS/PennState.

UNAIDS/WHO (2000, December). *AIDS epidemic Update.* Geneva: UNAIDS.

UNAIDS (2001). HIV/AIDS Updates. <www.unaids.org>

UNFPA-Kenya. (1994). Audience research and segmentation for population IEC. Unpublished Report. See also Pratt, C. Obeng-Quiadoo, I., Gikonyo, W., & Okigbo, C. Health-Information Sources for Kenyan Adolescents: Implications for Continuing HIV/AIDS Control and Prevention in Sub-Saharan Africa. Conference Paper Presented at the 1997 AEJMC Conference, Chicago, IL. 1997.

Ziegler, D., & Asante, M. (1992). *Thunder and silence: The mass media in Africa.* Trenton: Africa World Press.

Chapter 14

Health Promotion on HIV/AIDS in Africa

Karl Peltzer
Varghese I. Cherian
University of the North, South Africa

The European Office of WHO's International Working Group suggested a definition of health promotion: "The process of enabling individuals and communities to increase control over the determinants of health and thereby improve their health." In this chapter health promotion and health education are used interchangeably.

Sub-Saharan Africa is worst afflicted with the HIV/AIDS epidemic, and heterosexual transmission, the predominant means of the transmission accounts for as high as 90 percent of cases. In 1996 14 million people in sub-Saharan Africa were estimated to be infected with HIV. Eighty percent or higher of all HIV/AIDS cases worldwide are found in sub-Saharan Africa (Olayinka & Osho, 1997). Epidemiological information relating to HIV/AIDS in Africa contributes to the effective role health promotion can play in the following: increasing awareness of the need for an array of national and international strategies to decrease the epidemic in Africa; providing needed information concerning at-risk sexual behaviors and other possible correlates (e.g. stress) for HIV infection; and increasing self-efficacy, especially among at-risk groups such as women and adolescents (Livingston, 1993).

Changes in sexual behavior in response to the HIV epidemic among the general population are now being reported from African countries. The knowledge and behaviors of their populations are monitored and one can hypothesize whether prevention campaigns bear fruit, even though it is difficult to identify which specific action is accountable for which behavior change. This is partly due to the fact that very few studies enable proper assessment of interventions. Lagarde, Pison and Enel (1997) reports that on the basis of cross-sectional surveys performed between 1990 and 1994, AIDS-related knowledge increased and at-risk behavior decreased in a rural area in Senegal. Similarly, Olayinka and Osho (1997) found a decline in high risk sexual behaviors in southwest Nigeria as compared to those reported in previous studies.

The limited effect of interventions that provide information alone has been well documented, particularly with respect to AIDS education, indicating that health education strategies need to go beyond awareness raising to addressing shifts in social norms that support behavioral change (e.g. Fisher & Fisher, 1992).

Regarding health education on AIDS in Africa, Hubley (1988) indicated the need to address cross-cultural validity of health education models, use of fear appeals in persuasive communications, and the role of interpersonal communication and community participation. Scott and Mercer (1994) also refer to the importance of a full understanding of the cultural and social context of HIV/AIDS for global prevention efforts. In Africa, in particular, the following content of health promotion interventions have been identified as important: (i) changing government's attitude to accept AIDS problem and health promotion; (ii) how to avoid contracting HIV; (iii) dispel false beliefs about the virus; (iv) target different populations; (v) primary prevention (focused on prevention of HIV infection); (vi) secondary prevention (dealing with early diagnosis and with transmission from those found to be seropositive); and (vii) tertiary prevention (concerned with altering the progression of HIV natural history among those already infected). For example, regarding false beliefs about the infection, MacLachlan (1996) used the Nominal Group Technique (NGT) with Malawian students to achieve a consensus concerning which anti-health promotion ideas are most influential in terms of encouraging people to ignore health promoting messages such as "There is nothing you can do about AIDS" or "Some traditional healers can cure AIDS." Furthermore, in regard to targeting different populations O'Leary, DiClemente and Aral (1997) state that there is a need to identify the most effective interventions for a variety of at-risk populations.

Approaches to Health Promotion Interventions

Ziglio (1997) suggests that evidence-based health promotion interventions should not follow the strict criteria of "evidence-based" medicine of well-designed RCTs (randomised control trials) but a variety of research instruments for assessing process, outcome and economic evidence of the impact of health promotion are appropriate. Health promotion should be linked to wider public policy initiatives with strong socio-ecological orientations and their impact on processes to enable people to gain control over and improve their health. Health promotion should be positioned at the heart of social and economic development and be increasingly perceived as an investment strategy. Guidelines in the search for evidence process include the development of: a) a logic model about the logical connections among the various elements of a program including its activities, outputs, impacts, effects, objectives and goals; and b) an evaluation task group with the goal of actively involving the key stakeholders in the process of decision-making, providing a forum for the political and practical aspects to be taken into account, increasing commitment to the results, knowledge about evaluation, and ability to interpret the results. Therefore a multisectoral strategy for AIDS prevention at community level is proposed. AIDS prevention involves the modification of sexual activity, which raises sensitive social and cultural issues. The multisectoral AIDS prevention strategy involves carrying out community-defined initiatives by means of integrated, government and nongovernmental services (Elkins et al., 1996). Ng'weshemi et al. (1997) note that as AIDS matures, it is becoming clear that AIDS care and prevention of infections can no longer be seen as the sole preserve of the health sector providing a strong argument for a multisectoral approach in line with the primary health care strategy. Campbell (1997) proposes an integrated approach that combines public health, community and individual initiatives. Moses and Plummer (1994) highlights that influencing the underlying causes of the epidemic will do much more to control the spread of HIV infection than the best educational or counseling program. Governments, industries and donor agencies need to examine how policies might be changed to mitigate the social and economic causes of the spread of HIV infection.

A number of behavioral theories have been used as frameworks for intervention development. In STD/HIV risk reduction efforts, these have included the Health Belief Model (Rosenstock, 1966), the Theory of Reasoned Action (Azjen & Fishbein, 1980), and Social Cognitive Theory (Bandura, 1986). In addition, the "Transtheorectical" model, a description of the temporal process of change, and "Diffusion of Innovation" theory, which concerns the process of change caused by communications from people who influence each other (O'Leary et al., 1997).

The knowledge-attitude-belief-practice (KABP) model rest on the assumption that changes in knowledge levels, attitudes and beliefs lead to behavioral changes. Theory concerning the relationships between the four components is often drawn from two multidimensional health models: the Health Belief Model (HBM) and the Theory of Reasoned Action (TRA) (Joffe, 1996). Joffe (1996) refers to a social representational approach, which gives more attention to explaining AIDS-related thoughts and actions than the prediction of intentions. Knowing the social representation ascribed to by an individual may provide an indication of the behavior which can be expected. Programs with a theoretical grounding in social learning or social theories appear to have been the most successful in changing risk behaviors, although the changes obtained have usually been modest (Klepp et al., 1997). It is also seen as critical to publish well-done studies with null findings in addition to those that indicate significant intervention effects (O'Leary, 1997).

Socioculturally Informed Health Promotion Interventions

Airhihenbuwa (1989) informs that a conceptual model for health education in African countries must address cultural sensitivity and cultural appropriateness in program development. The proposed model consists of three dimensions of health beliefs and behavior that are dynamically interrelated and interdependent. They are: health education, educational diagnosis of health behavior and cultural appropriateness of health behavior. Similarly, Ulin (1992) states that AIDS prevention campaigns have not yet taken into account the cultural, social, and economic constraints on most African women's ability to comply with advice to limit partners and use condoms. In the light of the dominant role males have in sexual relations, health promotion campaigns must focus specifically on addressing at-risk culturally related sexual values and behaviors (Livingston, 1992). Laver, Van der Borne and Kok (1997) describe the utilization of social change theory and an ecological model for health promotion to develop a participatory intervention for HIV/AIDS prevention in farm workers in Zimbabwe.

Kawewe (1996) proposes a social-networking approach to combat HIV/AIDS in Zimbabwe that is culturally friendly and sensitive to Zimbabwean families. It is suggested that this approach will strengthen the currently isolated traditional family systems by informally connecting extended families with a large national community.

In South Africa, Toroyan and Reddy (1997/98) found on the basis of a photocomic AIDS intervention that the identification with the comic was stronger among coloured and African youth than that among their White counterparts, supporting the theory that involving the target group in developing health messages will result in a product that is most effective among that particular readership.

Janz, Zimmerman, Wren, Israel, Freudenber and Carter (1996) evaluated 37 AIDS prevention projects and identified the following sociocultural factors that facilitated intervention effectiveness identified by staff in the US: (i) design culturally relevant and language appropriate; (ii) embed AIDS information into broader contexts; (iii) provide creative rewards and enticements; (iv) build in opportunities for program flexibility; (v) promote integration into and acceptance by the community; (vi) repeat essential AIDS prevention messages; (vii) create a forum for open discussion; and (viii) solicit participant involvement. For example, designing culturally relevant and language appropriate interventions may include paying attention to the norms, values and traditions of the target population, combining vernacular with formal terminology to understand important terms and concepts, and solicited input and participation from the members of the target population. For instance, the South African government produced a manual on all HIV/AIDS related terms in all 11 official languages. These facilitating factors should be considered when designing and evaluating health promotion intervention programs in African sociocultural contexts. Attitude of participants towards the intervention activity may differ and has to be considered. For example, MacLachlan, Chimombo and Mpemba (1997) reported that Malawian secondary school pupils repeatedly enjoyed the educational AIDS board game and Bosompra (1991/92) found among Ghanaian communities that they preferred drama to songs as AIDS messages. Table 14.1 shows health promotion projects on HIV/AIDS carried out in Africa.

Case Example of Effective Intervention

One model AIDS education program in Tanzania for primary school children is described here in more detail, which is the first controlled,

Table 14.1: *Overview of Health Promotion Intervention Activities, Risk Populations,and Behavior Effected Changes in Africa*

Intervention Activity	*Target Population*	*Behavior Effected Change*
Awareness campaign (Wilson et al., 1989)	Teachers, adults, adolescents (Zimbabwe)	>knowledge
3-day course (Eagle & Brouard, 1995)	Health professionals (South Africa)	=knowledge, attitude
Workshop (Green et al., 1995)	Traditional healers (South Africa)	>knowledge >condom promotion
3-day workshops over 6 months for Imams and their lay assistants (Kagimu et al., 1998)	Muslim community (Uganda)	>knowledge >risk perception <risk behavior
Multifaceted (small group discussions, facts, creating songs and poetry, role plays, plays) (Klepp et al., 1997)	Primary school (Tanzania)	>knowledge >attitude PWA >behavioral intent
First AIDS kit, AIDS education (Kuhn et al., 1994; Visser, 1996)	Secondary school (South Africa)	>knowledge/ >attitude PWA/ “>” behavioral intent
Theatre, drama & open day (Dalrymple & Du Toit, 1993)	Secondary school (South Africa)	>knowledge, =attitude >attitude PWA
Drama & songs (Bosompra, 1991/92)	Rural & urban community (Ghana)	>behavior change
Puppetry & street theatre (one show only) (Skinner et al., 1991)	Community (South Africa)	>short-term knowledge
Photocomics (Toroyan & Reddy, 1997/98)	Urban youth (South Africa)	>knowledge, >attitudes >behavioral intention
Board game, repeatedly (MacLachlan et al., 1997)	Secondary school (Malawi)	>knowledge
Condom promotion (Moses et al., 1991) (Pickering et al., 1993)	Female prostitutes (Kenya) (The Gambia)	<HIV transmission =condom use
Voluntary HIV tests, individual Counseling (McKenna et al., 1997)	Married couples (Zambia)	<HIV transmission
Individual counseling (Peltzer et al., 1989)	HIV clinic population (Zambia)	<HIV transmission

multiple-community test of such type in a developing country (Klepp et al., 1997).

Aims

1. Reduce students' risk of HIV infection by delaying initiation of sexual intercourse.
2. To alleviate the consequences of HIV infection and AIDS in the community by reducing the stigma attached to AIDS.
3. Condom promotion was not assessed since the government was opposing condom promotion in primary schools at the time of the study.

Study Design

- Randomized controlled community trial

Participants

Sixth-grade students (mean age = 13.6 years) from all public primary schools in two regions in rural, semiurban and urban Tanzania. Those who had engaged in sexual activity at the time of study were excluded.

Theory

- Theory of Reasoned Action and Social Learning Theory

Baseline Survey (12-months follow-up)

AIDS information, AIDS communication, AIDS knowledge, Attitudes toward people with AIDS, Attitudes toward engaging in sexual intercourse, Subjective norms regarding sexual intercourse. Instruments were translated, peer reviewed for content validity and adapted to the local community by two local teachers, one local health educator and the investigators.

Local HIV/AIDS Education Program

Local teachers and health educators were given a one week training workshop. The intervention in the schools included teaching on factual information on HIV transmission and AIDS. Students created their own posters depicting their perceptions of HIV risk factors. Students wrote and performed songs and poetry about the danger of AIDS and how they can protect themselves. Small group discussions were held on how people are exposed to HIV risk, and what they could do to reduce such risk. Students wrote and performed role-plays, argued publicly, trying to convince each other about aspects of HIV risk behavior. Panel discussions with the community (elders, religious leaders and parents) were held at school on how the community could take action against AIDS. The intervention program was implemented over the course of a 2- to 3-month period, averaging about 20 school hours per class.

Outcome Measures

1. Repeated measure design (baseline and follow-up)
2. Process evaluation

Evaluation of Intervention Activities

Not many health promotion intervention projects have been done in Africa considering the extent of the problem and compared to industrial countries like the United States. The different intervention activities reported on Africa include more commonly awareness campaigns, distribution of educational materials, the development of new educational materials like photocomics or board game, drama and theatre, training of peers, condom promotion and less commonly training of professionals including traditional healers, HIV testing, small group discussions and individual counseling. Most intervention activities perceived to be most effective in this sample have also been found in other studies to result in knowledge, attitude, and behavior change (Janz et al., 1996). Drama, theatre and photocomics and multifaceted intervention activities have been reported as particularly effective in African contexts (Bosompra. 1991/92; Dalrymple & Du Toit, 1993; Klepp et al., 1997; Toroyan & Reddy, 1997/98). Learning theory suggests that people are more likely to learn when messages are presented in multiple formats using different communication strategies (Clark, 1987). Due to a lack of studies reported in the literature, no more detailed evaluation on the different health promotion intervention activities in Africa could be done.

However, several researchers have reported that a large body about HIV prevention, which has been applied to condom promotion campaigns and the reduction of sexual partners in developed countries, is available (Campbell, 1997; Janz et al., 1996). These approaches have not been used in a wide scale in African countries. Janz et al. (1996) evaluated 37 AIDS prevention projects in the United States identifying the following intervention activities as more effective: (1) Small group discussions [talk freely, repetition of messages, learn from each other and health educator, make social comparisons, building group norms, developing social support networks]; (2) Outreach to high risk populations (more in adults) [rewards & enticements with appropriate cultural cues]; (3) Training of peers and volunteers (more in youth) [behavioral and attitudinal role models, reinforcement and shaping group norms] and less effective: (i) Provision of safer-sex kits (more in adults); (ii) Large-group discussions; (iii) Support groups; and (iv) Individual counseling.

References

Airhihenbuwa, C. O. (1989). Perspectives on AIDS in Africa: Strategies for prevention and control. *AIDS Education and Prevention*, 1: 57-69.

Bosompra, K. (1991/92). The potential of drama and songs as channels for AIDS education in Africa: A report on focus group findings from Ghana. *International Quarterly of Community Health Education,* 12: 317-342.

Campbell, T. (1997). How can psychological theory help promote condom use in sub-Saharan African developing countries. *Journal of the Royal Society of Health,* 117, 186-191.

Clark, N. M. (1987). Social learning theory in current health education practice. *Advances in Health Education and Promotion*, 2: 251-275.

Dalrymple, L., & Du Toit, M. K. (1993). The evaluation of a drama approach to AIDS education. *Educational Psychology,* 13: 147-154.

Eagle, G. T., & Brouard, P. W. (1995). AIDS education for health professionals. *South African Journal of Psychology,* 25: 21-16.

Elkins, D. B., Kuyyakanond, T., Maticka-Tyndale, E., Rujkorakarn, D., & Haswell-Elkins, M. (1996). Multisectoral strategy for AIDS prevention at community level. *World Health Forum*, 17: 70-74.

Fisher, J. D., & Fisher, W. A. (1992). A general social psychological model for changing HIV risk behavior. *Psychological Bulletin,* 111: 455-474.

Green, E. C., Zokwe, B., & Dupree, J. D. (1995). The experience of an AIDS prevention program focused on South African traditional healers. *Social Science & Medicine,* 40: 503-515.

Janz, N. K., Zimmerman, M. A., Israel, B. A., Freudenberg, N., & Carter, R. J. (1996). Evaluation of 37 AIDS prevention projects: Successful approaches and barriers to program effectiveness. *Health Education Quarterly,* 23: 80-97.

Hubley, J. H. (1988). AIDS in Africa: a challenge to health education. *Health Education Research,* 3: 41-47.

Kagimu, M., Marum, E., Wabwire-Mangen, F., Nakyanjo, N., Walakira, Y., & Hogle, J. (1998). Evaluation of the effectiveness of AIDS health education interventions in the Muslim community in Uganda. *AIDS Education and Prevention,* 10: 215-228.

Kawewe, S. M. (1996). Social-networking Zimbabwean families: An African traditional approach to waging a war against HIV/AIDS. *Social Development Issues*, 18: 34-51.

Klepp, K. I., Ndeki, S. S., Leshbari, M. T., Hannan, P. J., & Lyimo, B. A. (1997). AIDS education in Tanzania: Promoting risk reduction among primary school children. *American Journal of Public Health*, 87: 1931-1936.

Kuhn, L., Steinberg, M., & Mathews, C. (1994). Participation of the school community in AIDS education: An evaluation of a high school program in South Africa. *AIDS CARE,* 6: 161-171.

Lagarde, E., Pison, G., & Enel, C. (1997). Improvement in AIDS knowledge, perceptions and risk behaviors over a short period in a rural community of Senegal. *International Journal of STD & AIDS,* 8: 681-687.

Laver, S. M. L., Van der Borne, B., & Kok, G. (1995). Using theory to design an intervention for HIV/AIDS prevention in farm workers in rural Zimbabwe. *International Quarterly of Community Health Education*, 15: 349-362.

Livingston, I. L. (1992). AIDS/HIV crisis in developing countries: the need for greater understanding and innovative health promotion approaches. *Journal of the National Medical Association*, 84: 755-770.

Livingston, I. L. (1993). HIV/AIDS control in Africa: The importance of epidemiological and health promotion approaches. *Health Promotion International*, 8: 189-198.

MacLachlan, M. (1996). Identifying problems in community health promotion: An illustration of the Nominal Group Technique in AIDS education. *Journal of the Royal Society of Health*, 116, 143-148.

MacLachlan, M., Chimombo, M., & Mpemba, N. (1997). AIDS education for youth through active learning: A school-based approach from Malawi. *International Journal of Educational Development*, 17: 41-50.

McKenna, S. L., Muyinda, G. K., Roth, D., Mwali, M., Ng'andu, N., Myrick, A., Luo, C., Priddy, F. H., Hall, V. M., Von Lieven, A. A., Sabatino, J. R., Mark, K., & Allen, S. A. (1997). Rapid HIV testing and counseling for voluntary testing centers in Africa. *AIDS*, 11: 103-110.

Moses, S., & Plummer, F. A. (1994). Health education, counseling and the underlying causes of the HIV epidemic in sub-Saharan Africa. *AIDS CARE*, 6: 123-128.

Moses, S., Plummer, F. A., Ngugi, E. N., Nagelkerke, N. J. et al. (1991). Controlling HIV in Africa: Effectiveness and cost of an intervention in a high-frequency STD transmitter core group. *AIDS*, 5: 407-411.

Ng'weshemi, J., Boerma, T., Bennett, J., & Schapink, D. (eds.) (1997). *HIV prevention and AIDS care in Africa: A district level approach.* Amsterdam: Royal

Tropical Institute.

Olayinka, B. A., & Osho, A. A. (1997). Changes in attitude, sexual behavior and the risk of HIV/AIDS transmission in Southwest Nigeria. *East African Medical Journal*, 74: 554-560.

O'Leary, A., DiClemente, R. J., & Aral, S. O. (1997). Reflections on the design and reporting of STD/HIV behavioral intervention research. *AIDS Education and Prevention,* 9 (Supplement A): 1-14.

Peltzer, K., Hira, S. K., Wadhawan, D., Kamamga, J., Ferguson, D. C. E., & Perine, P. L. (1989). Psychosocial counseling of patients infected with human immunodeficiency virus (HIV) in Lusaka, Zambia. *Tropical Doctor*, 19: 164-168.

Pickering, H., Quigley, M., Pepin, J., Todd, J. et al. (1993). The effects of post-test counseling on condom use among prostitutes in The Gambia. *AIDS*, 7: 271-273.

Scott, S. J., & Mercer, M. A. (1994). Understanding cultural obstacles to HIV/AIDS prevention in Africa. *AIDS Education and Prevention*, 6: 81-89.

Skinner, D., Metcalf, C. A., Seager, J. R., DeSwart, J. S., & Laubscher, J. A. (1991). An evaluation of an education program on HIV infection using puppetry and street theatre. *AIDS CARE*, 3: 317-329.

Toroyan, T., & Reddy, P. S. (1997/98). Participation of South African youth in the design and development of AIDS photocomics. *International Quarterly of Community Health Education*, 17: 131-146.

Ulin, P. R. (1992). African women and AIDS: Negotiating behavioral change. *Social Science & Medicine*, 34: 63-73.

Visser, M. (1996). Evaluation of the First AIDS Kit, the AIDS and lifestyle education program for teenagers. *South African Journal of Psychology*, 26: 103-113.

Wilson, D., Wilson, C., Greenspan, R., Sibanda, P. et al. (1989). Towards an AIDS information strategy for Zimbabwe. *AIDS Education and Prevention*, 1: 96-104.

Ziglio, E. (1997). How to move towards evidence-based health promotion interventions. *Promotion & Education*, 4: 29-33.

Chapter 15

Comprehensive and Integrated HIV/AIDS Prevention Campaigns: Potentials for South and Southern Africa

Keyan G. Tomaselli
Arnold Shepperson
University of Natal, Durban, South Africa

Warren Parker
Society of Family Health, South Africa

Worldwide, there is no single example of a national media campaign that has demonstrably reversed HIV infection trends, yet such campaigns remain the centerpiece of many government responses. At the core of the problem lies the assumption that knowledge and awareness lead to behavior change, and that, with careful attention to appropriate message-making, greater impact can be achieved. Media campaigns do readily achieve objectives of "knowledge and awareness", but it is the terrain beyond that awareness, that is harder to achieve.

The HIV pandemic, and the contexts that frame it are seldom understood within a theoretical whole. HIV is a complex disease with medical, socio-economic and cultural dimensions.

Behavior Change

The starting point for many campaigns is the notion of behavior change. This approach is based on the assumption that within each sector of society there are individuals whose existing sexual practices place them at risk of contracting HIV, and that through provision of information and education, alongside resources at local level, these individuals can be empowered to adopt safer sexual practices. Such notions of behavior change are problematic on a number of counts.

Firstly, many unsafe sexual practices take place within a complex interplay of socio-economic and cultural dimensions. These include, for example, diversities in language, poverty, unemployment, poor education, an inferior social position of women, rapid urbanization, labor migration, crime, political instability, rape and sexual harassment, sexual abuse of children, cultural practices such as dry sex and circumcision, limited health infrastructure, poor communications infrastructure, and the like. Sexual activity within such contexts is not always a matter of individual choice, nor simply a means for sexual gratification. Instead sex may occur by force, or as a means for economic survival, or as a function of distorted social contexts.

In South Africa there is growing concern around the high prevalence of rape and sexual harassment, where women are subjected to violent sexual assaults that expose them to HIV, other sexually transmitted diseases, and pregnancy. Labor migration has long been a cornerstone of economic life in South Africa, yet the social context that underpins it is a virtual recipe for HIV infection. Men and women are separated from their homes, families and loved ones for many months at a time, with the majority ensconced in single sex hostels near their places of work. Inevitably, leisure activities include the consumption of alcohol, cannabis smoking, and a prevalence of casual and unsafe sex.

Over and above potential infection in this milieu, wives and partners who remain at home are vulnerable to infection when their partners return. Similarly, economic activities such as commercial sex work (both formal and informal) and long-distance truck driving are internationally recognized and extensively documented as providing contexts for high-risk sexual activity. Rapid urbanization is often combined with limited access to adequate housing and employment. Burgeoning unsanitary and under-resourced shanty towns near urban centers tend to be framed by depressed social contexts that contribute to unsafe sexual activity. Furthermore, within such contexts the provision of resources such as condoms and resources for the treatment of sexually transmitted diseases, is often limited, thus sealing the fate of millions of people.

Clearly such contextual factors problematise the notion of behavior change. Within such contexts individuals are disempowered and have limited control over many aspects of life - sexual and otherwise. The prevention of HIV infection within such contexts requires a multi-faceted approach that emerges from theoretical and practical understanding of socio-economic and cultural contexts.

This is not a simple challenge, for it requires not only intervention at the level of knowledge and awareness, but also the timeous application of radical interventions that transcend the oft slow pace of change. Furthermore, such change can only occur within a consensual framework, and thus requires that all interventions have at their core, active participation and endorsement of the communities they seek to change.

A further problematic within the behavior change conundrum is that of the notion of risk. The vast majority of international campaigns have tended to focus on groups that are at high risk of infection. International data suggests that there is a certain inevitability in the infection patterns of these groups, with the vast majority becoming infected in spite of interventions. Much of this trend can obviously be attributed to the socio-economic and cultural contexts outlined above.

Depicted graphically, infections within such high-risk groups tend to grow exponentially, and then decline as the manifestations of the epidemic become tangible through visible illness and death within the community at risk. Infection levels peak and then gradually decline over time. Of urgent concern however, are the trends amongst the low-risk groups. With these groups there is a gradual but consistent rise in levels of infection, and trends suggest that this "second epidemic" amongst those at low risk may transcend the levels prevalent in high-risk groups. There is little theoretical clarity regarding which individuals, groups and communities constitute those at low risk. Obviously those who enjoy socio-economic and cultural contexts that are less compromised are included.

Analyzed in terms of sexual practice those at low risk would include individuals who practice serial monogamy, who use condoms relatively consistently, who have sex by choice rather than as a function of their contexts, and, importantly, those who are not yet sexually active. This latter group is particularly important in terms of understanding the notion of behavior change. Adolescents and young adults make up the majority of this group, and as a whole require somewhat of an inversion of the notion of behavior change. What is required is not behavior change, but rather a commitment to delayed onset of sexual activity, or to the establishment safer sexual practices from the onset of sexual activity.

It is well understood that behavior change is a complex process, defined both by contextual factors, and by personal commitment. Adoption of safer sexual strategies by adolescents and young adults is obviously also framed by contextual factors, for example limited access to condoms, that undermine concerted action, but does offer potential at the level of personal commitment.

Strategies can be led at national level, for example through the provision of "Family Life Education" in schools, but have to go hand in hand with adolescent friendly resources that allow easy access to condoms and other reproductive health resources. Research amongst adolescents in South Africa also suggests the importance of an integrated approach where educational and resource interventions should not focus only on HIV, but have a broader reproductive health focus that includes sexual biology, physical development, sexuality, pregnancy and contraception, HIV and STD prevention, and skills in accessing resources.

Broad-Based Strategies

National policy related to HIV in South Africa emerged through years of extensive negotiation amongst a coalition of AIDS organizations under the banner of NACOSA (National AIDS Convention of South Africa). Following the political transition a specialized directorate – the HIV/AIDS and STD Program – was established within the Department of Health in 1994. Key strategies recommended by NACOSA were integrated into the directorate. These included:

Life skills education targeted at youth:

- mass media campaigns to popularize prevention concepts and to reduce stigma and discrimination;
- improved STD care through appropriate treatment and management;
- increased access to barrier methods;
- the development of guidelines for the provision of appropriate levels of care and support.

These strategies obviously offer a viable framework for a prevention and care infrastructure. However their implementation over the 1995-1996 period was undermined by a range of constraints including staff limitations, poor management, inappropriate emphases, poor coordination within national government departments, amongst provincial governments and non-governmental organizations, and the influence of political imperatives.

In many ways these limitations can be attributed to insufficiencies in theoretical understanding, further undermined by limited capacity to deliver at a practical level. Obviously, failures need to be contextualized within the process of history, from which lessons learned can be integrated into subsequent strategies. There were however, some spectacular bungles, particularly within the media key strategy. A number of interventions were driven from ministerial level with little consultation. The most compromised of these was the pursuit of a "Broadway standard" stage play, *Sarafina II*, which sought to utilize the skills of internationally acclaimed South African playwright, Mbongeni Ngema. The political endorsement of this project, combined with overenthusiastic "fast-tracking" of financial procedures, poor accounting and monitoring procedures, and scant consultation with the HIV/AIDS directorate, nor the AIDS movement as a whole, resulted in unnecessary expenditure in the region of R10-million, and extensive compromise of the Department of Health, and AIDS prevention activities across all sectors.

Other interventions included the pursuit of an existing tender for billboards and the recruitment of a foreign video crew to produce a series of public service announcements. Both interventions were poorly contextualized within a broader strategy, and neither was able to make any significant contribution to awareness and prevention activities.

Activities in other key strategies were similarly constrained, and whilst discussion of these falls outside of the ambit of this chapter, it is worth recognising the potential for two further key strategies that may contribute to the development of a holistic overall strategy. These would be:

- training of health workers in issues related to the HIV/AIDS pandemic, and in the crucial area of non-judgmental and efficient service delivery;
- national coordination across all key strategies to ensure that national government departments, provincial governments, non-governmental organizations and other formations can act in concert.

Towards a Coherent Media Strategy

There are obviously no clear answers as to what a national government media campaign should be. At very least, what is required is the provision of a "backdrop" to the epidemic whereby public interest and awareness is maintained, without attempting to intervene at community level. The latter task is better served by provincial governments, non-governmental organizations and other formations that function closer to the "grassroots".

The role of local government cannot be ignored either, because this arm of government most directly represents and serves the people most at risk. Conversely, national government is the only agency sufficiently resourced to mount a national media campaign of requisite magnitude. This is not, however, a recommendation for independent activity. The content and emphases of such campaigns should allow for reflection and evaluation by key role-players nationally, with reference to on-the-ground activities.

Clearly, media campaigns can only be relevant when they contextualize a sound base of resources and services. Even if the cost and content of *Sarafina II*, for example, were deemed appropriate, the play would have had little relevance within the existing resource deficient context.

A Multilateral Approach

AIDS is an international problem compounded by high migrancy, at both sub-national and international levels. It is well understood that the HIV/AIDS pandemic ignores borders, and a media campaign run by any national government should ideally enjoy collaboration with neighboring countries. In South Africa this would include complementary strategies with the SADC countries (Zaffiro 1997).

Any media campaign should be conducted within the framework of an activated national strategy. This strategy should encompass at least the five actions of health promotion:

- development of healthy public policy;
- creating supportive environments;
- developing personal skills;
- supporting community action, and
- reorienting the health services.

Communication should be one aspect of this whole plan.

National campaigns must be developed in conjunction with provincial and local campaigns. Provincial and local campaigns should respond to local interpretive communities, but the key is to ensure that both the national and the respective provincial campaigns are conceptually interlinked in terms of a recognizable logo, jingles and the like which generate instant recognition of messages relating to AIDS.

Professional communicators should be contracted to undertake the campaign, particularly given that skills and resources to deliver key elements of the campaign are not present within the government infrastructure. It should also be recognized that there are numerous formations that actively promote awareness of HIV/AIDS and related issues. The impact of these formations needs to be recognized and should be seen as collaborative agencies that can be integrated into a broad national strategy.

Funds and resources should be devolved to small media producers at local level, i.e. a grassroots approach which empowers, for example, local drama groups, artists, musicians and cultural groups. Locally-based producers are also able to be more in touch with local communities, so at national level, messages may be standardized, but at local level these can be framed by local linguistic and socio-cultural perspectives.

Given that behavior change, or the adoption of safer sexual strategies cannot be brought about simply by access to information, but rather, are contextualized by the socio-economic and cultural milieu, it is clear that prevention activities need to be viewed on the longer term, with change being entrenched over a generation or more. Quite simply, there are no quick fixes.

But even generational change is contingent upon multi-media, multi-faceted and ongoing long-term integrated campaigns which directly connect media messages and educational campaigns with health delivery and comprehensive patient service. Furthermore, entrenched shifts in sexual activity can only be ensured if there are concomitant shifts within socio-economic and cultural contexts, and thus national efforts outside the direct parameters of reproductive health are equally important. Whether socio-economic phenomena such as migrant labor, commercial sex work and the like, can be modified timeously to achieve benefits in terms of entrenching lower risk sexual activities remains to be seen.

It is important to realize that at least three independent yet coordinated campaigns will have to be conducted simultaneously.

1. Orientive campaigns targeting children, adolescents and young

adults that reorient the socialization process towards critical awareness and empowerment around reproductive health, amongst other life skills.

2. Regulative campaigns for older adults, that may be more rhetorical in nature, but that also have an orientation towards critical awareness and empowerment, but that recognize the complexities of the socio-economic and cultural milieu.
3. Constitutive campaigns for communities within which traditional patterns of deference and respect are maintained. In these situations, the AIDS campaign must focus on ways in which these patterns can be reconstituted. The main issue here is traditional gender roles, privileges vested in authorities, and so on. Firstly, these may clash with the more democratic pattern of mutual rights needed for dealing with inculcating new patterns of conduct in the youngest generation. Secondly, a change in behavior in the second generation could redefine relations of authority which are (or are claimed to be) traditional. Again, mechanisms for promoting critical awareness and empowerment within communities would form part of such campaigns.

Within such campaigns, access to resources related to reproductive health are crucial. Two very basic requirements at national level are:

a. ***Condoms.*** The Department of Health procures millions of condoms annually for distribution through government clinics, hospitals, government run AIDS Training and Information Centers and some workplaces. For this to be effective considerable attention is required for condom logistics and distribution guidelines, "e.g. condoms should be transported and stored correctly; condoms should be distributed freely and non-judgementally by staff; training in correct use should be provided, etc. Complementary condom distribution is best achieved through social marketing "a non-governmental, non-profit approach that uses commercial infrastructures and marketing techniques to ensure availability of low-cost condoms in diverse outlets including pharmacies, doctors surgeries, supermarkets, cafe's, spaza shops, shebeens, bars, hotels and hair salons, amongst others.

In South Africa, social marketing of condoms is managed by the Society for Family Health, an affiliate of the Washington-based Population Services International (PSI). PSI run similar projects some 40 countries internationally, and successfully distribute millions of condoms and other health products each year. A basic infrastructure f or the provision of free female condoms in selected clinics has been pursued by the HIV/AIDS Directorate, but the successful implementation of this new technology requires considerable training of both users and service providers, and will take some years for effective integration as an optional barrier method.

b. ***Sexually Transmitted Disease Services.*** STD infection is losely associated with higher potential for HIV transmission. STD treatment is provided through state clinics, but is hampered by poor information support on the one hand, and the complexities of service delivery within a resource deficient context on the other.

c. ***National coordination across all key strategies to ensure that national government departments, provincial governments, non-governmental organizations and other formations can actin concert.*** In terms of a media campaign this approach suggests sufficient consultation and agreement on elements such as logos, key messages and strategies. At national level government would be tasked with providing a "backdrop" to the campaign with substantive foreground (grassroots) activities being provided through provincial, regional and local governments, organizations, and formations.

Campaign Expectations

The AIDS crisis in South Africa occurs in a context of broad societal and cultural transformation. There could be huge gains in linking AIDS provision campaigns to the mobilizing power of democratic values and human rights. This would increase people's ability to see the connection between a "rights issue" and their health, thus cutting across differences of heritage and culture. Similarly, the linking of HIV/AIDS and STDs to other reproductive health issues such as contraception, abortion, pre- and post-natal care, sexuality and sexual health, amongst others, will promote a framework for critical awareness and empowerment.

The cultural environment is more complex. Cultural dynamics tend to work in terms of generations, and action taken in the present will only have measurable impact in an indeterminate future. The campaign, therefore, cannot afford to make ANY kind of claim about what it will achieve. The watchwords are perseverance and adaptability. The campaign has to be open to understanding and acting upon relevant aspects of cultural transition. It has to be expected that certain groups will find that an emerging safer-sex culture clashes with their immediate interests, and will react by developing counter-measures. It is unlikely that every such interest-group can be identified now. Therefore it is necessary to build the widest possible flexibility into the strategy so that unexpected challenges can be met without undue stress to the overall policy.

The key to this flexibility lies in the extent to which the media component of the strategy meshes with the activity of non-health institutions Interest groups which perceive an effective AIDS strategy as a threat are likely to arise in unexpected sites which do not necessarily affect the health sector directly. Thus the major factor affecting the long-term success of the struggle against AIDS requires and institutionalized communications strategy. This involves the ongoing formal exchange of information between different institutional sectors.

Key Components to a Media Campaign

Conceptual Coherence

Current campaigns have been developed on an ad hoc basis by individual agencies working by themselves using various logos, media, messages, strategies and locations. Despite the excellent work being done by many of these agencies, there is little evidence of a coordinated campaign which draws on this local knowledge and experience. This does not rule out the participation of individual agencies: it simply points to the need f or all media sectors to act in concert.

Strategic Audience Targeting

State sponsored campaigns aimed its media at only one audience or interpretive community: the mass audience. This mass cannot be defined with any precision at all, as suggested by the unfocused campaigns centered on billboards, posters and *Sarafina II*. No audience research had been done, and no understanding of media consumption has been generated to measure the cost-effectiveness of this kind of ad hoc communication. Furthermore, campaign activities were uncoordinated within themselves. Communication/health groups which do offer media which start from the cultural, social an health assumptions of local and national communities is being done. This involves "small" media producers (video, pamphlets, booklets, posters, comics, puppets, participatory theatre, community radio programming), of in conjunction with health workers, social workers, teachers and the like, interacting with small groups which develop messages on a bottom-up basis by facilitating these forms of expression incorporating real messages. Examples include Dramaide participatory theatre, Action Media approaches to participatory development of small media undertaken by the Society for Family Health, and participatory development of illustrated and photo-comic books as undertaken by the Storyteller and Balisa groups.

Initiatives like *Soul City* television and radio series start with national big media (radio, TV) which reach mass audiences and then build their secondary campaigns using print media (comics, booklets, newspapers and so on.) While the structure and management of the *Soul City* campaign is big-media top-down, its message making is to some extent, bottom-up. Messages are developed through extensive consultation with organizations and other formations active in the field, and incorporate pretesting and review by target audiences.

The problem facing these civil society NGO media producers however, have include difficulties in obtaining funding and lack of integration into other national strategies. A campaign that sees national activities as providing a "backdrop" and small and localized media activities and functioning in the "foreground" could fund small media vis-a-vis national objectives, provided they are linked conceptually.

Initial activities require deep understanding of intended target audiences and interpretive communities: Who do we want to reach in each generational group? What are the linguistic and cultural characteristics of these audiences? What media and what kinds of messages are best suited to these audiences? What resources can these audiences access to entrench the validity of messages?

It is necessary to modify messages according to interpretive frames and ways of making sense of interpretive communities, each of which occupy diverse linguistic, geographic, economic and cultural milieu's. However, key elements of the national campaign such as logos, jingles and the like should be maintained.

It is obviously impossible to analyze interpretive communities and resources nationally. Rather this task should be devolved to provincial, regional and local structures that re-orient messages accordingly. This is no simple task, for it requires that resources be provided to facilitate the development of teams that might include health workers, media workers, sociologists, psychologists, anthropologists and other technical experts who are able to elicit the relevant data and act upon it timeously and efficiently.

Coherence Across Institutions

It is crucial that the media strategy be backed up by effective cooperation from all sectors. It is no good telling vulnerable women that they can and ought to say "no", when there is no institutional arm which can back up their right to refuse. Examples of this kind of co-ordination include:

- Social welfare: assisting women to manage without recourse to sexually exploitative relationships;
- Safety and security: credible response to, and protection against, rape, sexual harassment, child abuse and other forms of exploitation;
- Effective and coherent reaction to myths that typically distort and undermine effective prevention and management strategies;
- Provision of care and support for infected individuals that are practical in terms of health resources (e.g. home-based care);
- Demystifying and normalizing HIV infection, breaking down discrimination and secrecy around the disease;
- International links with immediate neighbors, continental and world bodies such as the Organization of African Unity (OAU), and various arms of the United Nations (UN);
- Interaction and formal/informal links with broad-based initiatives that seek to bring about change within the contextual milieu that facilitate HIV and STD infection.

Engagement with Social Reality

Media campaigns have to be developed around the reality of Southern Africa's social conditions. "Community" has to be understood in a non-romantic way, recognizing that people's mobility (for a majority, the mobility of labor migrancy) makes them members of many different groups across a variety of locations. This "membership" can place individuals in contradictory situations, creating a conflict between norms from one context to another.

Messages therefore will need to focus on the general democratic values of freedom and life. Freedom is the value in terms of which people are necessarily valued as ends in themselves, and not as mere means to the ends of another. Life is the value in terms of which people's endowments are raised into talents, in ways that protect, or even promote, the freedom of others. In a situation like that in South Africa, migrancy can lead to conflicting interpretations between different sets of local norms and rules.

Campaigns must thus incorporate the idea that fighting AIDS is a democratic obligation on the part of all.

Directness

Messages must stress the non-cultural nature of AIDS. AIDS is not some kind of race, class or party-political plot designed to disempower the poor. It strikes across all cultural boundaries and there is no cure. It is important to distinguish between different elements of media activity:

- awareness raising elements of media
- educational programs
- mass media
- small media.

A television series like *Soul City*, for example, contributes to awareness raising. Productions like this do not have the potential to change behavior without secondary reinforcement from other social formations.

Other media and direct education programs are required to build on the awareness created by such expressions, and require backup from resources on the ground.

Broad-based Definition of "Media"

The campaign has to avoid concentrating only on high-tech, high-cost national media systems like TV and radio. These are big media, and have the disadvantage of not always connecting with people's local experience and cultures. Thus the focus has to include small media which can be developed and in consultation and collaboration with target communities. The approach needs to be seen in terms of "broad" government, rather than the standard debates about "big" or "small" government strategies. At the national level, therefore, the message has to be formulated as a framework or "backdrop" rather than as a single campaign. National government's role is thus strategic and not pragmatic, directed more at facilitating than actually producing.

The national aspect of the AIDS campaign should be a coordinating one. This involves:

- keeping open the lines of communication between different agencies so that the relevant information is speedily available for use by media practitioners;
- maintenance of fiscal discipline by regional government; and
- acting as an agent of equity, topping up the resources of disadvantaged regions either directly from the fiscus or indirectly by transferring institutional resources on a more or less permanent basis.

There needs to be an approach at the regional level which curtails the possibility of ideological hijacking of the strategy in the form of campaigns which turn AIDS into a party-political football, or that are that are driven by political imperatives for perceived political benefit. The broad governmental approach has to incorporate the strengths of the American "politics of bipartisanship" in a multipartisan environment. Strategies must thus reflect a consensus nationally while permitting a plurality of message texts reflecting the realities of local contexts. Must also avoid the tendency for messages to become watered down in the reaching of consensus, as the price of accommodating interest groups" voting power. Both cultural and social issues are at stake here, and the politics has to reflect a future-directed task based in the human condition and not in sectional interest.

Constructing the Message

"One Message - Many Media"

The text containing a single message can be conceived in as many ways as there are creative practitioners in the media. Each media organization can therefore develop production approaches to the texts which most effectively use the relevant medium. Each media distribution organization – whether this is the same as the production organization or separate from it – can then present the transmitted message in the way that is most effective in its experience.

Campaigns are effective, however, to the extent to which those to whom messages are addressed actually change their attitudes and conduct. Thus the stress on "many media" takes into account the fact that people receive messages in many ways in their everyday lives, and furthermore, that messages should link individuals and groups to relevant resources. This can be achieved, for example, through telephone helplines, addresses and contact details of services formations active in their geographic location.

To the extent that there is a plurality of audiences at any one time, then, people will reconstruct a message in ways conditioned by what they are doing, where they are, and so on. Thus the way in which a given message is taken in by an audience incorporates an element of negotiation: people will talk about what they have heard and/or seen while they were busy, and come to some kind of consensus as to what the message was about. It is important therefore, that messages be understood as being largely subjective, with varying interpretations, and varying interpretive contexts with meaning being coalesced through a combination of dialogue, reflection, critical awareness and action.

The effectiveness or otherwise of the message becomes evident in the way people's conversation, conduct and so on form a social message which can be monitored by resource formations on the ground, and through formal research. This "chain of meaning" can only be marginally tracked on a large scale, because the specificities of local social message construction actually gives rise to a multiplicity of negotiation communities.

Smaller media make it possible for the perceived social meaning of a message to be conveyed directly (or almost directly) back into the creative side of the media development formation. Monitoring of the effectiveness of a campaign thus becomes easier, because local media formations can more readily develop and maintain contact with their audience(s) than a single centralized one. Local media formations are often made up of people who are part of the communities to whom they are broadcasting (printing, etc.).

Messages can thus be adapted, reconceived, reprogrammed, and so on, rapidly in response to actual events. The "teleported" text of any message in local – scale media is therefore more likely to reflect the impact of a campaign more readily than would be the case with mass texts disseminated nationally or provincially.

This kind of approach allows the strategic formulation of campaigns to focus on the relevant areas of orientation, constitution and regulation outlined above. For the youngest generation, the message is necessarily new, and is part of their encounter with the world. For the second generation, messages conform or clash with norms and rules of conduct which are part of their experience of the world. The form of the message is thus not discovery, but rhetoric. Finally, for the eldest generation (and the others to a lesser extent), messages have to mesh with or challenge people's intelligibility of the world they have both encountered and experienced in their lives. The message form is much more political and discursive in this instance.

Advantages of this Approach

The above approach offers the following benefits:
A balance between content reinforcement and identification, and variety across media so that the same message gets the exposure best suited to each medium:

- Instantly recognizable logo's and jingles across all media which link and reinforce all messages;
- Movement of the message closer to the target market without losing the character of the product. Repetition with freshness of variety, centered to a campaign which will always be recognizable no matter the audience;
- Newness and specificity – dynamic and tracked to keep campaign fresh and engaged with new developments arising from unexpected quarters;
- Local focus keeps message moving between two poles of identity on the one hand and aspiration on the other. The campaign must have role models who are both recognizable and aspirational – everyone wants to move up and out, but cannot move if the aspiration is not believable. It adds recognition of the "I" of reception, while clearly reinforcing the "we" of the target communities;
- Appeals to values greater than the individual – e.g. National priorities (AIDS is the new Struggle, etc.) It raises awareness that democratic values are limited to those of freedom and life, and that the plurality of democratic life lies in the non-contradictory interpretation of these values in the form of local or regional norms and rules. In many ways, the recent political transition in South Africa is extremely important in that it reinforces the notion that tangible and rapid change is realizable. In this way the socio-cultural context can be seen as malleable;
- Can include relevant life-skills and link individuals and groups to resources;
- Effectively avoids the mass-media tendency to pitch texts at the "lowest common denominator" definition of an audience;
- Should help the public construct the disease as a community

concept, not taking an individual victim blaming approach.

Kinds of Media

The choice of which media to use when and in what areas and communities is not an either/or choice. The different big and small media and programs need to be coordinated into a single campaign which have regional inflections and orientations. The media which could be used include:

Logo

A visual icon that that provides a linking mechanism between visual media products, that builds on existing iconic values (e.g. red-ribbon), or that derives meaning through application and repetition.

Jingles

One catchy tune and catchphrase immediately reinforces the logo across both big and small media.

Oramedia

Oral communication such as found in rural and informal settlement networks.

Group/Participatory Media

This includes innovative approaches such as Dramaide, which ensures high levels of participation in locally contextualized theatre/drama, or Action Media which employs focus group and participatory techniques to integrate local perspectives into the development of community-based small media. Within such approaches participants are able make their own messages while working with facilitators, and incorporates local linguistic and socio-cultural perspectives. Participants in message making, and their parallel interpretive communities are more likely to internalize messages because they are framed by reflection and critical awareness. Intensive message making and reception analysis is possible. Such activities often contribute to spontaneous peer awareness and resource access activities, and may develop an impetus that is independent of the initial intervention. Participants are more often drawn from adolescent and young adult groups and often evince strong commitment to behavior change or to the adoption of safer sexual strategies. These approaches draw on the educational theories of Paulo Freire and performance strategies of Augusto Boal. These approaches can be conducted by various formations active at local level, for example, non-governmental organizations active in health promotion, AIDS activists, staff within local government, and the like.

Face-to-Face

Like participatory theatre, face-to-face campaigns make a lasting impression, memorability and comprehension. This kind of communication continues in a more conventional format the groundwork established by participatory theatre. This involves health workers, teachers and religious workers in more intensive information-based campaigns in specific sites like schools, villages. In clinics, for example, this kind of communication relates directly to counseling and treatment protocols for client management.

In a similar way role model behavior is built into the dramatic dialogue and action in *Soul City* which creates awareness and legitimizes specific actions.

Drama/Theatre

Such big media interventions are not the same as participatory theatre. Participatory theatre is bottom-up, involving communities, is grassroots-oriented and empowering at local levels, usually within larger regions and administrative structures. This is a continuous process involving a variety of supporting agencies - health, educational, cultural and so on.

Big media drama tends to be top-down, authoritarian, non-involving and non-empowering, although can incorporate relevant and emotive artistic perspectives. Where participatory theatre is part of a process and confers agency upon its participants, big media drama is usually a once-off event. Whilst it may confer critical awareness during presentation, impetus of such awareness tends to diminish rapidly unless incorporated into local resources, formations and infrastructures.

Outdoor (Hoardings, Murals, Pavement Art, etc.)

Constant reinforcement of the prime nationally mediated message can be achieved through the ability of such media to provide visual reinforcement. Billboards offer immediacy, but are complex and expensive to produce. Within the South African context of competitive access to billboards, prime sites are not readily available. Murals and other art forms, when they incorporate local artists and other local participation, can express messages that are contextualized by local linguistic and socio-cultural milieu's and readily contribute to dialogue and critical awareness.

Pamphlets, Comics, Posters, etc.

These small media can be used to reinforce all of the media channels used. They have a longer life than radio and TV and have an appeal that is often independent of literacy and educational levels. Stories, narrative strategies and images can be inflected in terms of local or regional ways of making sense, cultural preferences and cosmologies.

Radio

Radio can be utilized across a range of geographic and contextual target areas. The medium provides for effective reach of the medium into both urban and rural areas and is extremely effective in delivering complex messages delivered through, for example, drama or dialogue, as well as the repetitive delivery of short key messages, jingles and songs.

Community radio is extremely effective in that allows for recognition of local linguistic and socio-cultural contexts and can provide an important linking role for locally available resources and infrastructures. For example, weekly call-in shows run by the Society for Family Health in Soweto have allowed for extensive locally contextualized dialogue around issues of sexuality and facilitated resource seeking by listeners.

Television

This complex medium offers the potential for complex messaging and high recall. Production of programming is costly and broadcasts are often once off. The *Soul City* series effectively harnesses this medium at national level to generate insights into a range of social issues including reproductive health. Benefits of such programming can be extended through localized playback (e.g. VCR) within formal or informal contexts and can be used to further stimulate reflection, critical awareness and action. Many government clinics, for example, have access to VCRs and would be able to play *Soul City* programs; mobile video units could be utilized to incorporate such programming into interactive events in resource deficient contexts where television is not available; and emerging initiatives around community television could incorporate elements of such programming to provide links to local resources.

Electronic Information Media

These intermediate media e.g. interactive CD-ROM and video programming offer potential to encourage problem solving and critical insights and can be seen as supplementary to other messaging.

Combined Media and Resources

There are few established formats but an interesting example of this approach initiated as part of the 1995 AIDS media campaign enjoyed considerable success. This involved the display of signage on minibus taxis combined with the distribution of free condoms within the taxis and training of drivers in basic HIV/AIDS and condom awareness. Commuters were thus able to engage drivers in dialogue, and were able to access the basic means for prevention. This approach was fairly costly in that signage space is rented, and only a small proportion of the national taxi fleet (400 out of an estimated 100,000 taxis) could be accessed. The process did however facilitate the normalization of condoms, and enjoyed considerable supplementary media coverage nationally and internationally as a result of the innovative approach.

Similarly, the provision of user friendly condom distribution boxes, combined with client friendly services at clinics, could facilitate condom normalization and utility.

Integrative Activities

Public relations approaches assign credibility to a brand or message, whilst at the same time providing access to supplementary channels and message interpretation.

Parallel activities such as research, and publicity around results, facilitates broad-based understanding and replication of successful approaches.

Other activities might include awards " for example the 'Soul Citizens" award offered under the auspices of *Soul City* " endorse proactive community based activities.

Conclusion

The AIDS Directorate of the South African Department of Health has tentatively accepted the above plan. However, the Ministry's work in the field still appears to be as directionless and uncoordinated as with the *Sarafina II* debacle. In the week that we completed this chapter, three Pretoria University academics received a standing ovation from the Cabinet and media accolades on their claimed dramatic new treatment for AIDS. The research community quickly established that these researchers had failed to adhere to ethical medical and research procedures and that the Minister of Health had failed to adhere to procedures established by her own Department in reacting to claims of cures or new treatments. Even the Minister's own AIDS Directorate knew nothing of this 'breakthrough'. Such are the continuing difficulties facing health promotion professionals. Governments look for quick fixes, but media scholars know that behavior reducing the chance of infection can take up to a generation to achieve. It is for this reason that the South African media strategy to combat AIDS is designed as an inter-generational campaign.

References

Epstein, E. (1996). The design, implementation and evaluation of a culturally and situationally appropriate STD education media programme in Hlabisa, KwaZulu Natal. M.A. Thesis.

Dramaide, Dramaide: Is Dramaide Making A Difference? Evaluations of the Dramaide Programme. 1996, 306 pp. Available from Prof. Lynn Dalrymple, Dept of Drama, UNIZULU.

Mann, J., & Tarantola, D. (1996). *AIDS in the World II.* New York: Oxford University Press.

Mthembu, M. (1995). An assessment of the effectiveness of radio information campaigns on HIV/AIDS awareness and behavior change in Swaziland. M.A. Thesis, 60pp.

Parker, W. (1996, September). A national media campaign – who makes the decisions and what is really needed. *AIDS Bulletin*, 5, 2: 14-15.

Parker, W. (1994). The development of community-based media for AIDS education and prevention in South Africa: Towards an action-based participation research model. M.A. Thesis, 170pp.

Tomaselli, K.G., & Tomaselli, R.E. (1984). Media graphics as an interventionist strategy. *Information Design Journal*, 4;2: 99-117.

Young, M., Walker, D., & Pather, P. (undated). *Evaluation of Dramaide in terms of Augusto Boal and Paulo Freire's Theories of Drama and Education*, 60pp.

Young, M. Gender dynamics and the role of participatory/development theatre in a post-Apartheid South Africa:The example of DramAidE. Research Essay, M.A., 35pp.

Zaffiro, J. (1996). Casting shadows on SADC: Policy in Southern Africa to the next century. *Africa Insight*, 26:4.

Chapter 16

Health Communication and Primary Health Care in Refugee Settings: Lessons and Promises

B.A. Jinadu
Department of Public Health, Country of Kern, California

Andy O. Alali
California State University, Bakersfield

Political independence from imperial powers has not produced as smooth a transition for most African countries as envisioned by most political observers. Clearly, the promises of democracy that were associated with political independence have been accompanied by widespread instability and conflicts in most of Africa. Ethnic violence and political conflicts, often escalating to war, are endemic on the continent, particularly West and Central Africa. These conflicts have public-health implications, which we will discuss later. For now, it is noteworthy to mention that the public health crises associated with conflicts pose new challenges for national governments, particularly in relation to health promotion and disease prevention efforts in most regions of Africa.

This chapter analyzes some of the decades of upheaval in Africa and the extent to which the conflicts have led to displacement of persons from their homes, thereby rendering a core segment of the population into refugee status. We also discuss the implications of displacement on public health and disease epidemics in refugee camps and settings. Our goal here is to articulate ways to effectively communicate healthy lifestyles in refugee settings and displaced-persons' camps. This is crucial to Africa's health, because refugees and displaced persons have no access to any kind of formal health care in their temporary residence. Without adequate health care, there is the possibility that upon re-entry to their domiciles with some of the infectious diseases they acquired in displaced settings, their communities could be devastated by the spread of such diseases. Also, the lack of government concern for these people and the people's lack of access to adequate medical care creates some serious health concerns. It is our belief that an effective health promotion program within refugee settings, nomadic environments, and during re-entry to homelands, can prevent, or at the least, mitigate the spread of infectious diseases. We hope our discussion in this chapter redirects policy issues that contribute to the institution of an improved and effective health promotion, as well as health care for those persons classified as refugees and internally displaced in most of Africa.

Understanding the Concepts of Refugees and Internally Displaced Persons

Before we proceed with our discussion, it is imperative that we define two concepts that feature prominently in this chapter: *refugees* and *internally displaced persons* (IDPs). Here, the term *refugees* refers to those who are classified under the 1951 United Nations (UN) Refugee Convention, the 1969 Organization of African Unity (OAU) Convention, in accordance with the United Nations High Commissioner for Refugees (UNHCR) Statute, as persons who fear persecution, in his or her home country, and who are granted a humanitarian status or who are granted temporary protection elsewhere. On the other hand, IDPs refer to those who are displaced within their country and to whom UNHCR extends protection and/or assistance pursuant to a special request by a competent organ of the United Nations.

The importance of defining these two concepts can be gleaned from a reading of the official position of most international and regional governing bodies, such as the UN and OAU. For example, the UN Refugee Convention in 1951 defines a refugee as someone who has involuntarily taken up residence outside of his/her own country and is unable to return to it as a result of a "well-founded fear of prosecution" in that country (UNHCR, 1968). The OAU Convention and the Cartazine Declarations' definitions of a refugee include anyone who sought refuge in other countries as a "result of aggression, occupation, generalized violence, and events seriously disturbing public order." The latter definition involving refugees/displaced people from Africa and other developing countries has tremendous implications on how statistics on refugees are kept, analyzed, and interpreted. It is the basis for the political enumeration of refugees, as well as classifications of IDPs.

Why the Politics of Enumeration?

As much as population displacements have reached epidemic proportions in most African countries, accurate assessment of refugee status has been almost impossible. Political imperatives appear to determine and impact on how persons who leave areas of conflict to a safer ground are classified and documented. Often, those referred to as IDPs are differentiated from those who may have found their way into a neighboring country, or may have been transported to more stable and developed countries of Europe and North America. Interestingly, the politics of differentiation appears to overshadow the fact that refugees and IDPs are in need of protection and/or assistance because of continued fear of persecution in their homeland and the absence of permanent settlement opportunities in their countries of asylum (Harrell-Bond, Voutira, & Kibreab, 1985). It is extremely important, to underscore that these are people at the worst moments of their lives, fleeing from danger, more than likely famished and emotionally distraught about their lost loved ones. Often, children are separated from their parents, husbands from their wives and the stability of their existence shattered. It is not uncommon that refugees and IDPs are in a state of flux, often moving back and forth across the borders, which also makes it difficult to produce an accurate number of those displaced.

Equally important to our discussion is the body of literature, which documents the limitations of maintaining an accurate number of refugees in conflict situations. It is the general belief that such statistical activity is uncertain, unreliable, tentative, and muddled in politics (See Table 16.1 – 16.2) (Kibreab, 1985; U.S. Department of State, 1991; Bilsborrow et al., 1997). In fact, the two main international agencies responsible for producing these numbers differ in their enumerations of the same condition. In many of the conflicts in Africa, which produce

Table 16.1: *Origins of Refugee Populations in Africa, 1999*

Country of Origin	Main Countries of Asylum	No. of Refugees
Burundi	Tanzania	568,000
Sudan	Uganda/ D.R. Congo/ Ethiopia/ Kenya/ C.A.R./ Chad	490,400
Somalia	Kenya/ Ethiopia/ Yemen/ Djibouti	447,800
Angola	Zambia/ D. R. Congo/Namibia	437,700
Sierra Leone	Guinea/ Liberia	400,000
Eritrea	Sudan	376,400

Source: UNHCR, Refugees by Numbers 2001 Edition

Table 16.2: *Principle Sources of Africa's Refugees and Asylum Seekers (as of December 31, 2000)*

Country	Number
Sudan	460,000
Burundi	420,000
Angola	400,000
Sierra Leone	400,000*
Somalia	370,000*
Congo-Kinshasa	350,000
Eritrea	350,000*
Liberia	200,000*
Western Sahara	110,000*
Rwanda	55,000*
Chad	53,000
Algeria	50,000*
Mauritania	50,000
Ethiopia	40,000*
Congo-Brazzaville	20,000
Uganda	20,000
Ghana	10,000
Senegal	10,000
Nigeria	7,000

*Sources vary widely in number reported

millions of refugees and IDPs, the difference between those enumerated by UNHCR, the United States Committee for Refugees (USCR) and the ruling governments of the affected countries are poles apart. In the case of the latter, refugees and IDPs are undercounted (often privatized) because huge numbers are indicative of the enormous impact of the conflict and, often, would serve as a source of embarrassment for the government in power, as well as to draw attention to the inhumane treatment to which IDPs may be subjected. And, even though the UNCHR (1968) has long acknowledged the limitations of its IDPs statistics, such agencies are regarded as authoritative sources of information, therefore, most people do not question the accuracy of the information nor their statistical representation of refugees in Africa (D'Souza, 1991).

While we struggle to cope with the limitations discussed above, it is our firm belief that refugees are often caught in the politics of enumeration. It is important to note that part of the purpose of counting refugees is to determine policy, planning, implementation and evaluating strategies for international humanitarian aid. It is also crucial that refugees are registered for future reunification, to plan budgets for donor states and, in the case of host countries, for national security purposes. Clearly, current enumeration (and it's limitations) of people who are in a displaced status often pitches them in the path of geopolitical definition of refugees and IDPs.

African Context of Refugees and IDPs

A reading of the literature about the refugee and IDPs crises in Africa would paint a realistic picture of a continent that is continuously embroiled in civil war, religious and political violence, and ethnic conflicts. Most of these conflicts and unrest have led to forced and massive population movements, both internally and across regional and international borders (see Tables 16.1, 16.2, 16.3, and 16.6). Currently, millions of Africans are either refugees or internally displaced from their homes. Provisional statistics from the UNHCR (see Figure 16.1) indicate that in 2000 alone, there were more than 3.4 million refugees and 1.1 million IDPs in Africa (PGDR/UNHCR, 2001). The USCR reports that "approximately 9 million people were already refugees or internally displaced in Central Africa and the Horn of Africa before 2001" (U.S. Committee for Refugees, 2001). And, as of July 31, 2000, millions of new displacements were identified in most African countries, including Burundi, Congo-Kinshasa, Eritrea, Liberia, Nigeria, Sierra Leone, Somalia, Sudan,

Figure 16.1: *Provisional Statistics of Refugee and Internally Displaced in Africa, 2000*

Country	# of Refugees (IDPs in parenthesis)
1. South Africa	15,063
2. Lesotho	-
3. Swaziland	1,007
4. Botswana	3,409
5. Namibia	17,740
6. Madagascar	50
7. Mozambique	207
8. Zimbabwe	4,127
9. Malawi	3,900
10. Zambia	250,940
11. Angola	12,086
	(257,508)
12. Zaire (DRC)	332,464
	(3,000)
13. Rwanda	30,118
14. Burundi	27,136
	(56,000)
15. Tanzania	680,862
16. Kenya	206,106
17. Uganda	236,622
18. Somalia	588
	(18,000)
19. Ethiopia	197,959
20. Eritrea	1,984
	(366,834)
21. Sudan	401,027
22. C. Afr. Rep.	55,661
23. Congo Brazz.	123,240
24. Gabon	17,982

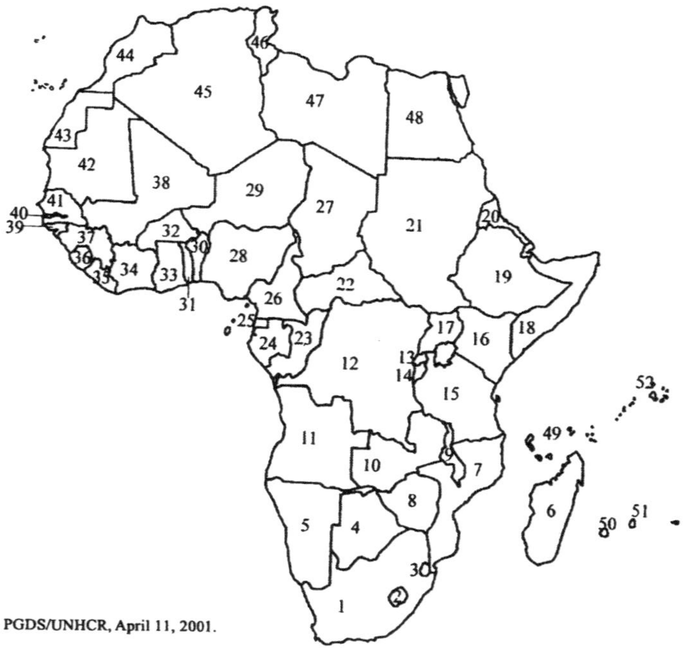

Country	# of Refugees (IDPs in parenthesis)
25. Equ. Guinea	-
26. Cameroon	43,680
27. Chad	17,692
28. Nigeria	7,270
29. Niger	553
30. Benin	4,296
31. Togo	12,223
32. Burkina Faso	696
33. Ghana	12,720
34. Ivory Coast	120,691
35. Liberia	69,315
	(110,686)
36. Sierra Leone	6,546
	(300,000)
37. Guinea	433,139
38. Mali	8,412
39. Guinea Bissau	7,587
40. Gambia	12,311
41. Senegal	20,766
42. Mauritania	-
43. Western Sahara	-
44. Morocco	-
45. Algeria	-
46. Tunisia	-
47. Libya	-
48. Egypt	-
49. Comoros	-
50. Reunion	-
51. Mauritius	-
52. Seychelles	-

Source: Adapted from Population Data Unit, PGDS/UNHCR, April 11, 2001.

and Uganda. As mentioned earlier, most of these displacements are a result of civil or border war, armed insurgencies, and political and religious violence (see Table 16.3).

Clearly, a detailed analysis of the figures we present here on refugees and IDPs suggests that the magnitude of these crises pose a serious threat to Africa's resources and development because most people who are unwillingly uprooted from their homes often need help and are not positioned to make positive or meaningful contributions to the affairs of the country of asylum nor to the economy of their respective nations. We do not say this out of a vacuum nor do we advance these perspectives because of our penchant to paint a bleak picture of Africa. Perhaps, an examination of the following few examples of Africa's refugees and IDPs crises, as documented by the USCR (2001) and other international agencies, would bolster our argument that Africa has a serious refugee and

Table 16.3: ***New Displacement in Africa (as of July 31, 2000)***

Source of Country	Newly Uprooted Population*	Cause
Sierra Leone	150,000	Renewed civil war
Liberia	30,000	Alleged insurgency, instability
Eritrea	700,000	Border war
Congo-Kinshasa	500,000	Civil war, foreign occupation
Sudan	10,000	Civil war
Uganda	50,000 – 250,000	Armed insurgencies
Burundi	65,000	Renewed civil war
Somalia	5,000	Civil war, lawlessness
Nigeria	50,000	Religious & political violence

* Includes combined estimates of refugees and internally displaced persons

Sources: *Refugee Reports*, Volume 21, Number 7 (2000); U.S. Committee for Refugees (August 2000)

IDP problem:

- At the beginning of 2001, more than a million Burundians were uprooted from their homes, including 400,000 Burundian refugees in neighboring countries and an estimated 600,000 internally displaced persons;
- Nearly 800,000 persons in Congo-Brazzaville were displaced during the 1990s and at the beginning of 2001 about 20,000 Congolese remained refugees in neighboring countries;
- At the start of 2001, some 300,000 to 350,000 Somali refugees continued to live in about two-dozen countries of asylum;
- Approximately 4 million Sudanese were internally displaced in neighboring countries at the beginning of 2001, including 360,000 refugees from other countries residing in Sudan;
- An estimated 400,000 persons have been forced from their homes in Uganda, of which 90,000 displaced persons reside in 46 camps;
- Over one million people are displaced from their homes in Sierra Leone;
- 750,000 Eritrean refugees fled their homes by the end of May 2000, even when Ethiopia claimed to have ended the war with Eritrea.

The magnitude of displacements in Africa has created a new class of individuals who are in constant need of aid and assistance.

Also, it is not uncommon for these refugees and IDPs to move across their national borders to neighboring countries. Indicative of this trend in population shifts is the data we present in Table 16.1, which shows the origin of African refugee populations and countries of asylum in 1999, as well as Table 16.4 that documents the ratio of refugees to host country population. A reading of these figures, particularly in Table 16.4, indicates that the ratio of refugees to total populations of host country range from 1-to-19 to 1-to-188. Unquestionably, this places enormous burden on host countries, as most are forced to redirect their scarce resources to sustain refugees and IDPs. Equally important is the data indicating that

Table 16.4: ***Ratio of Refugees to Host Country Population in Selected African Countries Listed by Host Country (as of December 31, 2000)***

Host Country	Ratio of Refugees to Total Population	No. of Refugees
Guinea	1 to 19	390,000
Congo-Brazzaville	1 to 22	126,000
Djibouti	1 to 27	22,000
Zambia	1 to 38	255,000
Liberia	1 to 41	70,000
Tanzania	1 to 65	543,000
Sudan	1 to 76	385,000
Uganda	1 to 101	230,000
Congo-Kinshasa	1 to 188	276,000

Sources: UNCHR, IOM, UNRWA, and USCR, 2002

Table 16.5: ***Principal Sources of Internally Displaced Persons, Africa (as of December 31, 2000)***

Country	Number
Sudan	4,000,000*
Angola	1,100,000–3,800,000*
Congo-Kinshasa	1,800,000*
Sierra Leone	500,000–1,000,000*
Burundi	600,000*
Uganda	500,000*
Eritrea	310,000
Somalia	300,000*
Ethiopia	280,000
Algeria	100,000–200,000*
Rwanda	150,000
Kenya	100,000*
Congo-Brazzaville	30,000
Liberia	30,000
Senegal	5,000

*Reliable estimates of displaced persons is unavailable

Source: U.S. Committee for Refugees, 2002

the principal sources of IDPs in Africa (Table 16.5) are not confined to one region. Rather, it is a problem that is endemic in Africa.

Beyond the regional implication of forced population movements on the economy, there are individuals in refugee settings and camps who do not have access to any kind of formal or adequate health care. It is likely that their new environment or condition would also have serious implications on Africa's health, as most are bound to either die from preventable diseases or host and facilitate the spread of infectious diseases.

Perhaps, what we want to impress on our readers here is that the context of Africa's IDPs and refugee crises is not without foundation. Clearly, the primary cause of displacement is the increasing number of civil wars and the political and religious conflicts that continue to ravage Africa (see Table 16.3). In the next section, we discuss some of the contexts of war and conflict, how they contribute to Africa's refugee status and the implication on public health, how to mitigate the public health crisis in refugee settings or camps, and the role health communication can play in this process.

Wars and Conflicts

Wars and conflicts are the main factors that contribute to refugees and IDPs in Africa. Clearly, the fact that over 25 million people have, at one point or another, been refugees or IDPs is indicative of the episodic socio-political unrest and destructive conflicts across Africa. There is hardly a region in Africa that is spared from conflicts and the dislocation of its population (see Table 16.3 and Figure 16.1). In 2000 alone, 20 percent of Africa's population and 14 countries were involved in wars and political and religious violence. Edmond J. Keller, a distinguished professor at the University of California, Los Angeles, once observed in a speech at an international conference that:

> Since 1960, Africa has witnessed more than a score of civil wars, and in just the past decade between 2 million and 4 million people have died in such wars. In 1993 alone, there were 5.2 million refugees and 13 million displaced persons in Africa (Keller, 1994).

These incursions range from what the U.S. Department of State (1999) refers to as large-scale wars to low-intensity conflicts. For example, in mid-1999 there were ongoing wars in Angola, Congo-Brazzaville, Congo-Kinshasa, Ethiopia, Eritrea, Rwanda, Somalia, and Sudan. During the same period, low-intensity conflicts plagued several African countries, including Burundi, Chad, Djibouti, Senegal, and Uganda. In 2000, these

Table 16.6: ***Major Displacement and Return in 2000, Africa****

Country	Displacement and Return
Angola	300,000 Angolans newly uprooted by continued civil war
Burundi	150,000 Burundians flee from civil war, atrocities, and forced displacement
Congo-Kinshasa	1 million flee war and atrocities
Eritrea	750,000 Eritreans flee because of border war with neighboring Ethiopia
Guinea	60,000 Guineans flee cross-border attacks by rebels from Sierra Leone and others
Liberia	50,000 Liberians flee insurgent attacks and retaliations by Liberian troops; 40,000 Liberians repatriate
Sierra Leone	210,000 Sierra Leoneans flee renewed civil war and rebel atrocities
Sudan	100,000 Sudanese forced from their homes by civil war and aerial bombings
Uganda	120,000 newly uprooted by insurgency and atrocities

*These numbers reflect movement during the year, not necessarily year-end totals.

Source: U.S. Committee for Refugees, 2002

conflicts resulted in the major displacements of over 2 million people in various parts of Africa (see Table 16.6).

The classification of these conflicts has also been discerned by Omoigui (n.d.) and suggests that African conflicts can be classified in terms of:

1. ethnic competition for control of state (for example, Nigeria);
2. regional or secessionist rebellions (for example, Sudan and Senegal);

3. continuation of liberation conflicts (for example, Angola, Western Sahara);
4. warfare arising from state degeneration or state collapse (for example, Somalia, Sierra Leone, Congo–DRC);
5. border disputes (for example, Ethiopia-Eritrea); and
6. protracted conflict within politicized militaries (for example, Congo–DRC, Sierra Leone, and Nigeria).

For further reading of the relationship between conflicts and refugees in Africa see: Abdulai, 1999; Englund, 1998; Ibeanu, 1998; Kalipeni & Oppong, 1998; Kloos, 1998; Downing, 1989; Ityavyar & Ogba, 1989.

An analysis of our discussion here would depict an indisputable, lucid picture that suggests that civil wars and political and religious unrest in Africa have led to the displacement of individuals who are in fear of their safety. The result of such fear is that citizens of the affected countries are either being displaced internally or most become refugees in another country. Often, these displacements are either across the border into a neighboring country or deeper within the region. For example, in the northwest corridor of Africa, where intractable conflicts in Sudan between the Sudanese People's Liberation Army (SPLA), the main rebel army, and the government and its allies persist, almost 500,000 people have taken up refuge in the neighboring countries of Uganda, the Democratic Republic of Congo, Ethiopia, Kenya, the Central African Republic and Chad (see Table 16.1). Interestingly, these countries are also embroiled in war and internal conflicts.

Also, it is useful to our discussion to mention that the unending Eritrean-Ethiopian conflict has divided and destroyed the Horn of Africa by producing millions of refugees, some of who have migrated to war-torn Sudan. The Great Lakes and Central parts of Africa, Congo, Zaire, Rwanda, and Burundi are all embroiled in wars and conflicts that have resulted in millions of refugees and IDPs. In East Africa are the Ugandans with countless insurgent groups and the resultant devastation and displacement of populations. The Somalian conflict, dating back to 1988, has overwhelmed the country and its neighbors, Kenya and Ethiopia. And, the ethnic conflict in Rwanda, between the Hutus and the Tutsis that received international attention, continues to create millions of refugees and displacement of persons in that region of the continent.

Other notable examples of conflict can be found in the West African countries of Liberia, Sierra-Leone, and Mali. There are also sporadic conflicts in other areas of the region, as in the occasional ethnic and religious flare-ups in Nigeria, a country that has not learned from the devastating effects of the civil war in 1960–1970. Interestingly, the problems in West Africa have also been punctuated by occasional border clashes between Nigeria and Cameroon, a conflict that has produced scores of refugees.

And, despite the dismantling of apartheid, the southern region of Africa is not without conflict. Countries such as Angola, Mozambique, South Africa, and Zimbabwe are caught up in the web of conflict and circle of violence that result in the displacement of populations within the region (see Figure 16.1; Table 16.1). There is no doubt that the series of war and conflict have not only led to chaos and displacement of individuals, but also have impacted public health in Africa. We devote the next section to a discussion of such impact.

Implications for Public Health and Disease

It is a well-known fact that political upheavals, violence, and wars carry with them tremendous challenges on how to maintain adequate public health for refugees and upon return to the homes they were forced to desert. There is ample evidence to support our contention here that the wars and conflicts that ravage Africa have placed enormous burden on existing infrastructure, as evidenced by population migration that leads to food shortages, economic deterioration, and the disruption of livelihood and social life; collectively, these problems serve as ingredients that affect the public's health. In this section, we discuss the contagion perspective of wars and conflicts on public health in Africa.

Disruption of Livelihood and Social Life

The start of a political strife or rumblings of civil war creates fear and uncertainties in the lives of the affected populations. As conflict escalates, mass migration begins, resulting in either internal displacement or migration across borders into refugee camps, disrupting livelihood and social life. Numerous examples and episodes of disruption of lives and livelihood that result from conflicts throughout Africa abound. A classic case in point is the Nigerian civil war during which there was mass exodus of the Ibos (Southerners) from northern Nigeria and other parts of the country to the secessionist Biafra. The abrupt relocation of the Ibos meant that they had to abandon most of their belongings and businesses that had been acquired over decades for relatively "safer grounds" of the South (Biafra).

Wars and the attendant displacement of victims dehumanize those affected because refugee camps are symbolic of helplessness and a center for handouts to erstwhile self-sufficient individuals. Families are dislocated and some of the children are abused both sexually and physically. Often able-bodied men become second-class citizens in their own countries because most are open to constant ridicule, taunting, and outright physical abuse. For the IDPs, there is a sense of loss of community and humanity as well as loss of their well-being.

There is no question that the psychological and symbolic impact of helplessness can adversely affect health, a point that has not gone unnoticed. In fact, this sense of loss of community and humanity has prompted post-emergency efforts to be directed at social reconstruction of trauma rather than on a medical approach to health care in some of the affected areas of Africa (Bracken, et al., 1995).

Food Shortage and Malnutrition

One of the other public-health effects of forced migration is malnutrition, due to food shortage. War and civil strife tend to aggravate an already decaying agricultural infrastructure, often brought about by preconflict corruption, neglect, and lack of planning, flood, or drought. A combination of political corruption and neglect, which often leads to discontent among civilians in the first place, becomes the "macular degeneration" phenomenon toward adequate planning (or lack thereof) for sufficient production and adequate or equitable distribution of food. Compound this scenario with natural or man-made disasters such as flood, crop infestation, or drought, and famine ensues with high malnutrition, especially in children, resulting in mortality and excess disease burden rates. While the immediate cause of death in those affected is usually a communicable disease, malnutrition produces a higher risk of mortality for those afflicted. Consequently, there is "increased case-fatality ratio (CFR) in the most common childhood communicable diseases, such as measles, diarrheal diseases, malaria, and acute respiratory infections (ARIs)" (CDC, 1992). However, "when malnutrition was not classified as an immediate cause of death, as in Sudan and Somalia conflicts, it was a major underlying factor accounting for the high CFR" (CDC, 1992).

Conflict-induced malnutrition was evident in the 1980s, as the world witnessed the plight of Ethiopians when the central government was engaged in an unrelenting military battle with opposition groups in Eritrea. Media coverage of the conflict, with associated pictures of malnourished women and children, led to a world-wide response and humanitarian efforts in the form of food donations and fundraising, such as the musical concert dubbed as "We Are the World." Besides the enormous expenditure of resources required to sustain refugees, the impact of these conflicts on public health is evidenced by the high levels of crude mortality rate (CMR) in famine-affected, internally displaced and refugee population in the Horn of Africa (CDC, 1992).

In the nomadic culture of Sudan and Mali, famine not only affected the herdsmen but also laid thousands of cattle to waste. It was estimated that two million civilians were displaced and experienced extensive hunger in 1992 as a result of "seriously diminished food production, continued fighting between rival warlords, and widespread looting and banditing" (Toole & Michael, 1995). This led to "Operation Restore Hope," a highly publicized humanitarian mission by the United States military personnel as well as troops from other nations. Clearly, we argue here to suggest that prolonged food shortage results in inadequate dietary intake and disease, which in turn, is the immediate cause of malnutrition. The most vulnerable are children, women of childbearing age, and the elderly. The consequences of malnutrition, particularly in children, include childhood morbidity, mortality, poor physical development and school performance (UN Report on World Nutrition Situation, 1997).

Reproductive Health

It is estimated that 75 percent to 80 percent of refugees and IDPs are women and their children. Women usually become titular head-of-household because the men either have been killed, conscripted into the army, or stay behind to care for their herds of animals. And, because women are occupied with providing food, shelter, and water for their children, reproductive health of women is often neglected. In a recent study of pregnancy outcomes in the Mtendeli refugee camp in Tanzania, it was found that reproductive-health-related deaths were the most common cause of death among women in the camp; maternal and neonatal deaths accounted for 16 percent of all deaths among these refugees.

Rape is also rampant and girls as young as 12 to 13 years of age are not spared. Often, this leads to unplanned pregnancy and illegal termination of the pregnancy to avoid cultural or religious ostracization. The pregnancies that come to term risk serious health problems due to the lack of early prenatal care, proper nutrition in the face of food scarcity, and malnutrition. The consequences of lack of prenatal care include increased risk of premature births, infant mortality, maternal mortality, and morbidity.

Health problems that affect reproductive health, including sexually transmitted infections, such as gonorrhea, syphilis, bacterial vaginosis, and trichomoniasis, are very high in these settings. It is estimated that more than 88 percent of the women in refugee camps had bacterial vaginosis, 28 percent had trichomoniasis and 67 percent had had at least one abortion. In areas of Africa where HIV/AIDS is endemic, the risk of contracting these deadly diseases are correspondingly high among refugees and internally displaced persons.

Communicable Diseases

Overcrowding in refugee camps and mass movements create conditions that predispose to communicable disease. For example, unsanitary conditions of refugee camps and the mass migration of internally displaced peoples result in diarrheal disease, which compounds the PEM status and accounts for high mortality. In 1997, a cholera outbreak was reported in 90,000 Rwandan refugees residing in three temporary camps and a total of 1,521 deaths were recorded in a 21-day period (March 30 – April 21), with the daily crude mortality rate CMR ranging from 7 to 14 per 1,000 people. Diarrheal diseases were responsible for between 25 percent to 85 percent of all mortality in Somalia between 1979 and 1981, Ethiopia in 1982, Sudan in 1985, Malawi in 1988, and Goma, Zaire in 1994 (Toole et al., 1988).

Mental Health

People in refugee settings or camps are often subjected to stress which results from being traumatized by the violence that placed them in their current situation. Virtually all of them have been displaced from their homes and most are separated from their families. They also find themselves in unfamiliar settings and are forced to witness murder. A majority of them, particularly women, have been subjected to abuse or rape that results in unwanted pregnancy. There is psychological trauma attendant with these conditions. Even though statistical data about mental health and refugee conditions in Africa are scarce, there is ample evidence of the role violence and trauma play on a person's mental state. For more discussion about mental health see Chapter 19.

Improving the Health Situation Among Refugees and IDPs

The refugee and IDPs crises that ravage Africa are deeply rooted in the ethnic conflicts and political dispensation that followed independence. Unfortunately, most governments of African countries are doing little to address the conflicts that result in displacements of their population. If anything else, it is imperative that interested parties, particularly governments and health professionals, continue prescribing and implementing health plans, as well as developing new ways to improve the health situation of refugees and IDPs. It is clear, as observed by J. P. Menu, director of emergency humanitarian efforts for the WHO, that "refugees have no easy access to health care, no easy access to sanitation [and] that makes them more vulnerable to disease" (Dube, 2002). There is an urgent need for improved health situations in refugee camps that cannot be ignored, as high prevalence of infectious diseases and lack of access to medical services continue to put peoples' lives in danger. At the same time, we would hope that efforts at disease control and prevention are not intended as solutions for people in "permanent" settlements, where refugees are now neglected and with no plan to return to their homes. We see this as crucial only to the control and prevention of diseases in the temporary setting of refugee camps. The goal here is to prepare the refugees to return to their homes with little or no disease. Therefore, health plans for refugees and IDPs must consider:

- the inclusion of immunization to control some endemic diseases, such as TB, measles, cholera (a waterborne disease), and typhus (a tick-carried disease);
- placing emphasis on women's health issues, particularly reproductive health;
- developing strategies for mental health care, without endearing the stigma and taboo associated with such disease;
- including oral health care, particularly as seen in the distribution of personal hygiene kits by the Red Cross;
- creating health posts and feeding centers, as seen in Southern

Somalia Refugee Camps (Downing, 1989, p. 1054);
- the distribution of daily rations that meet full nutritional needs;
- devising ways to truck in clean water and improve sanitation;
- peridomestic spraying of the refugee shelters with lambda-cyhalothrin (ICON) as a routine vector control measure in the camps; and
- emphasizing an integrated, camp-based system of care.

In addition, we recommend that responsible authorities should develop a surveillance system to monitor changes in health practices and behaviors as well as increase awareness of the causes of diseases in refugee camps.

Even though any health plan that is implemented should aim at reducing the health risks in refugee camps, the intended health outcomes cannot be realized if individuals in the refugee settings are not taught self-care. Self-care has been defined as "the range of behaviors individuals use to maintain or restore their health" (Hildebrandt, 1994, p. 247). This predicates that one's behavior materially affects health outcomes and that the link between personal actions to health outcomes is indisputable. Teaching people about self-care has the potential to help them internalize health practices that can restore their health and is complementary to their health because:

1. The performance or behavior of the individual is essential to health care;
2. It would help to conserve the limited resources available in refugee settings;
3. Self-care would empower people to make appropriate health decisions;
4. Self-care would engender refugee community participation; and
5. It would encourage information-seeking behavior to sustain self-help.

Sustaining the health of refugees and IDPs requires host governments to respect human rights and for a global commitment to solve conflicts before they escalate. Accordingly, the UN Secretary-General Kofi Annan, in a recent report on Africa to the UN Security Council, suggested that "an international mechanism should be established to help host governments maintain security and neutrality of refugee camps" (Africa: Secretary-General Report). Annan also recommended that such camps should be located away from borders; combatants should be separated from genuine refugees.

Finally, health plans in refugee camps must rely on oral, traditional communication networks that are easily recognized by refugees and adaptable to their cultural practices and folklores. Sometimes, the push to help people in desperate situations may blur perspectives on cultural practices that affect behavior. We say this to suggest that the communication of health in refugee camps must be situated within the cultural and communicative rules of the recipients of the health message. Disengaging and de-linking communication from the culture would adversely affect health outcomes. The goal here is to design communication strategies that situate health campaign messages within the contexts of the recipients. Therefore, we believe that the use of symbolism that is unique to the refugees' tradition would generate positive health outcomes.

References

Abdulai, N. (1999, April). Civil war in Guinea-Bissau. *Africa World Review*, 39-42.

Africa: Secretary-General's Report to the UN Security Council (n.d.). Posted on the web *(http://www.csih.org/papers/peacehealth.html)*.

Bilsborrow, R., et al. (1997). *International migration statistics: Guidelines for improving data collection systems*. Geneva: ILO.

Bracken, P.J., Giller, J.E., & Summerfield, D. (1995). Psychological responses to war and atrocity: The limitations of current concepts. *Social Science & Medicine*, 40;8: 1073–1082.

Centers for Disease Control (1992). Famine-affected, refugee and displaced populations: Recommendations for public health issues. *Mortality and Morbidity World Reports*, 41;RR-13: 6.

Downing, R. (1989). A tale of two clinics–Primary health care in refugee set tings: Lessons from Sudan and Somalia. *Social Science & Medicine*, 28; 10:1053–1058.

D'Souza, F. (1991). Who is a refugee? Definitions and assistance Disasters 5: 1473-5.

Dube, J. (2002, April 9). Refugees face 'Germ Warfare'. *ABCNews.com*.

Englund, H. (1998). Death, trauma and ritual: Mozambican refugees in Malawi. *Social Science & Medicine*, 46; 1165–1174.

Harrell-Bond, B., Voutira, E., & Leopold, M. (1992). Counting the refugees: Gifts, givers, patrons and clients. *Journal of Refugee Studies*, 5.

Hildebrandt, E. (1994). A model for community involvement in health (CIH) program development. *Social Science & Medicine*, 39;2: 247-254.

Ibeanu, O. (1998). Exiles in their own home: Internal population displacement

in Nigeria. *African Journal of Political Science,* 3; 2:80-97.
Ityavyar, D.A., & Ogba, L.O. (1989). Violence, conflict and health in Africa. *Social Science & Medicine*, 28; 7:649–657.
Kalipeni, E., & Oppong, J. (1998). The refugee crisis in Africa and implications for health and diseases: A political ecology approach. *Social Science & Medicine*, 46; 12:1637-1653.
Keller, E.J. (1994). African conflict management and the new world order. Paper presented at an international conference, "The End of the Cold War and the New African Political Order," held at the University of California, Los Angeles, February 7-11, 1994.
Kibreab, G. (1985). African refugees: Reflections on the African refugee problem. *Africa World Press*, 10.
Kloos, H. (1998). Primary health care in Ethiopia under three political systems: Community participation in a war-torn society. *Social Science & Medicine*, 46; 4–5:505–522.
Omoigu, N.A. (n.d.). Public health implications of conflicts in Africa. Posted on *http://www.gamji.com/nowa6.html.*
PGDS/UNHCR (2001, April 11). Population Data Unit. Geneva: UN.
Toole, M.D., & Michael, J. (1995, June). Infectious disease clinics of North America, 9.
Toole, M.J., Nieburg, P., Waldman, R.F. (1988). Association between inadequate rations, undernutrition prevalence and mortality in refugee camps. *Journal of Tropical Pediatrics*, 34: 218-20.
United Nations (1997). United Nations Administrative Committee on Coordination Sub-Committee on Nutrition. Third Report on the World Nutrition Situation. 1997.
United Nations High Commissioner for Refugees. (1968). *Convention and protocol relating to the status of refugees*. HCR/INF/29/Rev 3. UNHCR: Geneva.
United States Committee for Refugees (2001, October 2). More than half-million newly uprooted people in Central Africa and Horn of Africa in 2001. News Release.
United States Department of State (1999, July). Advisory issued by the Bureau of Intelligence and Research.
United States Department of State. (1991). *World refugee report*. GPO: Washington, D.C.

Chapter 17

Local Ideas on Prevention of Onchocercal Skin Disease: The Case of the Aowin-Suaman District of Ghana[1]

Albert K. Awedoba
University of Ghana, Accra, Ghana

This chapter examines the sets of ideas that some members of communities in which onchocerciasis is endemic hold on the prevention of onchocercal skin diseases. Social scientists have investigated at length issues concerning local aetiologies of specific illnesses and ill health generally. However, there has been little systematic research to date on local communities' views on the prevention of illness on the whole and least of all onchocerciasis which is only just beginning to engage the attention of social scientists. For example, Kleinman's concept of "Explanatory Models" of illness, which has influenced sociological and anthropological investigations of health issues, remains silent on prevention.[2] Johnson et al's (1994) discussion of knowledge and attitudes of some Malawian communities towards onchocerciasis makes no reference to local ideas on prevention of this disease or its symptoms, although there is mention of their knowledge of treatment sources for itching and nodules, two signs of onchocercal disease. Admittedly, the Kasl and Cobb (1966) concept of "health behavior" defined as "any activity undertaken by individuals who see themselves as healthy for the purpose of preventing disease or detecting it in an asymptomatic stage", cited in Ward et al (1997, p. 21), makes local behaviors on prevention of illness a valid research undertaking. [See also Ramakrishna et al. (1990) where prevention is accorded a role in the evolution of community control in Primary Health Care]. However, the bibliographical resources that were retrieved from databases on the subject of disease or illness prevention dwell almost exclusively on the strategies that the biomedical establishment offers. There seems very little interest in the layperson's behaviors and ideas of illness prevention. This is paradoxical given that prevention of ill health is the bedrock of primary health, as defined by the Alma Ata declaration of 1978, which, incidentally also seeks to empower local communities in the search for improved health status and well-being.

If we accept the point of view of social scientists themselves that health is holistic in character, then it is not just the recognition and assessment of signs and symptoms, therapeutic strategies and help-seeking behaviors and causes that should engage our attention but also the local strategies for maintaining health and ideas and behaviors on the prevention of illness and morbidity. Unfortunately, not even in the case of children's disease such as diarrhea and ARIs, which, because they are very common among children and threaten life, compel mothers and caregivers to adopt preventive measures, do we have information on illness prevention ideas and behaviors beyond the accidental observation. This hiatus in the knowledge and understanding of illness prevention behavior and ideology would seem to suggest that either local communities lack such ideas on the subject or that their notions and associated behaviors have no relevance for research agendas. Looking at the question from another perspective the omission of prevention from the discourse may be due to confusion or conflation of aetiology and prevention. If the latter is true then it is regrettable since cause and preventive need not coincide. One hopes that research objectives have not been too narrowly focused and tailored to prescribed biomedical intervention devised by the outside medical expert.

The Disease Onchocerciasis

Onchocerciasis is caused by a filarial worm, *onchocerca volvulus* and it is endemic in many parts of Africa. In Ghana it is found in many small-scale rural communities both in savannah and forest belts where the vector breeds. It is transmitted to humans through the bite of the simulium fly *(simulium damnosum)*, which breeds successfully near fast flowing rivers. The fly deposits its eggs on outcrops in the rivers and streams at depths not greater than 15 cm or 6 below water surface, to take advantage of the oxygen in the water as it foams and bubbles.[3] It is suggested that a velocity ranging from 60 to 250cm (2' to 8') per second is adequate. A female fly requires a blood meal to mature its eggs before oviposition and it takes this from humans though not exclusively (Samba, 1994). It is capable of flying up to at least 40 kilometers for feeding purposes, according to WHO (1966), and it can cover several hundred kilometers to establish colonies, especially when assisted by favorable wind.

In the human body the adult worm resides in subcutaneous nodules and its female produces millions of micro filarial worms. The dying of these in large numbers produces toxic effects that are responsible for the symptoms of onchocerciasis. These include blindness and a number of related conditions such as papular rashes, skin pigment changes, palpable nodules, hanging groins, skin atrophy and others. In addition it has been known to be associated with itching, which can affect any part of the body, weight loss, epilepsy, muscloskeletal pains and chronic poor health (WHO, 1987, p. 27; Duke, 1975).

Several kinds of treatment have been used for the disease, including chemotherapy. The drug Diethylcabarmacine (DEC) was once used, and probably still continues to be used by some individual Ghanaians suffering from itching. Currently, Ivermectin, a microfilaricide, is regarded as the drug of choice. Since 1987, its makers, Merck Corporation, have donated the drug for the treatment of the disease in endemic communities. In the West African zone the Onchocerciasis Control Programme has been engaged in controlling the disease through mass treatment of endemic communities, aerial spraying of river stretches where the fly deposits its eggs and entomological research on the vector, all in the attempt to break the transmission cycle of the disease and its eventual eradication.

Profile of Study Area

The findings discussed here derive from studies in Aowin-Suaman, one of the districts of the Western Region of Ghana. The area is forested with heavy annual rains that last for three quarters of the year. The area is drained mainly by the Tano river system, which includes numerous tributaries. Communities outside the main town, Enchi, lie close to the rivers that also serve as sources of drinking water. Communities are ethnically mixed due to the cocoa industry that has attracted migrants and capital from other parts of Ghana. The majority of people, constituting at least 80 percent in any settlement with a chief, are indigenous Brussa speaking a language of the Bia group. The main livelihood is cash crop agriculture concentrating on cocoa, palm oil and food crop cultivation. Farmers spend much of the day outside the village on the farms, which may be several kilometers from the main village. Some live in "cottages" on the farms during the cultivation and harvesting seasons. Over 40 percent of the sample have either no education or have spent less than six years in school. Study communities which have populations ranging from a few hundred to over three thousand in one case have a chief who is the traditional head assisted by a council of elders who represent kin groups and ethnic units. Village chiefs owe allegiance to the chief of Enchi, the paramount of the area. Indigenous Brussa, like their Akan neighbors, recognize matrilineal kinship, which is the basis for reckoning and tracing of jural ties and group memberships.

This part of Ghana, like much of the southwest, has been known to be endemic for onchocerciasis for some time. In fact, onchocerciasis was first reported in the region as far back as 1922 when J.F. Corson found *Onchocerca volvulus* in skin snips taken from prisoners in Sekondi, the regional capital (Patterson, 1978, p. 91; Hughes & Daly, 1951). However, it is only in recent years that endemic communities have received some treatment for onchocerciasis.[4] The remoteness of some communities, lack of logistic support, and sometimes unavailability of Ivermectin, have made it difficult to include all endemic communities in mass treatment programs. Apart from the District hospital at Enchi, communities lacked modern health facilities. One study community had portable water but the rest depended on the local streams for their supply of domestic water. This profile of the Aowin-Suaman study communities provides an essential backdrop to their ideas on prevention of onchocercal skin disease.

Study Design

The study sample is taken from four communities three of which are hyperendemic, with a nodule prevalence rate of 79 percent. Endemicity levels were based on rapid assessment procedures using nodule palpation. The respondents included 94 affected persons with visible lesions (nodules were not a criterion here) and 116 non-affected persons not known to have any of the symptoms of the disease. In each case respondents had to be at least over 16 years old, should have resided in the community for over five years and should consent to participate in the study.

The lesions of the affected were classified using the criteria developed by Murdoch et al (1993) and included the papular rashes: Chronic Papular Onchodermatitis (CPOD), Acute Papular Onchodermatitis (APOD), Lichenified Onchodermatitis (LOD) and Depigmentation (DPGM).

The information was collected using two semi-structured questionnaires for affected and non-affected respectively. In addition, two affected persons had in-depth interviews and eight focus group discussions were conducted with non-affected persons. While for the affected interviews were on the lesions diagnosed, for the non-affected two photographs for CPOD and DPGM respectively were used in conjunction with vignettes.[5] The study was aimed at investigating the psycho-social importance of onchocercal skin disease in a number of endemic African communities, using as guidelines Klienman's concept of explanatory model.[6] Interviews were conducted in the Brussa and Twi languages which respondents understood.

The Importance of Onchocercal Skin Disease (OSD)

In the study communities the vector fly was easily recognized and named as *ntumoa* (Twi term) and *nkontea* (Brussa term). Although there was no single term for onchocercal skin disease and the term "oncho" was by no means familiar to the people, nevertheless there were a variety of indigenous terms for onchocercal skin conditions such as *pclɛ* for nodule, *epini* and *nzooso* for LOD, *sabeng koko* or *kokole* for DPGM and *akele* and *asee* for APOD and CPOD. Non-affected respondents readily recognized CPOD and DPGM and not only did they say they had seen cases around some of them even thought the pictures shown them had been taken in the study village.

Most respondents view onchocercal skin conditions as serious. LOD and CPOD are regarded as much more serious that DPGM and APOD which are rated as milder illnesses. A greater percentage of the non-affected at the Ghanaian site, as the table above shows, consider the conditions as very serious.

In answer to an open-end question both affected and non-affected alike remarked that the skin conditions in question affected the quality of life. The appearance of the lesions caused shame to the affected, a view shared by affected and non-affected alike. The affected in particular were worried by the itching which results from the condition.

Table 17.1: ***Perception of Severity of OSD***

	Ghanaian Sample		African Sample	
SERIOUS	Affected %	Non-Affected %	Affected %	Non-Affected %
Not Serious	26.6	4.3	18.1	25.8
Moderately Serious	18.1	4.3	26.8	12.2
Very Serious	54.3	88.8	58.8	56.3
Uncertain	1.1	2.6	3.4	5.6
Total	94	116	626	655

For an affected 17-year old Ghanaian male, CPOD affected life thus: "It affects my life in the way that whenever people meet, I cannot go there as the scratching usually makes me ashamed." A 50-year old female with CPOD complains as follows: "it affects my life in the sense that when the itching starts I find it difficult to do any other thing. I am only grateful that it does not come very often."

The pattern is more or less the same for DPGM as the following comments from affected persons show. Thirty-five year old female remarks on the itching thus: "It at times interferes with my farming life in that sometimes in the midst of farming, I have to stop and scratch the place which itches" while her male counterpart, 65 years old man with DPGM complains thus: "It affects me serious for I cannot work very well. When I want to do some work and it starts to itch, then I have to abandon the work. Occasionally, I even experience pains in the body i.e. backache." One non-affected 22-year old Ghanaian female from a hyperendemic village interviewed about the effect of CPOD on life has the following to say: "When she sleeps, she will not have sound sleep because of the itching. The itching will also disturb her working ability because she will have to stop work to scratch. The appearance will also make her feel too shy to move with people."

Although it is not every affected person who complains, and there are a few of the DPGM cases that seemed not to be worried by the condition, for most people acquainted with onchocercal skin diseases, they are a great worry.

Causes of Onchocercal Skin Conditions

Altogether, many causes have been advanced by respondents to account for the disease. The most frequently mentioned causes include insect bites, drinking river water or bathing and swimming in it, particularly in the dry months when die water level in rivers is how, and contact with the vegetation, or contact with an infected person directly or indirectly by sharing toiletries. There were no significant differences on their perceived causes between the various onchocercal skin lesions, except perhaps for DPGM for which heredity was invoked.[7] While several respondents thought this condition was due to wounds received previously or a function of ageing, there were also a number who explained that itching affecting the limbs had led to intensive scratching which in turn produced sores which on healing heft behind the pigmentation changes. These views coincide with the expert opinion, which is stated thus: "It is probably the result of pruritus having led to scratching and to removal from parts of the skin of its melanin-bearing layers" [cited in WHO (1966, p. 22) on expert opinion about pigmentation changes].

Several researchers have remarked on the tendency in some Ghanaian societies to classify illness causation in terms of the dichotomy between natural and spiritual factors [see for example, Fosu (1981) and Wyllie (1994)], as far as onchocercal skin diseases were concerned, Ghanaian respondents discounted the possibility of there being a spiritual causative component. Thus, Ghanaian sites where only about one percent of respondents mentioned witchcraft as the cause of onchocercal disease, contrast with the other African sites, where the same study was conducted. In the hatter over 10 percent of the respondent sample considered witchcraft as a causative factor.[8]

In discussing the causes of the disease some respondents identified more than one cause, an immediate and a remote cause. This fact, perhaps confirms the uncertainty of local people about die exact causes of the disease.

Suggestions for Prevention of Onchocercal Skin Disease

To obtain respondents' views on how onchocercal skin disease might be prevented, both affected and non-affected were asked the following question: "What measures would you suggest to prevent this condition in the community". The question came at the tail end of the interviews. About 25 percent of the sample said they had no idea. Table 17.2 shows the findings.[9]

Table 17.2: ***Suggestions for Prevention of Onchocercal Skin Disease (All Samples from Ghanaian Skin Study Sites)****

	Affected		Non-Affected		Total	
Preventive	Freq	%	Freq	%	Freq	%
Treatment Affected Biomedically	27	24.5	26	20.6	53	22.5
Ensure Domestic Water is Good	15	13.6	35	27.8	50	21.2
Maintain Good Hygiene	13	11.8	26	20.6	39	16.5
Doctors Should Recommend	10	9.1	1	0.8	11	4.7
Prayers and Rituals	5	4.5	1	0.8	6	2.5
Not a Disease, No Prevention	4	3.6	0	0.0	4	1.7
Wear Protective Clothing	3	2.7	7	5.6	10	4.2
Spray and Eradicate Vector	3	2.7	4	3.2	7	2.9
Mass Treatment of Communities	3	2.7	4	3.2	7	2.9
Investigate Causes	1	0.9	4	3.2	5	2.1
Community Preventives	2	1.8	3	2.4	5	2.1
Don't Know	23	20.9	9	7.1	32	13.6
Others	1	0.9	6	4.8	7	2.9
Total	110	100	126	100	236	100

* Some respondents suggested more than one mode of prevention.

Illustrative Comments on Prevention of Onchocercal Skin Disease

The remarks of the following respondents show that it was not every respondent who could suggest preventives. A 41-year old male with DPGM and having had 10 years of elementary school education remarked: "I find it difficult to suggest any preventive measures because I can't tell apart from the discovery of the spots how the condition actually started. I therefore believe that doctors can be called upon to find a possible way of preventing it as well as curing those affected."

Those who do not perceive the condition as a pathological case did not offer any suggestions for it prevention. Among this group are a few DPGM and APOD cases like this 65 year old with 8 years of formal education who happens to have DPGM: "The condition needs no preventive measures because I have hived with my wives and children for years and none of them has got the condition." This comment is interesting, as it stands. It suggests that respondent is relying on his personal experience to debunk a conception of the condition as one that is transmissible from person to person. A 55-year old male with APOD remarks thus: "I don't know what to suggest as preventive measures because I don't think it is an illness. As already stated, I think it is *samanade gya* and I can't say how it can be prevented."[10]

Treatment of the Affected as a Preventive

The most common suggestion made was to have the affected sent to the hospital or some biomedical facility for treatment. The expectation behind this view is that if the affected were treated successfully, and most people held the opinion that the biomedical facility was the best source of treatment for the condition, then the community would be safe, the disease would cease to be transmitted to others through heredity or person contact.

Twenty-seven year old female with APOD and the benefit of 8 years of schooling maintains as follows: "Since I believe the cause is pregnancy related, I would suggest that every pregnant woman should be asked to visit the hospital in her pregnancy so that in case any such illness is inside her, it can be treated for her before it becomes a serious problem."

A non-affected person commenting on DPGM observes as follows: "I will suggest that since the condition is transferred from parents to children, then parents who have the condition should treat themselves of the condition in order not to pass it on to their children."

Comments on Local River Water Use

Those who believed that the water of the local rivers and streams was unwholesome and caused the disease thought people should not drink from these rivers and if they must, as for those without any other source of water supply, then the water should be boiled first, or as this respondent, a 34-year old male with LOD and elementary school background suggested medicine should be put into the streams: "We should stop drinking from the river. When the boreholes break down we should be given some medicines to put in the stagnant portions of the river Jensue which we drink from. This I believe will prevent the recurrence of the condition in the community." A 19-year old secondary school pupil diagnosed to have CPOD also does not recommend consumption of water from the local river: "We should stop drinking water from the Adwen River if we wish to prevent this condition from affecting people in this community."

It is the view of some that the quality of water in the local rivers leaves much to be desired in the dry months when the rivers become stagnant and that by using such water people place themselves in danger of getting the skin problems in question. This is exemplified by the view of a 20-year old illiterate man with CPOD who did not think the river water is safe in the dry season: "I believe we should be discouraged from swimming in the River Jensue especially when it dries up, because it can be contaminated by then. We should not use it as drinking water during that time. However we can use it during the wet season."

Maintaining Sanitation and Good Hygiene

A segment of the sample thought the skin conditions were due directly or indirectly to people maintaining poor personal hygiene. Poor hygiene however means different things to different respondents including not observing the basic rules of good sanitation, as remarked by this non-affected respondent: "We should be neat and cook with clean utensils. We should eat from clean plates and wash our hands before eating."

For some poor sanitation may include contact with an infected person. A male aged 38, with seven years of elementary school education who was diagnosed to have CPOD, would urge that the affected keep their distance: "People who have this condition should not have contact with those who don't have it, until they have been healed." His compatriot, a 25-year old female with LOD and four years of schooling, places the onus on the non-affected who should avoid using or sharing intimate personal effects such as toilet items with the affected: "To prevent this condition in the community, people should avoid using the towels, sponges, etc. of their friends and relation." The same point is echoed by another respondent thus: "I will suggest that people who are not affected should not eat with those affected and they should not use the same sponge and towel with those affected."

Wearing Clothing that Cover the Body

To prevent the bite of the black fly and other insects that are believed to be the potential causes of the disease some respondents advised that clothing that covers the body be worn. An affected respondent, aged 35 years with at least 12 years of basic education who has been diagnosed to have LOD is of that view: "I think people in the community should be advised to always wear long socks and long sleeved shirts so as to prevent the *ntmnbo* from biting them."

A non-Affected person remarks thus: "To prevent this condition in the community, people should be advised not to go about bare-footed. They should rather be advised to wear shoes or sandals to prevent worms from entering their bodies."

Prayers and Rituals

Rituals have always been one mode of healing as well as prevention, as Ebin (1994) illustrates with his account of *momome* rites.[11] Today individuals can do also go to the spiritualist churches and pray for healing and good health. Those who hold onto the spiritual cause of the condition are likely to seek spiritual means of preventing its occurrence or recurrence. This is the strategy of a 30-year old man with DPGM who has never been to school; he remarks as follows: "Since I believe witchcraft could have been the cause, I will suggest that as a preventive measure, we should all be prepared to undergo prayers so as to prevent evil spirits and demons and witchcraft being used to destroy people." However, there are also people who believe that whatever the cause of an illness, it can be dealt with through prayers. This 35-year old man with APOD and 10 years of basic schooling comments as follows: "I will attend church services and give myself to God for only God can help in this condition."

Eradication of Vector

Those who thought insects were responsible for the condition suggested that the offensive insects he destroyed. This is the opinion of a non-affected male: "I will suggest that to prevent this condition in the community, we shall have to find the insects. Later, such insects should be eliminated totally from the community." A 35-year old female unaffected respondent prefers, among other things, the use of powerful insecticides in the eradication: "Secondly, powerful insecticides should be used to spray the rooms and environment so that all the harmful insects can be killed."

Forty-two year old with LOD places the burden of controlling the flies on the government: "I suggest the Ministry of Health should also bring a sanitation team to our area to spray insecticides along the river banks, especially around August to kill the *ntummoa* or *memena* or *nkontea*." This respondent, not only knew the various local names for the black fly but also the time of year when the flies abound in the area. This information is coming from a man with 10 years of formal education.

Concerted Actions by Village

A number of respondents, both affected and non-affected, viewed the question of prevention as a collective enterprise that calls for community discussion and consensus. This strategy is exemplified by the comment of an 80-year old man with APOD: "We have to meet together with people hike the Assemblyman so that we can discuss about the preventive measures."

A non-affected interviewed on CPOD comments as follows: "I think we should beat the *gong gong dawuro* and summon all villagers to a meeting where we shall all debate the issue and come to a consensus as to what must be done to prevent the occurrence of these conditions."

As with the perceived causes of onchocercal skin disease, some respondents hike this 45-year old unaffected female, suggested multiple preventive measures. She urges education of people on the exact causes of the disease on the implied grounds that if they knew the causes individuals would adopt the necessary preventive measures: "Teachers should mount educational programs to educate the people on the causes. Communities like this one should be provided with pipe-borne water. The villagers should maintain good sanitation." Perhaps this approach is not surprising coming from a person with 14 years of education and a teacher by profession. It is representative of the perceived role of the village teacher as an opinion header in the community.

Discussion and Conclusions

This study is conscious of the fact that what local people say they do is not the same as what they actually do. As anthropologists, for example Beattie (1966), have long ago pointed out, what people say they do and what they say they ought to do are distinguishable but could be grouped under the emic to be set apart from what they actually do, the etic perspective. A parallax is inherent when the emic and the etic perspectives are compared. Secondly, saying, thinking and doing are not always the same. For example what people say is not the same as what they think, although these two are related. This study however attempts to combine an observer's perspective with some insider perspectives through the solicitation of views from affected and non-affected. The latter, in fact, stands between the outsider, the researcher and die true insider, and the affected, and by citing verbatim remarks attention is drawn not only to what is said but also how it is said and the context of the utterance.

Statistically, there are only slight differences in the proportions of affected and non-affected that favor specific prevention strategies, and the same is true of their verbal comments, nor do lesions influence the types of preventives that would be suggested. The only exception is attributable to DPGM, which is essentially a non-reactive lesion. A number of affected respondents who denied it a pathological status have ruled out the need for preventive measures. For some this attitude of denial derives from the perception that the lesion caused no pain but the possibility of denial constituting, as argued in Awedoba (1998), a potential strategy for coping with symptoms of a disease, which for some is associated with sigma, cannot be ruled out.

The impact of lesion type, gender, age group and education on ideas of prevention cannot be ruled out, however the data does not allow for conclusions on the role of such variables. Though educational level could conceivably influence ideas on prevention, however, some of the juxtaposed comments quoted above show people sharing similar ideas on prevention despite differences in educational attainment. Education is likely to become a factor shaping ideas on prevention in the case of tertiary education.

There is a concurrence in perception by both local communities and the biomedical establishment, as illustrated by the views of Cooper (op cit), that prevention, treatment and help-seeking causes are associated. These three sets of variables need to be distinguished however and each accorded its due significance in research schemes.

It cannot be doubted from the comments quoted above that perception of causes shape recommendations on prevention. Respondents themselves have often made the connection between knowing what the cause is and being able to suggest a preventive. This is illustrated by the comment of one 45-year old female with 10 years of education who had been diagnosed to have LOD: "Since I don't even know what caused it, I cannot suggest any measures aimed at preventing it. I believe doctors will be the right people to know the necessary measures to be taken for its prevention." This reminds one of Cooper's (1993, p. 397) remarks to the effect that "Prevention is the harvest of etiological research," made with epidemiological studies of risk exposure in mind. Some respondents however, imply by their response that knowing the immediate causes is not enough and that prevention should be based more on knowing the remote or underlying causes.

Important as knowledge of the causes may be, it does not always contribute to knowledge on prevention. Prevention is multi-faceted: it concerns future outcomes for the individual respondent (affected and non-affected alike), other individuals and the collectivity. Local knowledge of the causes does not necessarily point to what can or should be done to prevent illness and disease. The knowledge that the black fly causes the disease may be shared by many respondents, since respondents themselves remark on its bite inducing instant itching and a temporary rash. However, among those who attribute the problem to the black fly there are individual differences on what types of preventive to adopt. These differences may be due to the respondent's onchocercal status (i.e. whether affected or non-affected and if affected, what lesion), gender, age, education, religion, occupation and external experiences.[12]

Though knowledge of the cause might suggest ways of preventing the condition, it does not imply that the means or the will to go through with the preventive exists. A 50-year old illiterate woman with CPOD thinks the condition might be hereditary but she is at a loss as to how hereditary illness can be prevented: "I cannot say because I don't even know how I got the condition fully, even though I believe I go it from my mother." Conditions due to heredity and ageing, among others, defy prevention from the local point of view. This 38-year old woman with 9 years of education who was diagnosed to have CPOD thought it was caused by using soap obtained from the Republic of la Cote d'Ivoire but could not bring herself to say that people should for that reason boycott Ivoirian soaps.

> I cannot say. I could say that because I got the condition after I had used the Ivoirian soap to bathe people should not use soap made in Ivory Coast to bathe. However there are so many types of soap made in Ivory Coast and I have used some of the others (without causing harm to myself) so I don't know what to say. It is up to you people to know.

We see in these remarks an illustration that beliefs and behavior do not always tally, as Yoder (1997) recently pointed out.

Some affected respondents, on the other hand, especially people with DPGM have felt that the condition was not an illness and as such there should be no need to prevent it. If it is perceived as an issue which does not cause pain to the affected and is unlikely to impair bodily function or be transmitted to others, as one respondent remarks, a person might not appreciate the need to take preventive action, especially if that person also considers the illness as one that would not respond to treatment. It could be argued from one perspective that for stigma laden conditions like DPGM, the greater its prevalence within the community the lower the perceived stigma for the affected. It might thus be understandable why an affected person might not wish to prevent others from getting the condition.

In addition to knowing or not knowing the causes of the condition, knowing how or where to seek treatment seems to be an issue for some respondents. As we have seen from remarks displayed above, treatment is prevention for some respondents. Thus, not knowing an effective treatment for the condition can mean that prevention cannot be suggested. This view is shared by a 19-year old boy with LOD who has had 9 years of formal education: "I can't suggest since I have not got treatment for my condition. If I get treatment then I can use it as an example and suggest where and how I got treatment". A 54-year old man having DPGM and the benefit of three years of formal education feels this way too. "If doctors are able to treat mine, I can inform all others to seek medical advice and through that I believe everybody would be treated and the condition would thus be prevented," he remarks.

In conclusion, it can be seen that the responses assign a role and responsibility to both the individual on the one hand and the community on the other. Even the affected accept that they are responsible for ensuring that others do not get the disease. For the individual, multiple strategies were put forth:

- Individuals can avoid getting the disease by not exposing them selves to the perceived risk factors including avoiding intimate personal contact with those already affected. Good personal hygiene and sanitation was considered advisable.
- Drinking water should be boiled before being consumed, where there is no source of wholesome domestic water. However, where portable water exists, people should use it and not resort to the streams.
- The limbs should not be exposed to allow the vector fly or agent to bite people.
- The affected should seek treatment to remove the disease from the community.

In making the last suggestion, several respondents attached a proviso, namely that self-treatment should be sought where the financial means existed. This seems to suggest that though onchocercal disease is regarded as serious, it is not of the order to compel sacrifice of livelihoods or subsistence, a point worth taking into account at the intervention stage. In these communities hack of financial means inhibits the use of hospitals and biomedical facilities (see Awedoba & Hagan).[13]

From the community's perspective, it is suggested that collectively, people should keep the water sources clear of filth by not bathing or swimming in the streams or defecating near the banks of the rivers. The backdrop to this recommendation is the concern of southern Ghana communities to keep the living environment clean. This concern takes a religious and a practical dimension. At the practical level, communities provide for a collective pit latrine located some distance from the settlement. However, it is realized that some members of the community, especially children, might nevertheless prefer to attend to nature's call wherever more convenient, i.e. in the bushes and possibly near the banks of the rivers when river levels have subsided heaving open spaces with less vegetation. At the ritual level, Brussa communities performed "village sweeping rites" or *momome*, as they are known, and used white clay to demarcate the borders of the village settlement in times of epidemic and excessive rains to rid the community of the problem by returning and restricting it to the bush (Ebin, 1994, p. 131).

Respondents expect the government and the authorities to play their part in the prevention of the disease. Not only do they think the authorities, particularly the health authorities should investigate the source of the problem and come up with solutions they also perceive a role for the government in the solution of community problems.[14] The provision of portable drinking water seems to be one of the priorities of some of the study communities. At the time of the study, two of the communities had the infrastructure for portable water but unwillingness or inability of the people to meet the cost of maintaining the equipment[15] meant portable water could not be provide to the communities.

This study does not unfortunately answer all the questions focusing on the role of gender, education, religion, external experiences, etc, in structuring the views of respondents, since prevention was only a minor component of the study. It can however, be seen that the ideas for prevention tend to reflect local priorities such as the quest for good drinking water in communities that lack such a facility because of their inability to afford the expensive portable water delivery.[16]

The view that onchocercal skin disease has something to do with the river is not wrong. The intensity of bites tend to decrease with distance away from the rivers basins, the breeding sites of the vector fly, where oviposition takes place (WHO, 1987, p. 130; Hunter, 1981, p. 262). However, for what it is worth, educators may find it necessary to explain more clearly the connection between rivers, vegetation, water and the fly. Inadequate explanation can lead to local people drawing unintended conclusions, which might undermine intervention efforts. Clearly, local people have been educated previously on guinea worm and oilier water borne diseases. While it is good practice to seek the integration of health programs care should also be taken to avoid confusing local communities.

We find that all the measures suggested by respondents make health sense. They reflect local thinking and local priorities such as the quest for clean water. They show that there is a perception that it is not only recovery that should be of concern but equally communities have a role to play to protect the health of all. The importance of this is to be measured in the context of initiatives aimed at community owned and directed treatment programs. Given the perceptions of the disease in endemic communities and suggestions about prevention, it would be an urgent matter to educate endemic rural communities on the disease. In the case of community treatment of onchocerciasis, local communities must be persuaded to accept that though prevention in the short run may be the responsibility of the individual who is expected to cure the condition so that others do not get it the unaffected too have a contribution to make, if the transmission cycle of the disease is to be broken. In the absence of education, mass treatment of endemic communities is unlikely to find favor with those who do not see themselves to die affected.[17] This is likely to happen when it is remembered that those who test positive for onchocerciasis do not always exhibit the classical signs and symptoms of the disease.

The community should not be faulted for its view that the water and the rivers are the sources of the problem, but negative interpersonal attitudes suggested by some of the ideas on prevention need to be rectified. This can be achieved and the cooperation of communities gained by making it clear that the disease is not transmissible directly from person to person and that the bite of the fly, S. damnosum is responsible. There is suggestion that the best way to stem the disease is to distance those having reactive lesions from the unaffected. This not only undermines social relations unnecessarily, it stigmatizes those with lesions. This can be avoided with a simple explanation of the etiology, pointing out the connection between the fly, microfilariae (*mmoa* would be a satisfactory equivalent for microfilariae in Akan languages), rivers and lesions would be necessary.[18] It seems that association of the disease with the rivers may be due either to previous campaigns on guinea worm eradication or inadequate communication between some individuals who have sought treatment at health facilities and health personnel. Telling affected people that their rivers are the source of the problem does not go far enough. While professionals can understand what about the rivers accounts for onchocerciasis unless hay people are told precisely how the fly which breeds near fast flowing rivers plays its role in causing the disease, the villager who has previously known that the river water is responsible for diseases will conclude that it is the water as such which is to blame. This question of imprecision in communication of health information has been remarked upon by Sobo et al (1997, p. 317) in connection with AIDS misconceptions among runaway adolescents in Cleveland, Ohio.

Endnotes

[1]I wish to acknowledge the contribution of Dr. Maria Hagan, Head of the Eye Clinic at Korle Bu Hospital, Accra and principal investigator for the studies on onchocercal skin disease and the effect of Ivermectin on onchocercal skin disease and troublesome itching in the Aowin-Suaman communities. These studies were sponsored by WHO/TDR in the context of its multi-country African investigations on onchocercal skin disease. I hereby record my gratitude to the Takemi Program of the Harvard School of Public Health for a fellowship, which enabled me to examine the data and produce this and other materials on the subject. I also record my gratitude to Professor Obermeyer of the Harvard School of Public Health for her comments on a previous draft of this chapter.

[2]See Kleinman (1978, p. 256) where it is suggested that in the elicitation of patient's explanatory models, attention be paid to five issues: etiology; onset of symptoms; pathophysiology; courses of illness and treatment. There is no reference to the possibility that an explanatory model might include knowledge and behavior regarding prevention.

[3]WHO, 1966, p. 10.

[4]As recently as 1993, when we started researching in the Aowin-Suaman area, none of the communities in the District appeared to have been given mass treatment with Ivermectin, hence the choice of communities from this District for the study.

[5]The questionnaire was administered by the writer, two graduate students of the Institute of African Studies, University of Ghana and an employee of the District Health Office at Enchi. Interviews took place in April-May, 1994 and were preceded by a pilot study in December 1993.

[6]The study which was funded by WHO/TDR/World Bank grant was carried out in several African countries, including one site each in Ghana, Cameroon,

Uganda, Tanzania, and three sites from Nigeria. In this paper, the phrase "the rest of Africa" or "the other African sites" excludes Ghana from the total African sample.

[7]Given that in most of the endemic communities, most males of over 40 years has DPGM it is understandable that some respondents should think that the condition is hereditary or a function of aging.

[8]The questionnaires and procedures used in this study were similar to those employed in study sites in Nigeria, Uganda, Cameroon, and Tanzania, the rest of Africa sites.

[9]The statistics are derived from a search for themes in verbal comments made in responses to the question. No pre-coded categories had been prepared beforehand as there was no certainty how people would respond to the question.

[10]Respondent is here describing the lesion as a sort of birthmark.

[11]In the past, and probably even today, as Ebin suggests, in times of epidemics chiefs called upon the priests and priestesses to "sweep the dirt" way from the village hiving space. By so doing evil forces that are believed to have been responsible for ill health are banished to the forest.

[12]A 65-year old Brussa man diagnosed to have DPGM and with no educational background makes a suggestion that is interesting in the sense that it exhibits a level of knowledge about the causes of the disease, the vector and the conventional approaches used to control the disease by some programs in the past: "My suggestion for prevention would be for the government to spray the insects along the banks of the river with insecticide so as to get rid of them. These insects are very common in the seventh to the ninth month of the year and so they can be killed easily that time."

[13]Disparities exist between rural and urban center with regard to the cost of obtaining treatment at a hospital. Paradoxically, as Coleman (1997) indicates, it costs more in the district hospitals than in the regional hospitals. Respondents here do not only live far from the district hospitals, these are not perceived as helpful for the treatment of onchocercal skin conditions. Traveling to a regional hospital escalates the costs considerably not to mention the time spent in trying to present a case at a regional hospital.

[14]Since Ghana's independence village communities hike these have been wooed for their votes by making diem promises; consequently, villagers know they can expect governments to provide for some of their needs.

[15]It was suggested privately that people found the pipe water to be brownish and its taste unpleasant to the palate.

[16]It is no exaggeration to say that paying for water at the rate of 20 cedis per bucket of water makes water more expensive iii the rural areas than in the rural communities.

[17]In one of the study communities in the Aowin-Suaman District where the trial study of the effect of Ivermectin took place, one of the defaulters for the second round was traced and interviewed. His explanation for defaulting was that he needed the first treatment to cure his sore throat. Since that ailment no longer worried 1dm he felt there was no need to take the second dose which was given

after three months. Views and attitudes like these illustrate the need for education.

[18]In another endemic community in the Central Region of Ghana where this writer carried out a survey for OCP in 1996 there was considerable knowledge of how the disease came about and this was due to more effective education by FM radio.

References

Awedoba, A.K. (1997). Patterns of distress on onchocercal depigmentation in the Aowin-Suaman District of the Western Region of Ghana. *African Anthropology*, IV;1: 80-91.

Awedoba, A.K. (1998). Help-seeking behaviour and coping in relation to onchocercal skin disease in endemic communities in Southwestern Ghana. Takemi paper, Harvard School of Public Health, Boston.

Awedoba, A.K., & Hagen, M. (n.d). The burden of onchocerciasis and some rural Ghanaians' response: The case of the Aowin-Suaman District of the Western Region of Ghana.

Beattie, J.M. (1964). *Other cultures*. London: Cohen and West.

Coleman, N.A. (1997). The uneven implementation of user fee policy in Ghana. Research paper No. 138, Takemi Program in International Health, Harvard School of Public Health, Boston.

Cooper, R.S. (1993). Ethnicity and disease prevention. *American Journal of Human Biology*, 5;4: 387-398.

Duke, B.O.L. (1975a). Clinical manifestations and geographical differences. In Annon (1975), *Research and control of onchocerciasis in the western hemisphere* (pp. 25-29). Proceedings of an international symposium.

Fosu, G.B. (1981). Disease classification in rural Ghana: Framework and implications for health behaviour. *Social Science & Medicine*, 15B: 471-482.

Heggenhougen, H.K. (1991). The role of anthropological methods to identify health needs. In C.A.K. Yesudian (ed.), *Primary health care* (pp. 68-76). Bombay: Tata Institute of Social Studies.

Hughes, M.H., & Daly, P.F. (1951). Onchocerciasis in the Southern Gold Coast. In *Transactions of the Royal Society of Tropical Medicine & Hygiene* (pp. 243-252).

Hunter, J.M. (1981). Progress and concerns in the World Health Organization Onchocerciasis Control Program in West Africa. *Social Science & Medicine*, 15D: 261-275.

Johnson, K., Courtright, P., & Burnham, G. (1994). Knowledge and attitudes towards onchocerciasis in the Thyolo highlands of Malawi. *Trop Med Parasitol*, 4;45: 341-343.

Kasl, S., & Cobb, S. (1966). Health behaviour, illness behaviour and sick role behaviour. *Archives of Environmental Health*, 12: 246-266.

Kleinman, A., Eisenberg, L., & Good, B. (1978). Clinical lessons from anthropologic and cross-cultural research. *Annals of Internal Medicine*, 88;2: 251-258.

Murdoch, M.E., et al. (1993). A clinical classification and grading system of the cutaneous changes in onchiodermatitis. *British Journal of Dermatology*.

Patterson, K.D. (1978). River blindness in Northern Ghana, 1900-1950. In Hartwig, G.W., & and Patterson, K.D. (eds.), *Disease in African history*. Durham, NC: Duke University Press.

Ramakrishner, J., Brieger, W.R., & Adeniyi, J.D. (1990). Anthropology, health education, and the evolution of community control in primary health care. In Coreil, J., & Mull, J.D. (eds.), *Anthropology and primary health care* (pp. 278-301).

Samba, E.M. (1994). *The Onchocerciasis Control Programme in West Africa*. WHO: Geneva.

Sobo, E.J., Zimet, G.D., Zimmerman, T., & Cecil, H. (1997). Doubting the experts: AIDS misconceptions among runaway adolescents. *Human Organization*, 56;3: 311-320.

Ward H., Mertens, T.E., & Thomas, C. (1997). Health seeking behaviour and the control of sexually transmitted disease. *Health Policy Planning*, 12;1: 19-28.

WHO (1966). *WHO Expert Committee on Onchocerciasis, Second Report*. Technical Report Series 335. Geneva: WHO.

WHO (1987). *WHO Expert Committee on Onchocerciasis, Third Report*. Technical Reports Series 752. Geneva: WHO.

Chapter 18

Communication Strategies for Preventing Micronutrient Deficiencies in Africa

Andy O. Alali
California State University, Bakersfield

B.A. Jinadu
Department of Public Health, County of Kern, California

Micronutrient deficiencies are increasingly becoming a public health problem in African countries. Sub-Saharan Africa's 130 million children below six years of age (20 percent of its total population) are at-serious risk. Some of the children have already been devastated by the AIDS pandemic. War and civil conflicts increased the number of African refugees, as well as those internally displaced. (For more discussion on refugees and internally displaced persons, see Chapter 16). Nearly 30 million, or one-third, of the children in Africa are chronically malnourished. (For regional statistics on malnutrition in Africa, see Tables 18.1–18.5). This is due, in part, to inappropriate child-feeding practices, high morbidity, and poor child-caring practices. One of the consequences of persistent malnutrition is that 35 percent of the children in most African countries have developmental problems, including stunting, by age three.

Health surveillance of the continent shows that micronutrient deficiencies affect mostly women and children, and contribute to major health problems, high rate of morbidity and lowered productivity in adults.

TABLE 18.1: ***Percentage of Children Under Age 5 Suffering from Malnutrition in North African Region, 1990–1996***

Country	Percentage (%)
Algeria	10
Libya	NR
Morocco	10
Tunisia	9

Source: World Bank, World Development Report, 1998/99. Oxford: Oxford University Press, 1998, pp. 192–193.

TABLE 18.2: ***Percentage of Children Under Age 5 Suffering from Malnutrition in Central African Region, 1990–1996***

Country	Percentage (%)
Angola	35
Central African Republic	23
Chad	NR
Democratic Republic of Congo (Zaire)	34
Gabon	15
Equatorial Guinea	NR
Sudan	NR
Zambia	29

Source: World Bank, World Development Report, 1998/99. Oxford: Oxford University Press, 1998, pp. 192–193.

TABLE 18.3: *Percentage of Children Under Age 5 Suffering from Malnutrition in Southern Africa Region, 1990-1996*

Country	Percentage (%)
Botswana	NR
Lesotho	21
Namibia	26
South Africa	9
Swaziland	NR
Zimbabwe	16

Source: World Bank, World Development Report, 1998/99. Oxford: Oxford University Press, 1998, pp. 192–193.

In this chapter, we are interested in providing our readers and key constituents with an overview and status of the nutritional status in Africa, identifying some of the major micronutrient deficiencies and the factors that contribute to these deficiencies. Further, we articulate what we believe are appropriate communication strategies and framework for preventing micronutrient deficiencies in the affected areas of Africa. We believe our discussion here is an important contribution to Africa's health status because nutrition is a key development challenge facing the continent today. Some of the noticeable challenges include how to deal with the prevalence of underweight, stunting, and wasting among children under five years old. A more difficult challenge of nutritional deficiency facing Africa is how to reverse the tide of child morbidity because malnutrition accounts for up to 56 percent of a child's likelihood of dying within the first five years of life (Pelletier, et al., 1993). We hope our strategies can be embraced and applied for nutritional values. Before we discuss these strategies, it is important to paint the nutritional picture of the continent. In the next section we discuss the nutritional status of selected countries and some of their efforts to reduce micronutrient deficiencies.

Major Micronutrient Deficiencies in Selected African Countries

Evidence from nutritional surveillance programs indicates that micronutrient deficiencies are prevalent in Africa. The four most identifiable cases are: protein-energy malnutrition; vitamin A deficiency; iodine deficiency disorder (IDD); and iron deficiency anemia (IDA). In the next section we focus our discussion on the nutritional issues in five African countries, Burkina Faso, Ethiopia, Kenya, Tanzania, and Uganda and some of the programs aimed at reducing malnutrition. We chose these countries because of their comprehensive programs on nutrition and also with the hope that their approaches can serve as lessons we can apply to nutrition behavior change in other parts of Africa.

Burkina Faso

Burkina Faso, a country of 10.4 million people in West Africa, is characteristic of the chronic malnutrition problem in Africa. It is estimated that 33 percent of children under five years of age suffer from malnutrition (World Bank, 1998; see Table 18.4). Evidence from health surveys, particularly in rural areas of the country, suggests that "one-third of the children under five years of age have low weight for their age and one-third are stunted" (Gottert, et al., 1998, p. 3). Clearly, the low weight and stunting are evidence of chronic malnutrition, which is a consequence of unhealthy dietary practices in the country. Some of the dietary practices, as observed by Parlato and Seidel (1998), are a result of a host of factors based:

> on agro-ecological and market conditions, economic constraints, cultural preferences, intra household food distribution practices, beliefs about which foods are appropriate at which times and for whom, and traditional cooking practices and tastes (p. 2).

These conditions or constraints have placed some extra burden on an already inadequate and over-burdened health sector to develop and formulate nutrition behavior programs or strategies to reduce infant and child morbidity and mortality, a process that also demands focus on ways to improve maternal nutrition and infant feeding practices. Part of this effort in Burkina Faso has been demonstrated in specific strategic initiatives aimed at:

1. Improving the diet of pregnant and lactating women;
2. Promoting exclusive breastfeeding for up to six months of age, followed by consumption of nutrient-rich complementary foods;
3. Ensuring that children ate nutritious foods after being ill, espe-

cially with diarrhea; and

4. Encouraging prenatal visits and attendance at growth monitoring and nutrition promotion sessions at health centers (Gottert, Doumba, & Fishman, 1998, p. 4).

TABLE 18.4: ***Percentage of Children Under Age 5 Suffering from Malnutrition in West Africa Region, 1990–1996***

Country	Percentage (%)
Benin	24
Burkina Faso	33
Cameroon	15
Cape Verde	NR
Gambia	NR
Ghana	27
Guinea	24
Guinea-Bissau	23
Ivory Coast	NR
Liberia	NR
Mali	31
Mauritania	48
Niger	43
Nigeria	35
Soa Tomé and Principe	NR
Senegal	22
Sierra Leone	29
Togo	25

Source: World Bank, World Development Report, 1998/99. Oxford: Oxford University Press, 1998, pp. 192–193.

Ethiopia

The magnitude of micronutrient deficiencies in Ethiopia is equally alarming. Ethiopia is one of the oldest nations in the world and one of a few East African countries that was never colonized. With its population of almost 63 million and extremely low-income levels (GNP per capita of $100 U.S. dollars), it has one of the highest rates of infant, under-five, and maternal mortality. About 48 percent of children under five suffer from poor nutrition (see Table 18.5).

TABLE 18.5: ***Percentage of Children Under Age 5 Suffering from Malnutrition in East Africa Region, 1990–1996***

Country	Percentage (%)
Burundi	38
Comoros	NR
Djibouti	NR
Eritrea	NR
Ethiopia	48
Kenya	23
Madagascar	32
Malawi	28
Mauritius	15
Mozambique	47
Rwanda	29
Seychelles	NR
Somalia	NR
Tanzania	29
Uganda	26

Source: World Bank, World Development Report, 1998/99. Oxford: Oxford University Press, 1998, pp. 192–193.

Other evidence from national nutritional surveillance programs indicates that "39 percent of rural and more than 25 percent of urban children suffer from various forms of protein-energy malnutrition" (Haidar & Tsegaye, 1999, p. 181). Analysis of data from the same surveillance programs would show that the prevalence of wasting, stunting, and underweight in Ethiopia is the highest in the world. Interestingly, most of the micronutrient deficiencies are found in areas that are considered food surplus regions of the country.

Yet, even though it is not clear why these food surplus areas experience the most deficiencies in nutrition, a number of contributing factors have been identified. These include insufficient food production as a result of primitive agricultural practices, infectious diseases, recurrent drought and famine, as well as civil wars of more than a quarter of a century.

An equally visible occurrence is goiter, a consequence of IDD. It is estimated that the total goiter rate (TGR) and visible goiter rate (VGD) are 54 percent and 28 percent, respectively (Haidar & Tsegaye, 1999, p. 182). An associated part of micronutrient deficiency in Ethiopia is IDA. While IDA has not been classified as a public health problem in Ethiopia, there is evidence that shows a prevalence rate in approximately 10 percent of school children and 18 percent in pregnant and lactating mothers (Woldegabriel, 1992). Currently, World Bank projects, Ethiopian government initiatives, and numerous NGOs support nutritional programs in the country.

Kenya

Kenya, one of 15 countries in the East Africa region of the continent, is inhabited by almost 30 million people. With a population growth and life expectancy of 2.3 percent and 51 years, respectively, it is estimated that 23 percent of children under five are micronutrient deficient (see Table 18.5).

A report by the Green Africa Network (1999) suggests that the state of malnutrition in Kenya is on the rise. The report attributes this increase to "indebtedness, the economic structural adjustments programs (SAPs) imposed by donor countries, the HIV/AIDS scourge, rising poverty, and deteriorating infrastructure."

However, it is also obvious that numerous other factors contribute to micronutrient deficiency in Kenya. The most noticeable one is the inadequate intake of nutrients that pervades Kenya and most of the African continent. Other contributors, which are characteristics of the bundle of factors that cause nutrition problems in Africa are: disease; lack of food; wrong feeding practice; lack of water; inadequate health services; low incomes or purchasing power; lack of land for farming; inadequate or poor housing; poor hygiene; inequalities in the distribution of commodities and services; and lack of education and illiteracy. Additionally, there is evidence to suggest that the rapid population growth rates in Kenya have contributed to malnutrition because the number of people are increasing faster than food supplies. Clearly, the Kenyan population explosion has led to unequal distribution and control of resources that are necessary to create nutritional balance in the country.

As with other countries, numerous organizations, governmental and non-governmental, currently support nutritional projects aimed at improved health status. Typical of these is the promotion of breastfeeding for low birth weight (LBW) infants. This program, which is considered highly successful in the growth of LBW infants fed with human milk, has been achieved through education that "supports and encourages rooming-in, expression of breast milk, feeding breast milk to infants who cannot yet suck or swallow, and education of staff in supporting and teaching mothers to breastfeed" (The Consultative Group, 1989). This practice is facilitated through education, active participation of staff, and location of mothers within and near proximity of hospitals.

Tanzania

The nutritional status of children in Tanzania is as equally alarming as in the African countries discussed here (see Table 18.5). Evidence from WHO and UNICEF research indicates that the most prevalent types of micronutrient deficiencies in Tanzania are vitamin A deficiency (VAD), iron deficiency anemia (IDA) and iodine deficiency disorders (IDD). Because of the magnitude of micronutrient deficiencies in Tanzania, both the WHO and the Tanzanian medical community have classified nutrition as a clinical public health problem in the country.

The most recent international reports on micronutrient deficiencies in Tanzania estimate that over "10,000 children are likely to suffer from VAD-related blindness at any one time" (WHO & UNICEF, 1995; WHO, 1992; WHO, UNICEF, & ICCIDD, 1993). Also, the Tanzania Food and Nutrition Centre estimates that exophthalmia, a clinical eye lesion that lead to loss of sight, is the source of 2,000 to 4,000 cases of blindness every year (Kavishe, 1992). Surveillance reports collaborate the problems for public health as cases of clinical VAD have been identified in 0.6 percent of 3,177 preschool children, 45.3 percent of who had serum retinal (vitamin A) levels below the cut-off point [20 μg/dl] (WHO and UNICEF, 1995).

An equally widespread nutritional disorder in Tanzania is IDA, which affects 45 percent of children and lactating women (WHO, UNICEF, & ICCIDD, 1993). The severity of nutritional deficiencies is evidenced by the 30 percent of prenatal mortality in the country, most of which is attributed to IDA (Kavishe, 1994).

The nutritional problem in Tanzania has prompted renewed government policy to develop an adequate surveillance system that is disease-targeted and supplemented through public health care centers in the country. Also, the country has embarked on programs aimed at improving consumption of vitamin A-rich foods through combined communications/nutrition education (Gillespie & Mason, 1994).

Uganda

In Uganda, where more than 26 percent of the children under five years of age die of malnutrition, there are on-going efforts through community health programs (see Table 18.5). Heal the Nation has embarked on an ambitious program, among other health initiatives, at the cost of over $10,000 to reduce malnutrition and infant mortality rate. The program emphasizes training and supervising health workers to manage basic health programs that include nutrition and growth monitoring.

The Uganda experience also focuses on strengthening partnerships with the early childhood development caregiver in the family and at the community level. For example, the Uganda "program targets both mothers and fathers, primary caregivers (i.e. all those who are in touch with the child), community leaders, and community-based organizations" (Nyeko, 1997). In the past few years organizations such as Feed the Children — Uganda, have trained over 300 caretakers, 60 community-based organizations (CBOs) and have carried out home visits in over 52 families. In all, their efforts at capacity building aim to train the affected population in child-centered, activity-based methods; to promote mobilization for community-based organizations and women's groups for the provision of care for children; and to promote community participation.

The Uganda Ministry of Health has also reacted to the rampant malnutrition by asking the government to revisit its appropriations priorities and to increase the public health sector funding by more than 41 percent to 500 billion shillings annually (*New Vision*, 2001). It is expected that adequate dispensation of such funding would revitalize a neglected health sector.

Strategic Plans for Effective Nutrition in Africa

The changing global trends and challenges have led to new development problems and challenges for Africa. These changes, particularly those influenced by urbanization and industrialization, as well as increased rural-urban migration, have impacted family lifestyles and altered culturally appropriate solutions, patterns and practices to child development. One of the most visible areas of challenges relates to how Africa should deal with the nutritional deficiencies that plague the continent. We believe that the first step to solving this development problem is for the governments of Africa to acknowledge their levels of micronutrient deficiencies so as to forge and implement effective health and nutritional policies. Consequently, we suggest the following strategies that are classified within eight distinct, yet connected categories: emphasize research and data collection; develop appropriate channels of information for community-based nutrition efforts; build coalitions and social networks; emphasize the role of family; develop physical infrastructure; integrate strategies in development plans; embrace technology; and commit politically. Our discussion of the strategic points for effective health and nutrition gains follows.

Research and Data Collection

In the area of research and data collection, we must first begin with an understanding of the determinants of micronutrient deficiencies in the affected areas of Africa. Here, the focus should be on the totality of the population and within the context of their daily lives augmented by systematic collection of data at the household levels. This approach, we believe, would ensure the identification of the causes and consequences of micronutrient deficiencies and their relationship to other health problems (if any) within that community. This will also enable the formulation of health objectives that accommodate a contextual approach to facilitate shifts in attention from curative to preventive, and promotion of healthy nutrition practices. In fact, evidence from health research supports the notion that it is "more cost-effective to shift to preventive and health promotion programs than curative," because most of the health budget would now be spent on prevention rather than the expensive treatment of existing diseases (Garcia, 1984).

The emphasis on research also means that we can now identify primary target audiences, isolate behaviors amenable to change, and develop appropriate communication strategies for the primary target audiences. Clearly, the importance of research in formulation of communication strategies for nutrition health has already been proven in other settings. Illustrative of this is the Burkina Faso initiative where research focus on maternal nutrition and infant feeding practices identified specific determinants that influenced communication strategies on how to increase the production and consumption of vitamin A-rich foods (Parlato & Seidel, 1998). Here, the research identified specific elements that influenced the planned strategies for nutrition behavior change (p.5):

1. Most parents were poorly informed about the special nutritional needs of children and pregnant and lactating women;
2. Many fathers expressed an interest in doing more to improve their families' health and nutrition; and
3. Families had the necessary time, food resources, and economic flexibility to make positive changes.

Undoubtedly, the research in the context of nutrition health in Burkina Faso and elsewhere has produced localized knowledge that, ultimately, led to theoretical formulations and communication strategies designed to alleviate micronutrient deficiencies and preventable diseases. These strategies focus on integrated approaches that also recognize the different segments of the population.

Equally important is the fact that the research can enable inventory assessment of micronutrient deficiencies in each African country, as well as within the urban-rural axis. It is also an opportunity to analyze or measure the impact and outcomes of current programs – both institutional and logistical, as well as human resources. In the process, it would support institutional capacities, and perhaps, the development of a regional clearinghouse to link with state and national networks and enabling efficient information storage and retrieval apparatus. This is likely to have a positive impact on how nutrition information is collected, processed and reported as well as the feedback of such information within Africa.

Appropriate Channels of Information for Community-Based Nutrition Effort

A well-planned nutritional health promotion program must provide access to and encourage demand for health information so as to close the knowledge gap within the target population. In other words, there must be open channels of communication, between the wider community and service providers. Open communication encourages people to voice their opinions and enables feedback for health campaigns.

Also, a mechanism should be in place to provide accurate information of nutritional value of the different foods consumed within the local community. This can be accomplished through the use of available communication channels within the target population. Clearly, the channels selected should be sensitive to the community in which such media are applied. This is due, in part, to the differences in local media and where some African countries are located on the development ladder. Clearly, there are variations in the type of communication channels from community to community, and as one moves from the urban areas to rural settings. For example, the use of mass-media approach – radio, television, newspaper, billboards, and Internet – may not be as effective since these are considered elite communication forms in rural parts of Africa.

An equally important element is the fact that use of retail outlets as sources of information dissemination about nutrition would most likely work best in the urban areas where merchandising is more organized than in rural settings. Consequently, the choice of channels of information, whether at the marketplace or pharmacies, should be influenced by the observable contexts within the community that is targeted for nutritional campaign. (For examples of effective community-based nutrition communication see Parlato & Seidel (1998, pp. 5-8, 17, 26-29, 39-41).

Coalitions and Social Networks

Coalitions and community social networks are crucial in developing and supporting community-based nutritional programs. It is imperative that any formula devised within our proposed strategic plans include a method that engenders and facilitates effective coalition between private sectors, NGOs and social networks at the community level, including religious groups and schools. We believe that priority should be given to how the network of national, regional, and local leadership or opinion leaders can be integrated for involvement and actions at all levels.

Also, a key element of the strategy for effective nutritional health is the need to decentralize authority and responsibility for nutrition education, moving decision making to the local communities, coalitions and social networks. The one way to ensure such decentralization is to recruit and train volunteers at the local community level. They would serve as advocacy groups and leadership groups to answer questions. We believe the recruitment and training of these volunteers would be relatively inexpensive and beneficial to the poorer, rural populations. And, by decentralization, community participation and teamwork would be encouraged; it would empower communities to recognize and value nutritional information and dietary practices. Clearly, their active role in this regard would enhance project effectiveness and sustainability.

The Role of Family

It is equally important to recognize the importance of family in African societies, particularly in health contexts. (For further discussion on the role and influence of family on health decisions, see Chapter 12). The typical African is dependent on the family and because of the bond that emanates from this important relationship, the family often regulates the individual's behavioral system and orientation. Therefore, it is imperative that nutrition efforts, especially at the formative stages, target families and communities as a unit. After all, it is the collective behavior of family members that affect the nutritional health of its members.

Develop Physical Infrastructure

In most of Africa, very few health infrastructures are available to support nutrition at regional levels, urban centers, and rural areas. Nutrition infrastructure and resources development at all levels should be a priority of governments of Africa. The development of functioning nutritional health infrastructure in local communities and regional centers would secure the foundations for effective health promotion strategies and nutritional gains.

Integrate Strategies in Development Plans

As a matter of priority, African governments must develop effective nutrition policies and integrate them in their respective development plans. These policies must identify long-term goals and objectives for nutrition as well as focus on ways to ensure that each person in their countries has an adequate intake of nutrition.

Also, governments must formulate country-specific strategies, for monitoring and evaluating nutrition plans. The success of such policies and plans depend on an understanding of the immediate as well as the underlying and basic causes of malnutrition in Africa (Mwagi & Mwabu, 1986, p. 778). Some of these causes have already been identified in our earlier discussion in this chapter.

Once this new understanding and the resulting policies are fully integrated into the development plans, governments must appropriate funds to support nutrition programs at all levels and sectors. This also means that there must be equity in budgetary allocations to include, not only the urban areas, but also, the vast populated rural areas. It is through such a plan that Africa can develop a functioning system that is disciplined, financially sound, and maintains quality assurance and is accessible to the target population.

Embrace Technology

One of the major drawbacks in development projects in Africa pertains to the lack of or availability of, accessibility to, and application of technology. This is especially acute in the health sector, in which inoperable and antiquated systems or a staff that is not well trained to use modern technology predominates. It is equally important to note that, for so long, Africa has embraced turnkey (plug-in and operate) technology more than a focus on research and development (R&D) that would lead to modern technological innovations. Consequently, most countries in the continent are technologically dependent on the innovation of the West. However, with the proliferation of technologies such as the Internet, African governments ought to, as a matter of priority, embrace this newfound technology and apply it for immunization and effective case management of nutritional matters. We believe that with the effective application and management of available technology, Africa would be more exposed to existing disease control strategies and apply them to prevent "60 percent of childhood deaths – including those due to immunizable diseases, dehydration, malaria, and pneumonia" (USAID, p. 5).

Political Commitment

All of these intervention strategies would not work effectively without the commitment and support of the government whose policies enable people to make nutritional choices that may or may not improve their health. One area that needs urgent attention is a strong political commitment to improve the nutritional health of millions of displaced Africans, some of who are victims of conflicts and war in the continent. It is imperative that governments, especially those with displaced persons and refugees, commit themselves to develop mechanism for nutritional health in post-conflict situations.

Also, we believe that local efforts can be enhanced by the government's role in making available to these communities adequate advisory services. This will assist rural sectors in their ability to achieve nutritional balance; foster networking opportunities; increase capacity building; and fund local health promotion initiatives.

Conclusion

Even though micronutrient deficiencies are nearly a universal problem, it is more acute and a serious public health problem in Africa. Effective nutritional health involves an articulated marriage between nutrition behavior of the individual and institutional intervention and promotion efforts. We believe that the strategic points discussed here can provide direction for ensuring the delivery of high quality and effective nutritional programs to Africa.

First, this plan forces national governments to develop strategic nutritional plans to: identify the problem(s); formulate objectives; develop strategies; and define nutrition tasks. Second, our strategic points identify opportunities and mechanisms for collaborative work within and outside of target communities. The goal here is to empower communities to take active roles in planning their futures, particularly as it relates to nutritional health. We suggest that the importance of community involvement should not be de-emphasized because the faith and health of Africa's children lies in the hands of Africans – where it takes a village to raise a child. Third, the strategies we discussed earlier would facilitate the identification of individual and community barriers to nutritional health as well as the opportunity to explore ways they can be overcome.

Finally, these strategies are culturally sensitive because we recognize and respect traditional belief systems that drive the African mindset, which is commonly shared by Africa's diverse population. With these strategies, we hope to assist in the journey to improved nutritional health in Africa.

References

Garcia, D. (1984). The effect of ownership and control of health systems and the concept of health. Paper presented at a Workshop on Health Policy on Eastern and Southern Africa. Arusha.

Gillespie, S., & Mason, J. (1994). Controlling Vitamin A deficiency. *ACC/SCN State-of-the-Art Series, Nutrition Policy Discussion Paper No. 14.*

Gottert, P., Doumba, J.P., & Fishman, C. (1998). Integrating nutrition communication in a family health program. In Parlato, M., & Seidel, R. (eds.), *Large-scale application of nutrition behavior change approaches: Lessons from West Africa* (pp. 3-12). Published for the Basic Support for Institutionalizing Child Survival (BASICS) Project. Arlington, VA.

Green Africa Network (1999, July 6). *Sustainable rural health-care programme: Medical care for all.* Nairobi, Kenya.

Haidar, J., & Demissie, T. (1999, February). Nutrition situation in Ethiopia. *South African Medical Journal*, 89; 2:181–183.

Heal the Nations: Christian medical Missions. Posted on the web–(*http://www.healthenations.com/uganda.htm*)

Health needs sh500b annually. (2001, August 27). *New Vision* (Kampala). Posted on the web–*(http://allafrica.com/stories/200108270511.html)*

Kavishe, F.P. (1994, March). Control of iodine deficiency disorders: The Tazanian experience. *UN News on Health Care in Developing Countries*, 3/94; 8:27–32.

Kavishe, F.P. (1992, December). Preventing specific micronutrient deficiencies: A case study of Tanzania. Paper presented at the Micronutrient Break-Out Workshop at the International Conference on Nutrition, 1992. TNFC Report No. 1538.

Mwagi, W.M., & Mwabu, G.M. (1986). Economics of health and nutrition in Kenya. *Social Science & Medicine*, 22; 7:775-780.

Nyeko. J. (1997). Feed the children, Uganda. Presentation at ECCD Summer School, Windhoek, Namibia.

Parlato, M., & Seidel, R. (eds.) (1998). *Large-scale application of nutrition behavior change approaches: Lessons from West Africa.* Published for the USAID by the Basic Support for Institutionalizing Child Survival (BASICS) Project. Arlington, VA.

Pelletier, D.L., Frongillo, E., & Habicht, J.P. (1993). Epidemiologic evidence for a potentiating effect of malnutrition on child mortality. *American Journal of Public Health,* 83: 1130–1133.

The Consultative Group on ECCD. (1989). *Early childhood counts: Programming for early childhood care and development*. CD-ROM. Washington, D.C.: World Bank.

The Guardian (2001, December 20). Nigeria's population explosion worries PPFN, p. 7.

USAID. (undated). *An African framework for design and implementation of child survival interventions: Focused interventions for impact strengthened systems for sustainability*. USAID.

WHO (1992). *The prevalence of anemia in women: A tabulation of available information*. Geneva: WHO.

WHO & UNICEF (1995). Global prevalence of Vitamin A deficiency. *MDIS Working Paper #2*.

WHO, UNICEF, & ICCIDD. (1993, July). Global prevalence of iodine deficiency disorders. *MDIS Working Paper #1*.

Woldegabriel, Z. (1992). Micronutrient deficiencies in Ethiopia and their interrelationships. Ph.D. Thesis, Wageningen University, Netherlands.

World Bank (1998). *World Development Report, 1998/99*. Oxford: Oxford University Press.

Chapter 19

Providing Mental Health Care to Rural South Africans: Current Trends and Future Directions

Anthony L. Pillay
Carol-Ann Sargent
University of Natal Medical School and Midlands Hospital, South Africa

The notorious policy of apartheid which ruled South Africa until 1994 has left many legacies which its people have to deal with, and which, in many cases, are likely to take decades to repair. Currently the country has a population of 38 million, 86 percent of whom, merely because of their skin pigmentation, suffered racist atrocities and were deliberately disadvantaged in all spheres of life. Health care, education, housing, water and sanitation are among the major service deficits endured by apartheid's survivors (and those who unfortunately did not survive). Mental health care is one of the areas that has been both neglected and used in an abusive manner by governmental officials employed to uphold the discriminatory policies. Mental health has been affected by apartheid in two ways. Firstly, life for the country's black majority was mentally unhygienic, to say the least. The discriminatory policies of apartheid were described as "psychopathogenic" with the government jeopardizing the mental health of its oppressed millions (Dawes, 1985). Secondly, mental health services have been extremely poorly developed, more so for the black population.

Mental Health Care During the Apartheid Era

The treatment of mental health problems (i.e. curative care) was largely limited to two contexts, name y private practice and state-funded psychiatric hospitals. A very small percentage of the population was able to afford private consultations with psychiatrists or psychologists, either through direct payment or medical insurance. For this reason, virtually all private sector psychiatrists and psychologists were (and still are) based in the elite suburbs designated for white South Africans under the apartheid government's Group Areas Act. A survey in the mid 1980's showed that around four percent of the country's 803 clinical psychologists were black (Pillay, 1987).

The country had no more than 300 psychiatrists during its last few years of apartheid, many of whom were not in full-time clinical practice due to retirement or academic o administrative positions. It was around this time that the outspoken critic of apartheid and its psychiatric services, John Dommisse (1987), remarked how easy it was to calculate the ratio of psychiatrists to the population for black South Africa, since there was only one black psychiatrist and a population in excess of 23 million. Not only were the majority of psychiatrists and psychologists white, but virtually all were unskilled in the African languages used by the majority of the country's people.

Psychiatric hospitals in the country have been mainly state-funded institutions providing care fur acute and chronic mental health problems. Typically, these hospitals are housed in disused military buildings, at least one of which still has cannons on display on its grounds! This is an indication of the priority traditionally given to mental health in South Africa. It might interest the international reader to know that the country's first asylum for the mentally disordered was none other than Robben Island, which subsequently became a prison and gained fame (or rather notoriety) for housing the world's most famous political prisoner. Nelson Mandela, among other dissidents of apartheid. Of course, separate hospitals or sections of hospitals were used to accommodate black and white psychiatric patients. Needless to say, the facilities for black patients were usually in a poor, dilapidated condition and hardly conducive to the development of therapeutic milieu (Pillay, 1991). Facilities for white patients, on the other hand, were either modern constructions or extravagantly restored Victorian architecture. The internationally publicized report of the American Psychiatric Association (1979), following their inspection of psychiatric institutions in South Africa, was particularly critical of the sub-standard and sub-therapeutic facilities for black patients in comparison with those reserved for the white mentally ill. This finding was made despite the obvious superficial face-lifts given to some of the facilities just prior to the Americans' visit (since they had been expected)! The psychiatric care meted out to black patients was described as inferior, inadequate, violent and destructive. The World Health Organization (1977) was equally condemning of the South African psychiatric services, despite its decision not to undertake an inspection of mental health facilities in view of the apartheid government's refusal to allow unrestricted access and investigation.

Outpatient mental health services have also not been well developed. In the large metropolitan centers with academic health complexes, multidisciplinary mental health care has been available to differing degrees, depending on the city and it: informal reputation of being conservative or liberal. In the peri-urban and rural areas, however, mental health services have been virtually nonexistent. Of course, virtually all of the inhabitants of these outlying areas were black, with the exception of wealthy white farmers who could afford access to urban private practitioners. During the latter years of apartheid, visiting and satellite clinics were being implemented in the outlying areas, mainly from the region's psychiatric hospital. However, these clinics did not provide mental health care, as defined n modern times. Rather they were medication clinics, where patients were seen on a monthly basis to collect their psychiatric medication.

Until the time of preparation of this chapter, the psychiatric service situation had not changed substantially, but certainly not because of will or and problems inherited from the previous regime. Unraveling and undoing decades of apartheid is no easy task, as has been discovered by the newly elected government officials.

Epidemiology

Of the many difficulties facing planners of mental health services, the inadequacy of epidemiological data in South Africa is one of the most significant. While there have been numerous research studies over the years providing prevalence data, the methodological variations have made it largely impossible to draw accurate conclusions of national significance.

Investigations of clinic samples have reported rates of psychiatric morbidity around 10 percent (Freeman, Seris, Mathebula, & Price, 1991), even in neighboring Zimbabwe (Hall & Williams, 1987). Community based samples, however, have revealed psychiatric morbidity rates around 20 percent (Gillis, Lewis, & Slabbert, 1968), with rates up to 39 percent among the black elderly (Bester, Weich, & Gagiano, 1991; Ben-Arie, Swartz, Teggin, & Elk, 1983). A community sample in the mountain kingdom of Lesotho, landlocked by South Africa, showed a rate of around 22 percent, assessing only depression, panic disorder, and generalized anxiety disorder, suggesting a much higher rate of overall psychiatric morbidity (Hollifield, Katon, Spain, & Pule, 1990). The higher rates of conspicuous psychiatric morbidity noted in community samples compared to clinic samples is expected since there are likely to be individuals in the community with mental health problems which they (or their families) have not considered severe enough to warrant professional attention. This is verified by the National Institute of Mental Health study in the United States, which found that 28 percent of the general population had a definite mental health problem, but that only 8 percent sought treatment while 20 percent did not (Regier, Narrow, Rae et al., 1993; Narrow, Regier, Rae et al., 1993).

Despite the methodological issues the Southern African prevalence data are not substantially different to findings elsewhere in the world. An American rural primary health care study showed a psychiatric morbidity rate of 26.5 percent (Barrett, Barrett, Oxman, & Gerber, 1988), while the longitudinal collaborative study of the World Health Organization (WHO) conducted in 14 developed and developing countries revealed that 30 percent of people attending primary health care sites suffered mental disorders (Sartorius, Ustun, Costa et al., 1993). It is, of course, likely that the prevalence of mental health problems in South Africa is higher than that of developed and even some of developing countries, given its oppressive past and the current political violence in certain areas particularly the province of KwaZulu-Natal.

Economic Issues

Historically, it has been difficult to accurately ascertain the mental health bill for the nation. For example, it is evident that a little over 8 percent of the country's gross national product is spent on health (Mcintyre, Bloom, Doherty, & Briglal, 1985). However, the exact proportion of this budget spent on mental health services is unclear. A provincial analysis of this expenditure, undertaken for the Western Cape region, revealed that 8 percent of general health funds was devoted to mental health (Ensink, Leger, & Robertson, 1994). That study also found that 97 percent of those mental health funds was allocated to hospitals with the remaining three percent allocated to the community clinic services. While similar financial analyses are not available for other provinces, there is no reason to believe that the funding distribution is likely to be much different. In fact, since some of the other provinces have fewer hospital-based mental health services than the Western Cape, their overall mental health budgets may well be much lower. The allocation of around 3 percent of total mental health funds to community care is extremely low, even if one considers that a small portion of the hospitals' budgets is also spent on their own outpatient services. It is evident that the ratio of hospital-based mental health care to community care will almost need to be reversed if the government's plan of deinstitutionalization of the mentally ill is to be achieved (Natal Witness, 1998a).

Mental health expenditure at the primary care level is cited at around 0.6 percent of the total primary health care budget (Rispel, Price, & Cabral, 1996). This level of spending is disproportionate y low considering international findings that up to 80 percent of patients with psychological and psychiatric disorders are seen at the primary care level (Regier et al., 1993; Narrow et al., 1993). In addition, numerous studies have shown that in excess of 25 percent of primary care attenders show discernible evidence of mental health problems (cf Pillay & Lockhat, 1997). Also considering the national and international proposals favoring integration of mental health care into the primary care infrastructure (World Health Organization, 1978), it is essential that the mental health funding allocation to primary health care is drastically increased.

A further point of concern regarding the current mental health funding is that there is absolutely no allocation specifically for illness prevention and health promotion programs. It is vitally important that these aspects be formally incorporated into mental health care, and that administrators and providers instill an ethos of prevention and health promotion into the service. This needs to be achieved in order to avoid past (and even current) ways of thinking that have resulted in preventive and promotive programs being viewed as occasional appendages to health care.

Current Mental Health Situation in KwaZulu-Natal

Since the inception of democratic governance in April 1994, the previously fragmented health system has been integrated into a national department and nine provincial departments coinciding with the nine newly demarcated provinces (previously four). Functions of the former include national policy-making and the development of norms and standards, while the provincial departments have significant powers in the actual rendering of health services (Ntsaluba & Pillay, 1998). The province of KwaZulu-Natal, which is the focus of this paper, comprises an area of 92,180 km^2 along the eastern seaboard of South Africa. With a population of over 9 million people, KwaZulu-Natal is the second most populated province in the country. The majority of the population (62.4 percent) lives in rural areas where there is limited mental health infrastructure (Commission on Gender Equality, 1997).

The two major cities of Durban and Pietermaritzburg (80 km apart toward the east coast) provide inpatient mental health care in psychiatric hospitals and a few general hospitals (see Figure 19.1). In addition, a psychiatric hospital is situated in the far northwestern town of Newcastle. However, the large areas outside of these centers are without inpatient mental health facilities. The psychiatric hospitals in the three centers offer a total of 2,692 acute and long-term inpatient beds, which translates into a bed to population ratio of 29 to 100,000 including beds for mental retardation (KwaZulu-Natal Department of Health, 1997). When assessed against the WHO recommendation of 100 beds per 100,000 people, the deficit is substantial. As far as human resources are concerned, the ratio of public sector psychiatrists to population is in the order of 1 to 562,500 (considerably lower than the average ratio of about 1 to 14,000 found in many developing and developed countries) (Lin, 1983); public sector psychologists 1 to 209,302; and community psychiatric nurses 1 to 57,325 (Pillay, Bhana, & Petersen, 1994).

Community mental health services are provided to varying degrees within and from the three psychiatric centers in the province. While multidisciplinary services are available to residents of the two main cities of Durban and Pietermaritzburg, mental health care for many communities living in the rural areas of the province consists of medication dispensing points for ex-psychiatric hospital inpatients. This service may be provided by either a community psychiatric nurse or a district surgeon (a state-employed, non-psychiatrically trained medical practitioner). Within the private sector, diagnostic and curative psychiatric and psychological

FIGURE 19.1: ***Province of Kwa-Zulu Natal***

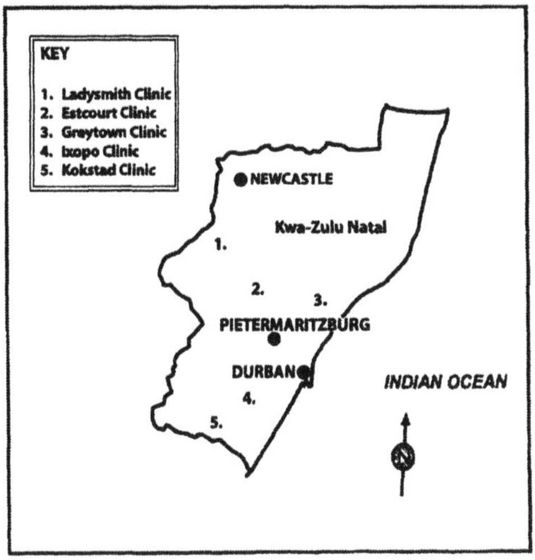

services are readily available in Durban and Pietermaritzburg, which also boast private hospitals offering limited inpatient care. In contrast to urban areas, rural and pen-urban populations are severely underserviced by both the public and private sectors.

The Midlands Psychiatric Complex in Pietermaritzburg is a large provincial teaching and service complex providing multidisciplinary inpatient care. This 1,668-bed complex comprises three separate hospitals. One 624-bed hospital provides custodial care for mentally retarded adults and children. Medical treatment, occupational therapy, industrial therapy, and very limited psychological services are available to inpatients. The remaining hospitals in the complex, which have approximately, 500 beds each, have historically been characterized by racial segregation: one hospital catering for white patients, and the other for black patients and for observation and custodial care of forensic patients. Treatment in these hospitals predominantly takes the form of medication and psychotherapy. Outpatient services are also available, but the threshold for using these services is geographical proximity to the hospital. Over the past few years, minor changes in the racial composition of hospital patients have been effected with true integration still to be achieved. With the exception of nursing personnel, all other professional and support staff are racially integrated. These issues are currently the focus of attention and debate at both administrative and grass-roots levels.

Midlands Psychiatric Complex has established a number of satellite clinics in outlying areas to provide follow-up care and management of patients who have been discharged to their communities. To this end, at least one community psychiatric nurse has been employed on a full-time basis in each of five rural or pen-urban clinics (see Figure 19.1). In addition, a team of three community psychiatric nurses based at the psychiatric hospital travel to outlying areas up to 250 km away to conduct monthly clinics. The follow-up care provided at these satellite clinics consists mainly of dispensing repeat medication to patients who have been stabilized whilst inpatients. New cases requiring involuntary hospitalization are usually referred to the local district surgeon to facilitate the process of committing the patient to a psychiatric hospital for further evaluation and treatment. In such cases the current Mental Health Act (1973) requires that the attending hospital psychiatrist or medical practitioner assesses the patient and compiles a report within a period of 72 hours from the time of detention. The Mental Health Act (1973) is currently being revised to meet human rights requirements set out in the new South African Constitution.

It is noteworthy that within the Midlands Complex (and other psychiatric hospitals around the country), significantly more black patients are committed under the Mental Health Act and fewer admitted as voluntary patients than white patients (Diedricks, personal communication). This finding is similar to that reported in the United States where proportionately more African-Americans are committed to public mental hospitals and receive diagnoses such as schizophrenia (Lindsey & Paul, 1989). In the South African context this may reflect a number of factors including the possibility that due to poverty, lack of transport and long distances to be traveled for mental health consultations, black patients only enter the mental health care system when they are severely mentally ill. Alternatively, the lack of outpatient mental health facilities in rural areas may result in the unnecessary committal of patients in order to ensure public transportation (albeit in an ambulance or police vehicle) to the distant psychiatric complex. Another important finding is that despite women comprising 52.7 percent of the province's population (KwaZulu-Natal Department of Health, 1997), the majority (75.84 percent) of patients admitted to the Midland Psychiatric Complex are men (Diedricks, personal communication). This is consistent with other African studies of admission rates to psychiatric institutions, and may be due to men's greater employment in the formal sector and hence access to health care; their greater physical aggression which may bring them to the attention of authorities; and women's preference for indigenous traditional healers and spiritual churches as sources of psychological solace (Kisekka, 1990). The last-mentioned hypothesis may account for the finding that the ratio of female to male admissions is significantly lower in the hospital treating patients of African descent than in that treating other cultural groups (1 to 3.8 and 1 to 2.3, respectively) (Diedricks, personal communication). In addition, these findings may reflect the health system's neglect of women - in particular black women - with mental health problems.

Examination of routine surveillance data from the five outlying clinics staffed by Midlands community psychiatric nurses suggests that community mental health services in the region are almost exclusively aimed at patients with major psychiatric disorders (psychosis, severe mood disorders). Table 19.1 shows the diagnostic distribution of adults attending these clinics at a specific point during 1998. The diagnoses are listed according to descriptive categories, rather than strict nomenclature, for ease of discussion. The majority of men are treated for schizophrenia (58 percent) and substance-induced psychosis (23 percent). Cannabis and alcohol, the most popular drugs of abuse are also commonly abused by male patients with schizophrenia. The high frequency of psychotic illnesses among the men (81 percent) receiving medication at these clinics must be seen in the context of the presentation of these conditions in most male patients. Families and society are far less likely to tolerate the positive symptoms during the active phase of schizophrenia (e. delusions, hallucinations, thought disorder, agitation) in males for fear of aggression and violence (even if there is none), than in females with this disorder. The women attending the clinics are mostly treated for schizophrenia (53 percent) and depression or anxiety (24 percent). The gender variations of disorders in this survey are consistent with studies in developed and developing countries which suggest that substance related disorders are more prevalent among men, and depression and anxiety more prevalent among women (cf de la Rey & Eagle, 1997; Nair & Pillay, 1997). In addition, the slightly higher rate of schizophrenia noted among males (the tender minority in the province) is consistent with recent hospital-based data showing higher rates among males (American Psychiatric Association, 1994).

A rather striking finding is the virtual absence of post-traumatic stress disorder (PTSD) at these clinics despite the political violence affecting several outlying areas of the province. Also, high levels of criminal violence are prevalent throughout the country to the point that risk of being

TABLE 19.1: ***Diagnostic Categories of Clinic Attendees***

	Male	(%)	Female	(%)	Total	Frequency
Schizophrenia	397	(58.38)	295	(53.44)	692	56.17
Substance-Induced Psychosis	153	(22.50)	13	(2.35)	166	13.47
Depression	34	(5.00)	85	(15.40)	119	9.66
Anxiety	6	(0.88)	50	(9.06)	56	4.55
Mental Retardation	35	(5.15)	16	(2.90)	51	4.14
Psychosis due to General Mental Condition	18	(2.65)	18	(3.26)	36	2.92
Bipolar Disorder	8	(1.18)	19	(3.44)	27	2.19
Epilepsy	10	(1.47)	16	(2.90)	26	2.11
Dementia	11	(1.62)	21	(3.80)	32	2.60
Brief Psychotic Disorder	0	(0.00)	7	(1.27)	7	0.57
Personality Disorder	0	(0.00)	5	(0.91)	5	0.41
Delusional Disorder	2	(0.29)	2	(0.36)	4	0.32
Schizophreniform Disorder	1	(0.15)	2	(0.36)	3	0.24
Amnestic Disorder	2	(0.29)	0	(0.00)	2	0.16
Post-traumatic Stress Disorder	1	(0.15)	1	(0.18)	2	0.16
Psychotic Disorder N.O.S.	1	(0.15)	1	(0.18)	2	0.16
Alcohol Dependence	1	(0.15)	0	(0.00)	1	0.08
Problems of Living	0	(0.00)	1	(0.18)	1	0.08
TOTAL	680		552		1232	100.00

murdered in South Africa is regarded as being amongst the highest in the world outside of known war zones. The excessive crime level is also cited as a major deterrent to foreign investment that is so desperately needed in the South African economy (*Daily News*, 1998). It is evident that the present finding reflects the lack of appropriate services rather then prevalence of the disorder A recent comparative study of urban and rural children's mental health problems revealed that PTSD was significantly more common among rural than urban clinic populations and that it was largely related to political violence (Pillay, Naidoo, & Lockhat, 1998). It is therefore likely that the parents of these children have also been affected in some way, but have not sought help or had their symptoms identified.

The estimated prevalence of conspicuous psychiatric morbidity in rural and urban community settings in South Africa ranges from 10 percent to 39 percent (Freeman, 1992). Based on research in other countries, it can be estimated that approximately 2.7 percent of the population presents for specialist treatment (Andrews & Teesson, 1994). Therefore, those with mental health problem: currently receiving specialized mental health care in KwaZulu-Natal comprise only a small proportion of the total population in need of mental health care. In sum, the unidisciplinary (medical) approach to community care, and the relative neglect of what appear to be minor psychiatric disorders (e.g., anxiety, depression, post-traumatic stress disorder) and psycho-social problems (e.g., substance abuse, woman and child abuse, rape violence, HIV epidemic), suggests that mental health care has been aimed *more* at protecting society than promoting mental health. This is a severe indictment of the mental health system which needs to re-examine its objectives. The health policy document of the African National Congress (1994) has emphasized, inter alia, health promotion, disease prevention, community empowerment and community care, and has prioritized vulnerable groups (e.g.. children, women and those affected by all forms of violence). It is important, therefore, that South Africa's developing mental health system move steadfastly in this direction.

Mental Health Needs

The existing system of mental health care in KwaZulu-Natal has clearly failed to meet the needs of the province's largely rural population. The discussion that follows outlines some of the neglected areas which urgently need to be addressed.

Caregivers

The current concepts of hospitalization as a means of stabilizing mentally ill patients, and community care as the dispensation of medicines post-discharge, means that the burden of caring for mentally ill individuals falls on relatives, and in particular aging and elderly women (Hamber & Eagle, 1997). This is not only the case in many developing countries (Leff, 1994; Murthy, 1998), but is also one of the consequences of the deinstitutionalization movement in developed countries (Goldman, 1982; Ascher-Svanum, & Sobel, 1989). Although Hamber and Eagle (1997) found that caregivers in South Africa uncomplainingly accept their role, there is a significant psychological, physiological and economic impact on these women's lives and the sense of subjective burden is high. Lefley (1987) aptly points out that care giving for one group at the expense of another is hardly a desirable mental health objective. The task of caregivers in KwaZulu-Natal is often more difficult because mental health resources are not easily accessible, and a number of families receive little or no information from mental health professionals about their mentally ill relative either during, hospitalization or on discharge. In fact, families should be treated as an essential component of mental health care, and multidisciplinary community interventions should address the needs of caregivers of mentally ill individuals (Murthy, 1998). This would, in turn, enhance their capacity to sustain their mentally ill relatives in the community. Interventions should include: provision of support and skills training to caregivers; education about the importance of medication compliance; provision of information about medication and possible side effects; suggestion of strategies for managing socially disruptive behaviors and other symptoms; education about the mental illness and early signs of relapse; and assisting families in networking (Petrila & Sadoff, 1992; Murthy, 1998). There may also be a need to involve other family members of both genders in the patient's support system (Ascher-Svanum & Sobel, 1989).

Substance Abuse

The high rate of co-morbidity of substance abuse and psychotic disorders in male patients presenting at the clinics in the KwaZulu-Natal Midlands is consistent with international research (Miller & Tanenbaum, 1989; Kovasznay, Bromet, Schwartz et al., 1993). However, while psychotic disorders are treated by means of medication, the problems of alcohol and substance abuse are largely neglected in the community clinics. This is particularly significant in view of the poorer treatment outcome among such patients. Weiss, Mirin and Frances (1992) point out that patients with co-morbid substance abuse disorders have a higher incidence of hospitalization, medication noncompliance, criminality, homelessness and suicide. In fact, alcohol and substance abuse are important psychological disorders which should be addressed by mental health professionals. This is evident in the National Health Department's decision, following the new government's inception, to extend the National Mental Health Directorate to include Substance Abuse. The country's previous national Health Policy did not include substance abuse under the umbrella of mental health. Finally, while the government's intention to curtail tobacco and alcohol use is certainly positive. South Africa's re-entry into world markets has exposed the country to international drug trafficking, with the result that hard drugs are now more accessible in urban and rural areas than ever before.

Common Disorders

Community mental health efforts are currently concentrated on severely mentally ill individuals. However, Andrews and Teesson (1994) point out that depression, substance use and anxiety disorders a e the most common disorders. Although few studies of prevalence and incidence o these psychological disorders in community setting have been conducted in South Africa, the reported African prevalence for depression ranges from 14 percent to 49 percent (Reeler & Todd, 1994). In view of the high rate of political and sexual violence, criminal victimization, woman and child abuse, and poverty in the KwaZulu-Natal Midlands, higher rates of disorders such as anxiety, depression and post-traumatic stress disorder may be expected. However, the clinic data indicates that these disorders are not being identified and treated. This finding is unfortunately not unique to South Africa or developing countries. An American study found that only a minority of patients with depressive and anxiety disorders were diagnosed and treated by means of psychiatric or psychological interventions (Simon, Ormel, Von Korff, & Barlow, 1995). The importance of identifying and treating these disorders is highlighted by findings in primary care settings, in both developed and developing countries, that disability and functional impairment are more strongly associated with mood, anxiety and somatoform disorders than with most medical illnesses (Abas & Broadhead, 1994; Thurston-Hicks, Paine, & Hollifield, 1998).

Violence

Political violence in KwaZulu-Natal has had a huge impact on the lives of adults and children alike, It is estimated that over 13,000 people have died and half a million rendered homeless as a result of the political violence in the province between 1985 and 1996 (Stavrou, 1998a). As far as sexual violence in KwaZulu-Natal is concerned, 8,639 rapes were reported to the South African Police Services in 1997 (SAPS Quarterly Report, 1998), and it is estimated that only I in 35 rapes/attempted rapes are actually reported (Commission on Gender Equality, 1997). In fact, the Edendale valley in the greater Pietermaritzburg area has recently been branded the "rape capital" of South Africa (Natal Witness, 1998b). Published findings to date suggest that exposure to war, sexual assault and other types of trauma are *likely* to lead to elevated symptomatology (Kessler, Sonnega, Bromet et al., 1995; Bromet, 1996). Post-traumatic stress disorder amongst men is most commonly associated with combat exposure or witnessing someone being badly injured, while amongst women it is associated with rape and sexual molestation (Kessler et al, 1995). The increased probability of other lifetime disorders among people with lifetime post-traumatic stress disorder (ibid), underscores the importance of increasing the limited community mental health services to include trauma counseling for survivors of violence. The government has acknowledged both the needs of survivors of criminal and political violence and the lack of sufficient services, by developing a National Crime Prevention Strategy (NCPS) which promotes a victim-centric approach to crime prevention through the Victim Empowerment Programme (VEP) (Prozesky & Kotze, 1998; Stavrou, 1998b). However, although the NCPS was released in 1996, health-led projects envisaged by the VEP have still to be implemented.

HIV Infection and AIDS

The growing epidemic of HIV infection and AIDS poses another problem for mental health in the province. There is an estimated prevalence of HIV infection among women attending antenatal clinics in KwaZulu-Natal of 19.9 percent (KwaZulu-Natal Department of Health, 1997). This places increased demands on the mental health system since counseling is viewed as critical to the prevention of HIV transmission and to the reduction of the psychosocial impact of HIV infection and AIDS (Lindegger & Crewe, 1997). Moreover, HIV infection and AIDS are associated with an increased incidence of psychological difficulties and psychiatric disorder (ibid).

Suicidal Behavior

Self-destructive behaviors are becoming increasingly common among all cultural groups in South Africa, despite being historically viewed as a more culture-specific problem. Women are regarded as a high-risk group, especially those women who are subjected to domestic violence by substance-abusing husbands (Pillay, Van der Veen, & Wassenaar, 1998). In the urban areas patients presenting with suicidal ideation or behaviors are able to access health care at most general hospitals and mental health care at some institutions. However, for suicidal individuals in outlying areas, there is there is no mental health care available. This is particularly disconcerting considering the level of distress and feelings of hopelessness endured by the affected individuals during the state of heightened crisis. Research has demonstrated the effectiveness of psychological interventions in reducing the intensity of these pathological processes, and thus decreasing suicidal risk (Pillay & Wassenaar, 1995). The neglect of this, the most seriously life-threatening of the mental health problems, needs to be addressed in the rural communities, both in terms of management and prevention.

Child Development

Child development and psychopathology constitute significant areas of need in the disadvantaged communities. Recent research has emphasized the deficiency in the detection of childhood disorders in rural and pen-urban communities (Pillay, Naidoo, & Lockhat, 1998). Treatable conditions such as attention deficit/hyperactivity disorder (ADHD) are not identified mainly as a result of the over-crowded classroom situations in rural areas, making detection by school teachers (who are often less qualified than urban teachers) more difficult. The significantly higher rate of post-traumatic stress disorder (PTSD) noted in rural children in that study was attributed to the high levels of political violence in some of the rural areas. Children have often witnessed brutal atrocities, including the murder of their family members, and gunshot injuries in children have become commonplace (Hadley & Mars, 1998). Although non-governmental organizations have attempted to meet these needs, it is time for the government to respond to the mental health needs of children and youth. In addition, the importance of child development and support programs for the prevention of mental health problems, particularly for impoverished families, has been documented (McGuire & Earls, 1991). The national mental health and substance abuse sub-directorate of Child, Youth, Women and Family Health has prioritized the mental health of children and youth, and is currently drafting policy guidelines (Tzhotzho, 1998).

The Elderly

The mental health needs of older adults have been severely neglected, particularly within the black population (Ferreira & Gillis, 1997). It has been suggested that at least 20 percent of people over the age of 65 years will have mental health problems, especially dementia, delirium and depression (ibid). In KwaZulu-Natal, elderly black people are thought to constitute a greater proportion of rural than urban populations. Rural elderly are often more vulnerable to mental health problems because their families have usually migrated to towns and cities to seek employment, leaving them with less social support. Elderly women in particular are a high-risk group, since they are expected to carry the burden of managing household tasks, rearing grandchildren and caring for mentally or physically ill relatives. In some areas the elderly are displaced from their homes by political violence, and are forced to seek refuge in informal settlements on the periphery of urban areas. In addition to psychological trauma, they are forced to cope with substantial economic, social and personal losses. It is therefore not surprising that Gillis and colleagues (c.f. Ferreira & Gillis, 1997) found a prevalence of depressive symptomatology in older residents of a newly-settled shack township of 44 percent for women and 17 percent for men. Detection, diagnosis and treatment of depressive symptomatology in elderly patients is imperative, as is support for caregivers of demented older persons, and the facilitation of social networks and support groups for the elderly.

Mental Retardation

In South Africa mental retardation has been viewed as a static lifelong condition requiring either special schooling or long-term institutionalization (in more severe cases). Historically, access to these facilities has been dependent on race, with the result that special schools and institutions providing custodial care are characterized by a predominantly white population (Molteno, 1997). Consequently, the majority of black children with mental retardation do not attend school and are cared for by their families (more so in rural areas) with minimal support (community care by default). Community tolerance of individuals with mental retardation is generally high in rural areas and the simple ways of life allow for valued community participation (Murthy, 1998). However, in South Africa rural black families caring for handicapped children or adults also have to contend with poverty. Although individuals with mental retardation are eligible for a monthly government grant, there has historically been inequity between the races as far as grant amounts were concerned. In addition, many rural individuals have no access to psychological services and, therefore, have not been diagnosed as having mental retardation, thus not qualifying for state grants. There is a certainly a need for community based services which would develop the capacity of caregivers to meet the needs, and develop the potential, of individuals with mental retardation.

Addressing Mental Health Needs in South Africa

There are several possible ways of approaching the problems and deficiencies in the country's mental health services. However, some of these ideas are neither immediately helpful nor economically feasible, for example, training more mental health professionals and/or creating more rural facilities. Clearly the traditional mental health model has failed the people of South Africa (with the exception of a select few). What is needed instead is an approach that is able to deliver at least basic mental health care to all who need it, regardless of geographical location or other discriminatory factors. The two models that could answer this call are the Community Mental Health and Primary Health Care models. The present authors are of the opinion that both of these paradigms have valuable strengths and could be applied in the South African situation. However, there are also difficulties envisaged in the use of one of these approaches to the exclusion of the other.

The Community Mental Health Model

The community mental health model has its roots in the deinstitutionalization lobby of the 1960's, and favors the provision of mental health services at community level, mainly through outpatient and day-clinic facilities. However, history has demonstrated in several countries that the community mental health movement may have focused over-enthusiastically on emptying psychiatric hospitals and insufficiently on providing the after-care and support programs necessary to sustain affected individuals in the community (Barham, 1992). This is one of the reasons why many mentally ill people are among the homeless on the streets and subway stations in these countries.

The community mental health model has a strongly humanistic ideology, seeking to entrench the rights of the mentally ill. The major thrusts of this model may be summarized as follows:

(i) Hospitalization in a psychiatric institution is kept to an absolute minimum, with strict control over involuntary admission and discharge policies.
(ii) Mental health care is provided at community mental health cen-

ters located in or around residential areas. In other words, mental health care must be available where people live, and not in institutions far removed from society.

(iii) More centers, smaller in size provide care for smaller sections of the populous, than the traditional psychiatric hospitals.

(iv) Individuals with mental health problems are managed within the context of their families and friends, and more importantly in familiar surroundings. Only if problems cannot be managed at this level, will hospitalization be considered, firstly in a general hospital mental health unit, and thereafter at a psychiatric hospital.

(v) The centers focus solely on mental health care, using specially trained mental health professionals (e.g. community psychiatric nurses, psychologists, psychiatrists, social workers), but adopt a generalist approach, i.e. providing care to all mental health problems. The human resource element is not intensive (may comprise only a community psychiatric nurse), but is specialized.

(vi) The community is encouraged and expected to take an active role in "owning" the center and its service. This helps make the service user-friendly, unlike traditional mental health structures where consumers feel like intruders.

(vii) This model has a strong emphasis on illness prevention and health promotion, which must be considered vital aspects of any mental health system in the country.

The Primary Health Care Model

The primary health care (PHC) approach was originally conceived with the intention of providing physical health care at grass-roots level for socioeconomically disadvantaged communities. However, it is being increasingly employed, even in developed countries, mainly due to its reputation of providing relatively low cost care to those unable to afford private health care. Notwithstanding its popularity, the PHC model was born out of the dichotomous mind-body model and, as a result, has focused exclusively on physical health problems. In this respect an interesting conceptual shift was mooted by the WHO (1978) in its Declaration of Alma Ata, calling for the integration of mental health care into the PIJC system.

Epidemiological research has revealed that the PHC infrastructure may be the most appropriate level at which to deliver mental health care, since up to 80 percent of those with mental health problems are seen at these health sites (Regier et al., 1993). The implications of providing mental health care at this level may be summarized as follows:

(i) Mental health care would be available to all communities at the most basic level in the state-funded health system.
(ii) The stigma attached to receiving care at a special mental health clinic is avoided, since a wide range of illnesses (mainly physical) are addressed at PHC clinics.
(iii) A truly holistic approach is possible, incorporating focus on both physical and mental health.
(iv) Earlier identification of psychological problems is possible during routine or other visits for physical problems. This is especially important in the case of developmental problems in children, as well as prodromal stages of psychotic disorders in adults.
(v) The easier accessibility to PHC centers would result in fewer barriers and resistances to treatment that often plague people with mental illnesses.

The South African government has adopted a new national health policy which is driven by the PHC approach. In accordance with the three-tiered (national, provincial and local) system of governance introduced in the new South African Constitution, the National Health White Paper for the Transformation of the Health System (gazetted on 16 April 1997) delineates areas of responsibility for the development and delivery of health services. It provides for a district health authority system which will function at the local level to provide comprehensive primary health care services (including mental health care). The PHC policy adopted by the national government also calls for the deinstitutionalization of psychiatric hospitals and a shift toward community-based care (Natal Witness, 1998a). While it is recognized that primary mental health care may be the only mental health care available to certain sectors of the population, there are a number of practical difficulties which may result from the integration of mental health into primary health care to the exclusion of more specialized mental health care at a community level.

South Africa's primary health care system is still in the developing stage. Despite limited primary health infrastructure and personnel, free health care for children and pregnant women was introduced in June 1994 in an attempt to improve accessibility to health care. In June 1996, the cost barrier was eliminated completely, and free primary health services were extended to all South Africans (Ntsaluba & Pillay, 1998). This has led to overcrowding in health facilities, to the point that the primary health care system is unable to meet the demands placed on it by physical problems. For example, in the Western Cape, 32,000 health workers treat 3 million outpatients per year (Rasool, 1998). The shortage of PHC personnel means that health care is currently being provided tinder extreme time constraints. Thus, the integration of mental health services into PHC could mean a collapse of mental health services, which are likely to be allocated a back-seat to physical health care. This is a realistic concern since mental health care has historically occupied the position of a neglected stepchild in the general health care family.

An Alternative Approach

The delivery of mental health services at the PHC level is an important route that needs to be taken in providing mental health care to rural communities. However, if this approach is used in the absence of more specialized community mental health care, it is the authors' contention that apartheid (or a close relative) could be back in business! People living in rural areas (who are virtually all of African descent) will once again be short-changed by being given limited and lower grade care. That is to say, in other developing countries with scarce resources the integration of mental health into PHC has been practically translated into the medical care of people with schizophrenia, affective disorders and epilepsy (Freeman, 1992). While it is acknowledged that it is not possible to provide tertiary level specialist and super-specialist care in the outlying areas, it is vital that mental health services are appropriate, effective and accessible to all those requiring mental health interventions.

Unlike many developed countries, where general medical practitioners and nurses staff PHC clinics, PHC clinics in South Africa are essentially conducted by general nurses. The delivery of mental health services at these clinics will therefore necessitate the extension of the clinical role of nurses to include detection and treatment (basic counseling and pharmacotherapy) of mental health problems. Appropriate training of these personnel is an essential first step toward the integration of mental health into PHC. However, this is a major task and even *with* training, only some conditions may be identified and effectively managed at this level (Reeler & Todd, 1994; Tarrier, Tantam, & Gater, 1994; Lambert & Hartley, 1998). In South Africa the application of effective mental health treatment will be even more difficult given the excessively large numbers of physically ill patients presenting at PHC clinics. For these reasons, the onus of providing mental health care to millions of rural South Africans should not rest solely on PHC personnel. The need for active, intensive support of PHC nurses must be recognized and included in this approach.

The establishment of community mental health centers or specialist points at district level would ensure the provision of support for PHC nurses, among other functions. The staffing and size of these specialist points or centers would vary, depending on geographic location and population density. The minimum human resource requirement should be a community psychiatric nurse (CPN), i.e. a registered nurse who has received specialized training in psychiatry. Under ideal circumstances a clinical psychologist and a psychiatrist (or medical doctor with some psychiatric training) should either be available or provide a visiting service. This community-based multidisciplinary mental health team should be functionally distinct from the specialist teams staffing the secondary (regional) and tertiary (provincial) inpatient units, since caseloads and time constraints of secondary and tertiary personnel would interfere with their capacity to provide adequate support to PHC workers.

The minimum requirement of a CPN in each health district would ensure a consultative and support service for PHC nurses in the provision of primary mental health care, and a referral source for more complicated problems. The CPN, in turn, would have the opportunity to refer difficult cases to the resident (or visiting) clinical psychologist or psychiatrist should the need arise. It is also essential that the role of the CPN be extended to include the promotion of psychosocial well-being, and the implementation of prevention and rehabilitation programs in the health district (something which the overburdened PHC workers will certainly not have time for). In addition, the CPN would facilitate self-help groups in the community, and network with non-governmental and community-based organizations to develop the capacity of communities to meet the mental, physical and social needs of individual members. In other words, the CPN would not focus exclusively on people with mental disorders, but would also provide either direct or non-direct services to other vulnerable groups with mental health needs, for example, caregivers of mentally ill patients, survivors of sexual, domestic and political violence, substance abusers and people with HIV/AIDS. Collaboration with traditional healers is also imperative since they play an important role in the mental health care of many individuals residing in rural areas, particularly women.

Concluding Comments

This chapter has examined the current nature of psychiatric disorders and mental health care in rural areas of South Africa in the context of formulating appropriate mental health services. While the government's PHC and deinstitutionalization policies are acknowledged as representing important steps towards providing community-based mental health care for all South Africans, there is a danger that these policies may maintain the status quo at best, or result in the collapse of mental health services at worst. However, this may be avoided if deinstitutionalization is not viewed as a cost-saving exercise, but rather as a progressive therapeutic strategy. This would mean deploying some of the mental health specialists currently employed in institutions to service PIIC sites and communities at a district level.

References

Abas, M., & Broadhead, J. (1994). Mental disorders in the developing world. *British Medical Journal*, 308: 1052.

African National Congress (ANC). (1994). *A National Health Plan for South Africa*. Johannesburg: ANC.

American Psychiatric Association. (1979). Report of the committee to visit South Africa. *American Journal of Psychiatry*, 136: 1498-1506.

American Psychiatric Association. (1994). *Diagnostic and statistical manual of mental disorders* (4th edition). Washington, DC: APA.

Andrews, G., & Teesson, M. (1994). Smart versus dumb treatment: services for mental disorders. *Current Opinion in Psychiatry*, 7: 181-185.

Ascher-Svanum, H., & Sobel, T.S. (1989). Caregivers of mentally ill adults: a women's agenda. *Hospital and Community Psychiatry*, 40: 84 -845.

Barham. P. (1992). *Closing the asylum: The mental patient in modern society.* London: Penguin. Barrett, J. B., Barrett, J.A., Oxman, T.B., & Gerber, P.D. (1988). The prevalence of specific psychiatric disorders in a primary care practice. *Archives of General Psychiatry*, 45: 1100-1106.

Ben-Arie, O., Swartz, L., Teggin, A.F., & Elk, R. (1983). The Coloured elderly in Cape Town - A psychosocial, psychiatric and medical community survey: Part II. Prevalence of psychiatric disorders. *South African Medical Journal*, 64: 1056-1061.

Bester, F.C.J., Weich, D.J.V., & Gagiano, C.A. (1991). Mental disorders of elderly blacks in the Orange Free State. *The Journal of Age Related Disorders*, 3: 13-16.

Bromet, E.J. (1996). Impact of trauma. *Current Opinion in Psychiatry*, 9: 153-

157.
Commission on Gender Equality. (1997). Report of the Commission on Gender Equality information and evaluation workshop, KwaZulu-Natal Province. *Daily News* (1998). Durban, August 26, (p.19).
Dawes, A. (1985). Politics and mental health. *South African Journal of Psychology*, 15: 55-61.
de Ia Rey, C., & Eagle, G. (1997). Gender and mental health policy development. In D. Foster, M. Freeman, & Y. Pillay (eds.), *Mental health policy issues for South Africa*. Pinelands: Medical Association of South Africa.
Dommisse, J. (1987). The state of psychiatry in South Africa today. *Social Science & Medicine*, 24: 749-761.
Ensink, K., Leger, P., & Robertson, B. (1994). Public sector mental health services in the Western Cape. In Y. Pillay, A. Bhana, A. Bhagwanjee, A. Parekh, & I. Petersen (eds.), *Proceedings of the Primary Mental Health Care Workshop*. University of Durban-Westvile, September, 1994.
Ferreira, M., & Gillis, L. (1997). The elderly. In D. Foster, M. Freeman, & Y. Pillay (eds.), *Mental health policy issues for South Africa*. Pinelands: Medical Association of South Africa.
Freeman, M. (1992). Providing mental health care for all in South Africa - structure and strategy. Paper No. 24. Johannesburg: Centre for Health Policy. University of the Witwatersrand.
Freeman, M., Seris, N., Mathebula, E., & Price, M. (1991). *An evaluation of mental health services in the South Eastern Transvaal*, Vol. 10. Johannesburg: Centre for Health Policy, University of the Witwatersrand.
Gillis, L.S., Lewis, J.B., & Slabbert, M. (1968). Psychiatric disorder amongst the Coloured people of the Cape Peninsula. *British Journal of Psychiatry*, 114: 1575-1587.
Goldman, H.H. (1982). Mental illness and family burden: A public health perspective. *Hospital and Community Psychiatry*, 33: 557-560.
Hadley. G.P., & Mars. M. (1998). Gunshot injuries in infants and children in KwaZulu-Natal - An emerging epidemic. *South African Medical Journal*, 88: 444-447.
Hall, A., & Williams, H. (1987). Hidden psychiatric morbidity Part 1: A study of the prevalence in an out-patient population at Bindura Provincial Hospital. *Central African Journal of Medicine*, 33: 239-243.
Hamber, B., & Eagle, G. (1997). Psychiatric outpatients: Family burden and implications for mental health policy. Paper presented at the 3rd Annual Congress of the Psychological Society of South Africa. Durban, September 1997.
Hollifield, M., Katon, W., Spain, D., & Pule, L. (1990). Anxiety and depression on a village in Lesotho, Africa: A comparison with the United States. *British Journal of Psychiatry*, 156: 343-350.
Kessler, R.C., Sonnega, A., Bromet. E., Hughes, M., & Nelson, C.B. (1995). Posttraumatic stress disorder in the national comorbidity survey. *Archives of General Psychiatry*, 52: 1048-1060.
Kisekka, M.N. (1990). Gender and mental health in Africa. In E. D. Rothblum,

& B. Cole (eds.), *Women's mental health in Africa* (pp. 1-13). London: Harrington Park Press.

Kovasznay, B., Bromet, B., Schwartz, J.E., Ram, R., Lavelie, J., & Brandon, L. (1993). Substance abuse and onset of psychotic illness. *Hospital and Community Psychiatry*, 44: 567-571.

KwaZulu-Natal Department of Health. (1997). Health Informatics Bulletin.

Lambert, D., & Hartley, D. (1998). Linking primary care and rural psychiatry: Where have we been and where are we going? *Psychiatric Services*, 49: 965-967.

Leff, J. (1994). Cultural influences on psychiatry. *Current Opinion in Psychiatry*, 7: 197-201. Lefley, H.P. (1987). Aging parents as caregivers of mentally ill adult children: an emerging social problem. *Hospital and Community Psychiatry*, 38: 1063-1069.

Lin, T.Y. (1983). Mental health in the third world. *Journal of Nervous Mental Disease*, 171: 71-77.

Lindegger, G., & Crewe, M. (1997). HIV/AIDS: Managing the madness. In D. Foster, M. Freeman, & Y. Pillay (eds.), *Mental health policy issues for South Africa. Pinelands*: Medical Association of South Africa.

Lindsey, K.P., & Paul, G.L. (1989). Involuntary commitments to public mental institutions:

Issues involving the over-representation of blacks and assessment of relevant functioning. *Psychological Bulletin*, 106: 171-183.

McGuire, J., & Earls, F. (1991). Prevention of psychiatric disorders in early child hood. *Journal of Child Psychology and Psychiatry*, 32: 129-153.

McIntyre, D., Bloom, G., Doherty, J., & Briglal, P. (1985). *Health expenditure and finance in South Africa.* World Bank and the Health Systems Trust, Durban.

Miller, F.T., & Tanenbaum, J.H. (1989). Drug abuse in schizophrenia. Hospital and Community Psychiatry, 40, 847 - 849.

Molteno, C. (1997). Beyond "mental handicap". In D. Foster, M. Freeman, & Y. Pillay (eds.), *Mental health policy issues for South Africa.* Pinelands: Medical Association of South Africa.

Murthy, R.S. (1998). Rural psychiatry in developing countries. *Psychiatric Services*, 49: 967-969.

Nair. M.G., & Pillay, S.S. (1997). Psychiatric disorder in a South African general hospital - prevalence in medical, surgical and gynecological wards. *General Hospital Psychiatry*, 19: 144-148.

Narrow, W.E., Regier, D.A., Rae, D.S., Manderscheid, R.W., & Locke, B.Z. (1993). Use of services by persons with mental and addictive disorders: Findings from the National Institute of mental health, epidemiological catchment area program. *Archives of General Psychiatry*, 50: 95-107.

Natal Witness. (1998a). Pietermaritzburg, July 21, (p. 2).

Natal Witness. (1998b). Pietermaritzurg, August 28, (p.3).

Ntsaluba, A, & Pillay, Y. (1998). Reconstructing and developing the health system - the first 1000 days. *South African Medical Journal*, 88: 33-36.

Petrila, J.P., & Sadoff, R.L. (1992). Confidentiality and the family as caregiver.

Hospital and Community Psychiatry, 43, 136-139.
Pillay, A.L. (1987). Pediatric psychology: Relevance in South African health care. *Newsletter of the Society of Pediatric Psychology (American Psychological Association)*, 11: 9-11.
Pillay, A.L. (1991). Presenting problems in black children referred for outpatient psychological consultation in South Africa. *Perceptual and Motor Skills*, 72: 1135-1138.
Pillay, Y., Bhana, A., & Petersen, I. (1994). Mental health policy initiatives at the provincial level with specific reference to KwaZulu-Natal. In Pillay, Y., Bhana, A. Bhagwanjee, A., Parekh, A., & Petersen, I. (eds.), *Proceedings of the Primary Mental Health Care Workshop*. University of Durban-Westvile, September, 1994.
Pillay, A.L., & Lockhat, M.R. (1997). Developing community mental health services for children in South Africa. *Social Science and Medicine*, 45: 1493-1501.
Pillay, A.L., Naidoo, P., & Lockhat M.R. (1998). Mental health problems in urban and rural/peri-urban children. Paper presented at the 4th Annual Congress of the Psychological Society of South Africa, Cape Town, September 1998.
Pillay, A.L., Van der Veen, M.B.W., & Wassenaar, D.R. (1998). Gender and suicidal behaviour in South Africa. Paper presented at the 2nd Pan-Asia Pacific Conference on Mental Health. Beijing, October 1998.
Pillay, A.L., & Wassenaar, D.R. (1995). Psychological intervention, spontaneous remission, hopelessness and psychiatric disturbance in adolescent parasuicides. *Suicide and Life Threatening Behaviour*, 25: 386-392.
Prozesky, J., & Kotze, S. (1998). Crime prevention through development and restorative justice. *Social Work Practice*, 1: 4-7.
Rasool, E. (1998). Health care achievement and challenges in the Western Cape. *South African Medical Journal*, 88,1: 30-31.
Reeler A.P., & Todd. C.H. (1994). An overview of psychological disorders and psychiatric services in Zimbabwe. In Pillay, Y., Bhana, A., Bhagwanjee, A., Parekh, A., & I. Petersen, I. (eds.), *Proceedings of the Primary Mental Health Care Workshop*. University of Durban-Westvile, September 1994.
Regier, D.A., Narrow, W.E., Rae, D.S., Manderscheid, R.W., Locke, B.Z., & Goodwin, F.K. (1993). The de Factor U.S. mental and addictive disorder service system: Epidemiologic catchment area prospective 1-year prevalence rates of disorders and services. *Archives of General Psychiatry*, 50: 85-94.
Rispel, L., Price, M., & Cabral, J. (1996). *Standards and guidelines for primary health care in South Africa*. Technical report. Johannesburg: Centre for Health Policy, University of Witwatersrand.
Sartorius, N., Ustun, T.B., Costa, E., Silva, J.A, Goldberg, D., Lecrubier, Y., Ormel, J., Von Korff, M., & Wittchen, H.U. (1993). An international study of psychological problems in primary care. *Archives of General Psychiatry*, 50: 819-823.
Simon, G., Ormel, J., Von Korff. M., & Barlow, W. (1995). Health care costs

associated with depressive and anxiety disorder in primary care. *American Journal of Psychiatry*, 152: 352-357.
South African Police Services. (1998). Quarterly Report.
Stavrou. P. (1998a). Caring for survivors of violence. A community mental health care model: The south coast hospice trauma counselling network. *Social Work Practice*, 1: 31-42.
Stavrou, P. (1998b). The South African government's victim empowerment programme. *Social Work Practice*, 1: 25-30.
Tarrier. N.. Tantam, D., & Gater, R. (1994). Social, community and public health psychiatry. Editorial comment. *Current Opinion in Psychiatry*, 7: 165-166.
Thurston-Hicks, A., Paine, S., & Hollifield, M. (1998). Functional impairment associated with psychological distress and medical severity in rural primary care patients. *Psychiatric Services*, 49: 951-955.
Tzhotzho, Z. (1998). Consultative workshop facilitated by the National Mental Health and Substance Abuse Sub-Directorate of Child, Youth, Women and Family Health, September, Pietermaritzburg.
Weiss, R.D., Mirin, S.M., & Frances, R.J. (1992). The myth of the typical dual diagnosis patient. *Hospital and Community Psychiatry*, 43: 107-108.
World Health Organization. (1977). *Apartheid and mental health care*, MNH/ 77.5 World Health Organization, Geneva.
World Health Organization. (1978). *Alma Ata. Primary Health Care Report.* World Health Organization, Geneva.

Part V

Health Communication and the New Media

Chapter 20

Selected Internet Resources for Health Information and Communication in Africa

Andy O. Alali
California State University, Bakersfield

B.A. Jinadu
Department of Public Health, County of Kern, California

Following is a selected list of websites our readers are likely to find useful in their study and research about current health issues and health communication initiatives in and about Africa. Over the past few years profit and not-for-profit organizations have relied on the Internet as a source for documenting or archiving health information as well as repository for health surveillance data.

We purposefully chose these sites for the following reasons. First, we present sites that we believe have been screened for quality so as to avoid the minefield of misinformation associated with web-based health issues. Second, we felt that our readers in the continent would benefit from a ready access to website of their choice without incurring the additional expenses associated with navigating the Internet in their respective countries. Lastly, we seek to create a marketplace of ideas where researchers, students and practitioners can obtain and share information about health issues related to Africa. Also, we recognize that our aim at objective selection of these sites might be seen as subjective, we hope that this endeavor contributes to a healthy Africa.

Following is a list of organizations and websites:

Academy for Educational Development; supports projects in Africa on health and related issues. This independent non-profit organization maintains health and human resources data on Africa.

Address: http://www.aed.org/sara/

ACC Network; database of African nutrition status.

Address: http://www.accnetwork.net/en/themes/Adec98be.html

AF-AIDS; a regional HIV/AIDS information network with over 200 organizations working in or with African countries.

Address: http://www.hivnet.ch:8000/africa/af-aids/

Africaland: Sao Tome and Principe; provides information about basic social sector, including health and population issues, in Sao Tome and Principe.

Address: http://www.focusintl.com/saotomep.htm

African Council of AIDS Service Organizations, AfriCASO; a network of non-governmental organizations, community based organizations, groups of people living with HIV/AIDS (PWAs) and other interested groups; maintains a county-by-country directory of African HIV community based health care.

Address: http://www.africaso.org/

Africa - Health; links to health journals, resources, and organizations in Africa.

Address: http://www-sul,stanford.edu/depts/ssrg/a...

African Journal of Reproductive Health; a publication of Harvard University's School of Public Health. Articles are primarily written by African health workers and deal with complexities of women's reproductive health, including general information on reproductive rights.

Address: http://www.hsph.harvard.edu/ajrh/current.htm

African Medical and Research Foundation (AMREF); based in Nairobi, Kenya with offices in Tanzania, Uganda, and South Africa. The organization runs the Flying Doctor's Service and offers programs in environmental health, sexual health, child health, health policy, and publishes manuals and books on primary health care for Eastern Africa, as a medical and health workers journal.

Address: http://www.amref.org/

Africa Nutrition Chartbooks; downloadable PDF files of surveys on nutritional status of children in Africa.

Address: http://www.measuredhs.com/pubs/chartbooks/start.cfm?

Africa Programme for Onchocerciasis Control (APOC); offers detailed description of river blindness, as well as background on treatment and the Onchocerciasis Control Programme in West Africa (OCP).

Address: http://www.who.int/ocp/index.htm

Africa Tobacco Documents - UICC GLOBALink; repository of reports on tobacco in Africa.

Address: http://www.globalink.org/tobacco/docs/af

African Networks for Health Research & Development; an electronic conference for various health networks across Eastern and Southern Africa.

Address: http://www.healthnet.org/afronets/index

Afro-Nets, African Networks for Health Research & Development; discussion forum focusing on health research and development in the Eastern and Southern African Region. Ministries of Health in Africa can also be linked through this site.

Address: http://www.healthnet.org/afronets

Amazon Africa Aid Organization; offers medical and dental volunteer opportunities in Brazilian Amazon and Africa.

Address: http://www.amazonafrica.org

Autism Africa; links to resources on autism in Africa, including information in English and French.

Address: http://www.autism-alabama.org/africa

AVSC International; nonprofit organization dedicated to making reproductive health care accessible to women and men around the world, including family planning issues in Africa

Address: http://www.avsc.org/

Body, An AIDS and HIV Information Resource, The; maintains database of information on AIDS care in Zimbabwe.

Address: http://www.thebody.com/index.shtml

Cancer Links; provides comprehensive informative cancer URLs.

Address: http://www.cancerlinks.org

Carter Center's River Blindness Program; describes organization's role in the treatment of river blindness.

Address:http://www.emory.edu/CARTER_CENTER/health.htm#rblind

Centers for Disease Control & Prevention; primary U.S. government public health agency that maintains extensive information on health situations around the world, as well as in North, West, Central, East, and

Southern Africa.

Address: http://www.cdc.gov/travel/index.htm

Center for Communication Programs; a Johns Hopkins University center that promotes healthy behavior worldwide through communication.

Address: http://www.jhuccp.org/

Cornell Food and Nutrition Policy Program; examines nutrition issues in Africa, particularly on education, impact and implications on health.

Address: http://www.nutrition.cornell.edu/cfnpp.html

CRIA - Community Research Initiative on AIDS; a community-based organization that studies new treatments for HIV and AIDS-related diseases and conducts a comprehensive treatment education program.

Address: http://www.criany.or

Department of Health, South Africa: HIV/AIDS and STD Directorate; provides information about HIV/AIDS and STDs in South Africa.

Address: http://www.health.gov.za/hiv_aids

Doctors Without Borders/Medecins san frontiers/MSF; nonprofit, international organization which provides medical aid to populations in crisis worldwide, and carries information about health issues in Africa.

Address (U.S.): http://www.dwb.org/index.htm
Address (International): Address: http://www.msf.org

EQUINET; Network on Equity in Health in Southern Africa is a network of research, civil society and health sector organizations working towards and influencing equity in health in Southern Africa.

Address: http://www.equinet.org.zw

Ethiopian Journal of Health Development; an official journal of the

Ethiopian Public Health Association. Full-text of published articles on health in Ethiopia are accessible online.

Address: http://www.cih.uib.no/journals/EJHD/EJHD-main-page.htm

Family Care International; working on improving women's sexual and reproductive health and rights in developing countries, particularly in Francophone Africa.

Address: http://www.familycareintl.org/work/work_

Ghana Health Foundation; the foundation is an alliance of health care professionals and others concerned with current health issues in Ghana.

Address: http://www.ghanahealth.org

Global Alliance for Africa; a not-for-profit organization that developing community-based health care programs for impoverished people of Africa, with emphasis on local participation.

Address: http://www.globalallianceafrica.org

Global Reproductive Health Forum: West Africa Project: Information Technology Africa: Projects and Initiatives; The West Africa Project at the Global Reproductive Health Forum (GRHF) at Harvard University collects works found on the Internet, on reproductive health, gender, population, HIV/AIDS, family planning, and demography.

Address: http://www.hsph.harvard.edu/Organization

Green Africa Network: Sustainable Rural Healthcare Programme; repository of information about reproductive health, diseases control, child nutrition, indigenous medicine and AIDS awareness in Africa.

Address: http://members.spree.com/greenafrica/Rur

Harvard School of Public Health; provides public health education through learning, discovery, and communication. It's an important resource center for current research on health in Africa.

Address: http://www.hsph.harvard.edu

Heal the Nation: Christian Medical Missions; Christian medical organization sponsoring community health programs in Uganda.

Address: http://www.healthnation.org/uganda.htm

Health and Human Resources Analysis for Africa (HHRAA); a project of USAID's Bureau for Africa to increase the utilization of research, analysis, and information to improve health, nutrition, education, and family planning strategies, policies, and programs in Africa. Abstracts and full-text reports are accessible online.

Address: http://www.info.usaid.gov/regions/afr/hhraa

Health and Nutrition; monitors health issues, including nutrition, family planning, sanitation, and AIDS education. It created the first Portuguese-language AIDS education program in Africa.

Address: http://www.africare.org/about/annualreport/healthnut/healthnut.html

Health and Nutrition in Tanzania; discusses Tanzanian nutrition policy and outreach strategies.

Address: http://www.unicef.org/trans/trans05.html

Health Care Project for Mothers and Children, Mali; a project of Novartis Foundation for Sustainable Development (NFSD) aimed at improving the health of women and children in Mali.

Address: http://www.foundation.novartis.com/health

Health Effects; documents health issues, including blindness, impotence, breast cancer, and effects of smoking.

Address: http://www.health.usyd.edu.au/tobacco/su

Health Index on Africa; links to Africa-specific health topics, AIDS resources, health studies, emerging diseases and population statistics.

Address: http://www.africaindex.africainfo.no/pages/Subject_pages/Health

Health Information & Organizations on Africa; provides links to journals, research, conferences, and publications for African health issues.

Address: http://www.cc.columbia.edu/libraries/

HealthKenya.com; Kenya health news.

Address: http://www.healthkenya.com

HEALTHLINK; a project of the Health Systems Trust to help meet the communication and information needs of health workers in South Africa.

Address: http://www.healthlinks.org.za/hlink/main

HealthNet; provides information on heart problems with emphasis on prevention.

Address: http://www.healthnet.org.uk

HealthNet Africa; provides comprehensive and contact information about health. Links to country health issues.

Address: http://www.healthnet.org/hnet/africa.html

Healthnet International, Inc.; provides news, research and information on health and wellness.

Address: http://www.healthnetint.com/healthnet/de

Health – Search Beat; The World Wide Beat offers information about health by geographic region, as well as on individual towns and localities.

Address: http://www.searchbeat.com/Regional/Africa

HELINA-L; Health Informatics in Africa; provides a comprehensive e-mail list on health in Africa, as well as an archive of messages and conference information.

Address: http://www.uku.fi/english/organizations/

HIV/AIDS Net: Southern Africa Directory; a directory of HIV/AIDS sites relevant to Southern Africa.

Address: http://www.safaids.org/dirweb.html

HIV InSite – University of California, San Francisco; covers policy and statistics on HIV. Has section on Sub-Saharan Africa with country profile and links to full-text articles.

Address: http://HIVInSite.ucsf.edu/

HOPE for Kids Children's Health Education Program; provides information about children health education.

Address: http://www.hopeww.org/Kids/kids1.html

Independent Group for Health in Africa; a watchdog group that monitors health problems, policies, strategies and programs, including research, in Africa.

Address: http://users.harare.iafrica.com/~gtz-hsr/igha.htm

Information, Education and Communication; provides regional IEC family planning training for paramedical, auxiliary and community personnel.

Address: http://www.devassoc1.com/iec.html

Lungwena Child Survival Study; details of study on maternal and child health in a rural community.

Address: http://www.uta.fi/~blpeas/lcss

Malaria and Infectious Diseases in Africa; an English and French publication with abstracts and links to information and discussion lists on malaria, tropical diseases and health in Africa.

Address: http://www.chez.com/malaria/

Malaria Foundation International; provides news summaries and general background information on current medical research on malaria.

Address: http://www.malaria.org/

Malaria Network; a collaborative project of the World Bank and the WHO that serves as a repository of recent articles, reports, and resources on malaria.

Address: http://www.rbm.who.int/

Malaria Prevention and Control from the WHO Division of Control of Tropical Diseases; provides background information, including an overview of the disease itself and statistical and progress reports on WHO programs.

Address: http://www.who.int/ctd/html/malaria.html

Management Sciences for Health (MSH); a nonprofit organization working in public health areas to strengthen health care management and improve access to critical health care services worldwide, including maternal/child health and family planning.

Address: http://www.msh.org

Mapping Malaria Risk in Africa; a South African site that provides an atlas of malaria in Africa. It is available in both French and English.

Address: http://www.mara.org.za/

MEASURE DHS + – Demographic and Health Services; assists in the collection and use of data to monitor and evaluate population, health, and nutrition programs in developing countries. Has extensive datasets for African countries on fertility, early childhood mortality, maternal and child health, maternal and child nutrition, AIDS and other STDs.

Address: http://www.measuredhs.com

MEDLINE – Pub Med. U.S. National Library of Medicine; allows users to search the National Library of Medicine's database of over 8 million citations to articles in 3,800 biomedical journals on medicine, dentistry, veterinary medicine, and health care.

Address: http://www.ncbi.nlm.nih.gov/PubMed/

Mesob.org; directory of Ethiopian NGOs, and HIV/AIDS education organizations in Ethiopia.

Address: http://www.mesob.org

Middles East News Online; provides news about health and medicine in the Middle East, including Libya.

Address: http://www.middleeastwire.com/libya/health

Nigeria AIDS.org; an NGO by Journalists Against AIDS (JAAIDS) Nigeria. It provides discussion, monthly bulletin, *AIDS News Service*, statistics and full-text of the HIV/AIDS Emergency Action Plan (HEAP); also covers issues related to other countries of West Africa.

Address: http://www.nigeria-aids.org

Nigeria Family Health Services; covers information on major projects to improve the health of Nigerians through public health medicine.

Address: http://elmer.jsi.com/JSISearch/oldweb/99

Nutrition; links to programs and policies to promote the optimal nutrition of women and children in South Africa.

Address: http://www.uct.ac.za/depts/chu/nut.html

Nutrition and Orphans; resources fro nutritional rehabilitation in Africa.

Address: http://www.worldmedicalfund.org/Nutrition.html

Nutrition Documents and Links; this joint effort of the United Nations and the World Bank houses the Africa Nutrition Database (ANDI), which provides data, research and information on nutrition in Africa.

Address: http://www.foodaid.org/nutrition.html

Nutrition Society of South Africa; devoted to nutritional issues in Southern Africa.

Address: http://www.nutritionsociety.co.za/

Office of Global Health; a CDC unit aimed at increasing the Center's ability to increase its ability to respond to the new realities of global public health.

Address: http://www.cdc.gov/ogh

Organization of African Traditional Healers (OATH); a non-profit organization for the promotion of African traditional religions.

Address: http://www.mamiwata.com/OATH.html

Outbreak; provides free access to information about the world's latest emerging infectious diseases. Has extensive information on the Ebola virus.

Address: http://www.outbreak.org/

Penn Library-Communication/Health Communication; access to health information on Africa, as well as link to Health AFRO-NETS.

Address: http://www.library.upenn.edu/resources/s...

Pharmnet; a comprehensive information and communications channel for the pharmaceutical profession in South Africa. It provides access to accurate and up-to-date pharmaceutical and related information to all uses and easy communication with their colleagues, other healthcare workers and the public.

Address: http://www.pharmnet.co.za

Pioneering Partnership in Nutrition Communication; provides important health messages to children about nutrition.

Address: http://www.nutrition.tufts.edu/feature

Population Communications International; publishes a monthly online newsletter on health issue, including population growth rates, and sexual and reproductive health.

Address: http://www.population.org/

Population Council; maintains database and operates programs on reproductive health, HIV/AIDS, with full texts reports.

Address: http://www.popcouncil.org/

Population Information Network (POPIN) - Africa; provides population and reproductive health information resources in the form of software, journals, and bibliographies.

Address: http://www.un.org/Depts/eca/divis/fssd/popin/

Pretoria Urology Hospital; includes mission, medical topics, contact details, doctors, facilities, news and health information links in South Africa.

Address: http://www.urology.co.za

Primary High School Nutrition; an evaluation of South Africa's primary high school nutrition program.

Address: http://www.hst.org.za/pubs/psnp/

Public Health - Africa; an annotated directory of Web sites dealing with African health, as well as information on individual countries.

Address: http://www.ldb.org/vl/geo/africa/index.htm

Public Health Reports; a journal of the U.S. Public Health Service. Covers issues such as tobacco control, teenage violence, occupational disease and injury, immunization, drug policy, and other health issues.

Address: http://phr.oupjournals.org

Pub Med (MEDLINE) - U.S. National Library of Medicine; provides free access to MEDLINE's database of over 8 million citations to articles in 3,800 biomedical journals on medicine, dentistry, veterinary medicine, and health care.

Address: http://www.ncbi.nlm.nih.gov/PubMed/

PubMed Central; has full text articles on traditional healers, TB, and HIV in South Africa.

Address: http://www.pubmedcentral.nih.gov/

Research Triangle Institute; an independent research organization that serves government and industry clients throughout the world.

Address: http://www.rti.org

Réseau africain de recherché sur le SIDA, RARS; maintains a directory and online list of periodicals.

Address: http://www.refer.org/sngal_ct/rec/rars/

Safe Motherhood; a general resource, as well as Africa-specific section on maternal health and the causes of maternal death.

Address: http://www.safemotherhood.org/

SANGONeT; links to medical publications, journals, and libraries, including online rural health care and information in Southern Africa.

Address: http://wn.apc.org/health

SatelLife; provides electronic communication and health information in the developing world.

Address: http://info.isoc.org/isoc/whatis/confere

Satellife, Healthnet; provides an electronic network for health professionals in Africa and other countries. Services include e-mail, discussion forums, publications, and exchange programs.

Address: http://www.healthnet.org

SD Development Newsletter; a quarterly publication of U.S. Agency for International Development's projects in Africa, including health issues.

Address: http://www.usaid.gov/regions/afr/abic/sdindex.htm

Social Sciences and Medicine Africa Network; a network of scientists, institutions and agencies working in health and social sciences in Africa.

Address: http://users.harare.iafrica.com/~gtz-hsr

Solidarité Médicale Bourbonnais Sénégal; provides information on health projects and for travelers to Senegal.

Address: http://assoc.wanadoo.fr/senegal.bourbonnais/

SOMA-Net, the Social Science and Medicine Africa Network; a network of scientists, institutions and agencies working in Health and social sciences in Africa.

Address: http://users.harare.iafrica.com/~gtz-hsr/somanet.htm

South Africa's Integrated National Disability Strategy; discussions on how majority of disability can be prevented in South Africa serve as a model for the rest of Africa.

Address: http://www.independentliving.org/LibArt/

South Africa Online, Health - Organizations; a link to health organizations in South Africa.

Address: http://www.southafrica.co.za/health/org

South African Natural Health Network; lists therapies, practitioners, forums, news and workshop on natural health in South Africa.

Address: http://www.naturalhealth.co.za

Straight Talk Foundation; online access to newspapers of reproductive health, safe sex practices, sexuality for children and young adults in Uganda.

Address: http://www.swiftuganda.com/~strtalk

SynergyAIDS - The Synergy Resource Center; a technical resource for health program planning and design, and monitoring and evaluation.

Address: http://www.synergyaids.com/resources.php

The Communication Initiative - Communication Interventions for Sustainable Development; access to communication information and interventions on development.

Address: http://www.comminit.com/

The Luke Society of Uganda; provides community health education, AIDS counseling and medical care in Kampala, Uganda (also provides services in other parts of Africa).

Address: http://www.lukesociety.org/profiles/uganda

The South African Beyond Awareness HIV/AIDS Campaign; promotes access to HIV/AIDS communication tools in South Africa.

Address: http://www.aidsinfo.co.za

The World-Wide Web Virtual Library: Public Health - Geographical Locations (Africa); links to public health sites in Africa.

Address: http://www.ldb.org/vl/geo/africa

Tools for Life; a comprehensive health communication kit for health workers and educators in Anglophone Africa.

Address: http://www.jhuccp.org/tools/about.html

UNICEF - Progress of Nations; provides access to information on sanitation, health, education, as well as statistical tables comparing population, birth, mortality, and more.

Address: http://www.unicef.or/pon

United States, Army War College, Strategic Studies Institute; has full text medical reports on Africa.

Address: http://carlisle-www.army.mil/usassi/ssipubs/catalogs/africa.htm

United States, Census Bureau, HIV/AIDS Surveillance; has country profiles and database on HIV/AIDS.

Address: http://www.census.gov/ipc/www/hivaidsn.html

University of Pretoria - School of Health Systems and Public Health; offers programs in tropical medicine and public health, as well as other public health disciplines.

Address: http://www.up.ac.za/academic/medicine/sh

University of Zimbabwe Medical Library; access to health related resources on health research, HIV/AIDS, and teaching hospital projects in Zimbabwe, including annotated bibliography and articles/information from Zimbabwe discussion list on health.

Address: http://www.medguide.org.zm/

USAID in Africa; an Internet resources on health in Africa.

Address: http://www.info.usaid.gov/regions/afr/ab

WHO Initiative on HIV/AIDS & Sexually Transmitted Infections (HSI); provides important country-specific, as well as general information about HIS.

Address: http://www.who.int/asd/

WIDNET Africa; Women Development Network's page of resources on Africa. Contains information about communication, health, and nutrition.

Address: http://www.focusintl.com/r1aafriq.html

World Bank Global Partnership to Eliminate Riverblindness; highlights efforts and activities of the Onchocerciasis Control Programme (OCP) and the African Programme for Onchocerciasis Control (APOC) aimed at eliminating river blindness.

Address: http://www.worldbank.org/gper/

World Health News; weekly stories on public health issues from around the world published by the Center for Health Communication of the Harvard School of Public Health.

Address: http://www.worldhealthnews.harvard.edu

World Health Organization; has extensive information on Africa, as well as statistical information on incidences of diseases by region. Has online information on travel and health, health hazards, malaria and drug resistance bacteria. Other health issues covered include Guinea-worm disease, schistosomiasis, onchocerciasis, sleeping sickness, and other diseases. Has must recent data on HIV/AIDS and sexual behavior.

Address (main site): http://www.who.int/
Address (regional Office of Africa): http://www.whoafr.org/

WWW VL Public Health: Africa - Lesotho; provides links to resources on public health in Lesotho.

Address: http://www.ldb.org/vl/geo/africa/1les.html

INDEX

I

About the Editors

Andy O. Alali, Ph.D., is Professor of Communications and Founding Chair of the Department of Communications at California State University, Bakersfield. The author of several refereed journal articles and book chapters, Dr. Alali has written and edited/co-edited five books, including the well-received *HIV/AIDS in public schools: A handbook for curriculum development, teacher education, and the placement of affected students*. His research focus is on health communication as well as issues related to intercultural and interpersonal communication, social support and health decisions in African health context. He is completing a project on media, violence, and terrorism in Africa sponsored by the United Nations Education, Scientific, and Cultural Organization (UNESCO).

B.A. Jinadu, M.D., MPH, is a board certified pediatrician, and is currently the Health Officer and Director of Public Health for the County of Kern, California. Dr. Jinadu has been at the forefront of public health issues for more than a decade, with a primary focus on health promotion, disease control and prevention efforts at the county, state, national, and international levels. He is also the author of several articles and has made numerous presentations on issues related to public health at national conferences.

About the Contributors

E.S. Ataudo, now deceased, was affiliated with the Division of Medical Sociology and Biopsychosocial Health, Department of Community Health, University of Calabar, College of Medical Sciences, Calabar, Nigeria.

Albert K. Awedoba, D.Phil., is a Senior Research Fellow at the Institute of African Studies, University of Ghana. He served as the Takemi Fellow in International Health at Harvard School of Public Health from August 1997 to August 1998. His research interests are in the areas of medical anthropology, social relations, and languages. Dr. Awedoba participated in several health research projects on onchocerciasis, acute respiratory infections and diarrhea diseases sponsored by WHO and other organizations. He is completing a book on the *Burden of onchocerceal skin disease in endemic communities*.

Freddy Batundi has worked in Rwanda as a Prosthetic Technician, later managing a recreational program for children with disabilities. Currently, he is affiliated with Christian Blind Mission as Supervisor of Kigali Community Based Rehabilitation Program in Rwanda. He began his professional life as a teacher and later, worked in refugee prosthetics programs and care of mentally handicapped children.

Varghese I. Cherian, Ph.D., is Professor and Head of the Department of Psychology of Education at the University of the North in South Africa. His areas of specialization are educational psychology and social psychology. He is a researcher who contributes frequently to international journals.

Andrea Crystal lectures in the Department of Communication at the Rand Afrikaans University, Johannesburg, South Africa. She specializes in integrated marketing communication, and is currently completing her doctorate in the field of health communication. Her interest in health communication grew from a research visit to Emerson College in Boston, in 1997.

Igbo N. Egwu, DrPH, is Professor and Director of the Graduate Program in Public Health at the University of Calabar, Nigeria. Dr. Egwu received his Master of Public Health and Doctor of Public Health degrees from the University of Michigan, Ann Arbor, Michigan. He served on the WHO Expert Advisory Committee on Health Education/Promotion from 1996 to 1999.

Bernice N. Ezeilo is affiliated with the Department of Psychology at the University of Nigeria, Nsukka, Nigeria.

Arglenda Friday is Executive Director of the African-American Research Library and Cultural Center in Broward County, Florida. She previously held appointments as a tenured Librarian at San Jose State University, San Jose, California, and an HIV/AIDS instructor.

Leah Gilbert, Ph.D., MPH, is Associate Professor in the Department of Sociology at the University of Witwatersrand, Johannesburg, South Africa.

Gwendolyn J. Lusi, M.Sc., is Administrator of the Continuing Medical Education Program in Africa for Doctors on Call for Service. Previously, she worked as Administrator of Nyankunde Hospital, Congo, and later as Director of the Community-Based Rehabilitation Program in Kigali, Rwanda. She has over 25 years experience in development of higher education, hospital administration and program management in Congo-Zaire, Kenya and Rwanda.

Ogom Peter Nwosu, Ph.D., is Professor of Intercultural and International Communication at California State University, Sacramento, and a consultant on multicultural issues, training, and development. His research interests focus on human communication processes and patterns across cultures. He has published in various journals and is co-author of *Transcultural realities: Interdisciplinary perspectives on cross-cultural relations* and *Communication and the transformation of society: A developing region's perspective*.

Carol A. Okigbo teaches courses in mathematics, research design, and educational statistics in the Department of Multidisciplinary Studies at Minnesota State University, Moorhead. She has conducted field research on AIDS communication campaigns in Kenya, and was formerly community organizer at the Lutheran Social Services of North Dakota.

Charles C. Okigbo, Ph.D., teaches communication at North Dakota State University, and was formerly Executive Coordinator of the African Council for Communication Education (ACCE), Senior Lecturer in mass communication at the University of Nigeria, Nsukka, and Executive Registrar of the Advertising Practitioners Council of Nigeria. He has been health communication consultant to UNICEF, WHO, and UNAIDS.

Warren Parker is an M.A. graduate of the Centre for Cultural and Media Studies, University of Natal, Durban, South Africa. He developed the Department of Health's media strategy relating to AIDS prevention. He currently works for the Society of Family Health in South Africa.

Karl Peltzer, Ph.D., is Professor of Psychology in the Department of Psychology at the University of the North, South Africa. He has written books on *Psychology and health in Africa* and *Counseling and psychotherapy of victims of violence in sociocultural context*, and his research interests are in psychology and health in Africa.

Anthony L. Pillay, Ph.D., is Associate Professor and Principal Clinical

Psychologist at the University of Natal Medical School and Midlands Hospital, South Africa. His research interests include child and adolescent disorders, and community mental health.

Carol-Ann Sargent, M.Sc., is a Senior Psychologist and Lecturer at the University of Natal Medical School and Midlands Hospital, South Africa. Her reserach interests are in community mental health and neuropsychology.

Arnold Shepperson is a Researcher at the Centre for Cultural and Media Studies, University of Natal, Durban, South Africa. He co-authored the Department of Health AIDS Media Plan.

Keyan G. Tomaselli is Director and Professor at the Centre for Cultural and Media Studies, University of Natal, Durban, South Africa. He serves as the media expert on the Department of Health Advisory Committee on AIDS/STDs.

Sonja Verwey, Ph.D., is Chairperson of the Department of Communication at the Rand Afrikaans University, Johannesburg, South Africa. She specializes in organizational communication. Professor Verwey is the Editor of *Communicare, Journal of Communication Sciences* in South Africa, and serves on the editorial committee of several scholarly journals. Dr. Verwey's special interest in health communication was influenced by the health status of South Africa and the challenges posed by the growing AIDS pandemic in the country. She is widely published in the area of health communication.

Susanne L. Williams, Ph.D., is an Assistant Professor of mass communication and Assistant to the President at Minnesota State University Moorhead. Dr. Williams teaches courses in health communication, public relations, and gender and media. She completed her doctorate and master's degree in communication at Wayne State University, and a Bachelor of Arts at the University of Nebraska-Lincoln.

www.ingramcontent.com/pod-product-compliance
Ingram Content Group UK Ltd.
Pitfield, Milton Keynes, MK11 3LW, UK
UKHW040227290926
15471UKWH00001B/39

9 780761 824077